T0249441

Diseases of the Esophagus

Editor

JOHN O. CLARKE

GASTROENTEROLOGY CLINICS OF NORTH AMERICA

www.gastro.theclinics.com

Consulting Editor
ALAN L. BUCHMAN

December 2021 • Volume 50 • Number 4

ELSEVIER

1600 John F. Kennedy Boulevard • Suite 1800 • Philadelphia, Pennsylvania, 19103-2899
http://www.theclinics.com

GASTROENTEROLOGY CLINICS OF NORTH AMERICA Volume 50, Number 4
December 2021 ISSN 0889-8553, ISBN-13: 978-0-323-83548-0

Editor: Kerry Holland
Developmental Editor: Hannah Almira Lopez

Gastroenterology Clinics of North America (ISSN 0889-8553) is published quarterly by Elsevier Inc., 360 Park Avenue South, New York, NY 10010-1710. Months of issue are March, June, September, and December. Business and Editorial Offices: 1600 John F. Kennedy Blvd., Suite 1800, Philadelphia, PA 19103-2899. Customer Service Office: 6277 Sea Harbor Drive, Orlando, FL 32887-4800. Periodicals postage paid at New York, NY and additional mailing offices. Subscription prices are $365.00 per year (US individuals), $100.00 per year (US students), $945.00 per year (US institutions), $391.00 per year (Canadian individuals), $100.00 per year (Canadian students), $997.00 per year (Canadian institutions), $463.00 per year (international individuals), $220.00 per year (international students), and $997.00 per year (international institutions). Foreign air speed delivery is included in all *Clinics* subscription prices. All prices are subject to change without notice. **POSTMASTER:** Send address changes to *Gastroenterology Clinics of North America*, Elsevier Health Sciences Division, Subscription Customer Service, 3251 Riverport Lane, Maryland Heights, MO 63043. **Telephone: 1-800-654-2452 (U.S. and Canada); 314-447-8871 (outside U.S. and Canada). Fax: 314-447-8029. E-mail: journalscustomerservice-usa@elsevier.com (for print support); journalsonlinesupport-usa@elsevier.com (for online support)**.

Reprints. For copies of 100 or more, of articles in this publication, please contact the Commercial Reprints Department, Elsevier Inc., 360 Part Avenue South, New York, New York 10010-1710. Tel. 212-633-3874, Fax: 212-633-3820, E-mail: reprints@elsevier.com.

Gastroenterology Clinics of North America is also published in Italian by Il Pensiero Scientifico Editore, Rome, Italy; and in Portuguese by Interlivros Edicoes Ltda., Rua Commandante Coelho 1085, 21250 Cordovil, Rio de Janeiro, Brazil.

Gastroenterology Clinics of North America is covered in *MEDLINE/PubMed (Index Medicus), Excerpta Medica, Current Contents/Clinical Medicine, Science Citation Index, ISI/BIOMED,* and *BIOSIS*.

Contributors

CONSULTING EDITOR

ALAN L. BUCHMAN, MD, MSPH, FACP, FACN, FACG, AGAF
Professor of Clinical Surgery (Gastroenterology), Medical Director, Intestinal Rehabilitation and Transplant Center, The University of Illinois at Chicago/UI Health, Chicago, Illinois

EDITOR

JOHN O. CLARKE, MD, AGAF, FACG, FACP, FASGE
Director, Esophageal Program, Clinical Professor of Medicine, Division of Gastroenterology & Hepatology, Stanford University School of Medicine, Redwood City, California

AUTHORS

NITIN K. AHUJA, MD
Assistant Professor of Clinical Medicine, Division of Gastroenterology and Hepatology, University of Pennsylvania, Philadelphia, Pennsylvania

LEE M. AKST, MD
Associate Professor, Division of Laryngology, Department of Otolaryngology–Head and Neck Surgery, Johns Hopkins School of Medicine, Baltimore, Maryland

YEWANDE ALIMI, MD, MHS
Clinical Scholar, Department of Surgery, Stanford University School of Medicine, Washington, DC

DAN E. AZAGURY, MD
Department of Surgery, Stanford University School of Medicine, Stanford, California

RICHA BHARDWAJ, MBBS
Department of Internal Medicine, Lenox Hill Hospital, New York, New York

JOHN WILLIAM BLACKETT, MD, MSc
Division of Digestive and Liver Diseases, Columbia University Irving Medical Center, New York, New York

DUSTIN A. CARLSON, MD, MS
Division of Gastroenterology and Hepatology, Department of Medicine, Northwestern University, Feinberg School of Medicine, Chicago, Illinois

WALTER W. CHAN, MD, MPH
Director, Center for Gastrointestinal Motility, Division of Gastroenterology, Hepatology and Endoscopy, Brigham and Women's Hospital, Assistant Professor of Medicine, Harvard Medical School, Boston, Massachusetts

KAREN CHANG, DO
Department of Internal Medicine, University of California, Riverside School of Medicine, Riverside, California

JOHN O. CLARKE, MD, AGAF, FACG, FACP, FASGE
Director, Esophageal Program, Clinical Professor of Medicine, Division of Gastroenterology & Hepatology, Stanford University School of Medicine, Redwood City, California

SHUMON I. DHAR, MD
Assistant Professor, Division of Laryngology, Department of Otolaryngology–Head and Neck Surgery, Johns Hopkins School of Medicine, Baltimore, Maryland

NIELSEN Q. FERNANDEZ-BECKER, MD, PhD
Clinical Associate Professor, Department of Medicine, Stanford University, Redwood City, California

SHAI FRIEDLAND, MD
Stanford University, Stanford, California; Veterans Affairs Palo Alto Health Care System, Palo Alto, California

C. PRAKASH GYAWALI, MD, MRCP
Professor of Medicine, Division of Gastroenterology, Washington University School of Medicine in St. Louis, St Louis, Missouri

CHRISTIAN S. JACKSON, MD
Section Chief, Section of Gastroenterology, Loma Linda VA Healthcare System, Loma Linda, California

DANIELA JODORKOVSKY, MD
Division of Digestive and Liver Diseases, Columbia University Irving Medical Center, New York, New York

ANTHONY N. KALLOO, MD
Chairman, Department of Medicine, Maimonides Medical Center, Brooklyn, New York; Professor Emeritus, Johns Hopkins School of Medicine, Baltimore, Maryland

ABRAHAM KHAN, MD
Medical Director of Center for Esophageal Health, Department of Medicine, NYU Langone Health, New York, New York

RITA KNOTTS, MD, MSc
Center for Esophageal Health, Department of Medicine, NYU Langone Health, New York, New York

AMANDA J. KRAUSE, MD
Division of Gastroenterology and Hepatology, Department of Medicine, Northwestern University, Feinberg School of Medicine, Chicago, Illinois; Division of Gastroenterology and Hepatology, Department of Medicine, University of California, San Diego, La Jolla, California

ANNE LIDOR, MD, MPH
Department of Surgery, University of Wisconsin-Madison School of Medicine and Public Health, Madison, Wisconsin

KRISTLE LYNCH, MD
Associate Professor of Medicine, Division of Gastroenterology, University of Pennsylvania Perelman School of Medicine, Philadelphia, Pennsylvania

CAROLYN NEWBERRY, MD
Assistant Professor of Medicine, Director of Nutritional Services, Innovative Center for Health and Nutrition in Gastroenterology, Division of Gastroenterology, Weill Cornell Medical Center, New York, New York

SAOWANEE NGAMRUENGPHONG, MD
Assistant Professor of Medicine, Division of Gastroenterology & Hepatology, Johns Hopkins Medicine, Baltimore, Maryland

NOREEN C. OKWARA, MD
Department of Medicine, Brigham and Women's Hospital, Instructor in Medicine, Harvard Medical School, Boston, Massachusetts

SYDNEY POMENTI, MD
Division of Digestive and Liver Diseases, Columbia University Irving Medical Center, New York, New York

WILLIAM J. RAVICH, MD
Associate Professor of Medicine, Section of Digestive Disease, Yale School of Medicine, New Haven, Connecticut

BENJAMIN D. ROGERS, MD
Assistant Professor of Medicine, Division of Gastroenterology, Washington University School of Medicine in St. Louis, St Louis, Missouri; Division of Gastroenterology, Hepatology, and Nutrition, University of Louisville School of Medicine, Louisville, Kentucky

GRACE SNOW, MD
Clinical Instructor, Division of Laryngology, Department of Otolaryngology–Head and Neck Surgery, Johns Hopkins School of Medicine, Baltimore, Maryland

KENNETH J. VEGA, MD
Professor and Chief, Division of Gastroenterology and Hepatology, Augusta University Medical College of Georgia, Augusta, Georgia

MIKE T. WEI, MD
Stanford University, Stanford, California; Veterans Affairs Palo Alto Health Care System, Palo Alto, California

LINDA Y. ZHANG, MBBS
Advanced Endoscopy Fellow, Division of Gastroenterology and Hepatology, Johns Hopkins Medicine, Baltimore, Maryland

CHRISTOPHER J. ZIMMERMANN, MD
Department of Surgery, University of Wisconsin-Madison School of Medicine and Public Health, Madison, Wisconsin

Contents

of esophageal motility disorders. The update incorporates application of complementary testing strategies during HRM, such as provocative HRM maneuvers, and recommendation for barium esophagram or functional luminal imaging probe (FLIP) panometry to help clarify inconclusive HRM findings. FLIP panometry also represents an emerging technology for evaluation of esophageal distensibility and motility at the time of endoscopy.

Endoscopic findings in early esophageal cancer are often subtle and require careful inspection and meticulous endoscopic examination. When dysplasia is suspected, we recommend performing 1 or 2 targeted biopsies of the abnormal area and review with a pathologist specialized in evaluating gastrointestinal diseases. In the case of adenocarcinoma, after resection of any visible cancer, residual Barrett's can be treated by ablation. Endoscopic resection can offer the opportunity for patients to avoid surgery. Further studies are needed to evaluate the optimal management of circumferential and near-circumferential lesions as well as tools and techniques to facilitate the performance of endoscopic submucosal dissection and endoscopic mucosal resection.

Approximately, 10% to 15% of patients in the United States experience gastroesophageal reflux symptoms on a weekly basis, negatively affecting the quality of life and increasing the risk of reflux-related complications. For patients with symptoms recalcitrant to proton pump inhibitor (PPI) therapy or those who cannot take PPIs, surgical fundoplication is the gold standard. The preoperative workup is complex but vital for operative planning and ensuring good postoperative outcomes. Most patients are highly satisfied after fundoplication, though transient dysphagia, gas bloating, and resumption of PPI use are common postoperatively. Multiple newer technologies offer safe alternatives to fundoplication with similar outcomes.

Eosinophilic esophagitis (EoE) is an antigen-mediated esophageal disease defined by the presence of esophageal eosinophilia and symptoms of esophageal dysfunction. The pathophysiology involves an allergen-driven Th2 T cell response that triggers infiltration of eosinophils into the esophagus leading to inflammation, remodeling, and fibrosis. This results in disruption of esophageal function and accompanying symptoms – most notably dysphagia. Effective therapies target inflammation or fibrostenotic complications and include proton pump inhibitors, swallowed topical steroids, dietary exclusion, and dilation. Clinical trials testing promising biologic therapies are ongoing.

Functional chest pain, functional heartburn, and reflux hypersensitivity are 3 functional esophageal disorders defined by the Rome IV criteria. Specific criteria, combining symptoms and the results of objective testing, allow for an accurate diagnosis of these conditions. Management may include medications targeted at optimizing acid suppression or neuromodulation, as well as a host of complementary or alternative treatment options. Psychological and behavioral interventions, such as cognitive behavioral therapy and hypnotherapy, have displayed substantial benefits in the treatment of functional chest pain and functional heartburn. Acid suppression and focused neuromodulation are key evidence-based treatment options for reflux hypersensitivity.

Patients with obesity who present with gastroesophageal reflux disease (GERD) require a nuanced approach. Those with lower body mass index (BMI) (less than 33) can be counseled on weight loss, and if successful may be approached with laparoscopic fundoplication. Those who are unable to achieve weight loss or those who present with a BMI greater than or equal to 35 should proceed with laparoscopic Roux-en-Y gastric bypass (LRYGB). Conversion to LRYGB from sleeve gastrectomy is a safe and effective way to manage GERD after sleeve gastrectomy.

Laryngopharyngeal reflux (LPR) is frustrating, as symptoms are nonspecific and diagnosis is often unclear. Two main approaches to diagnosis are empiric treatment trials and objective reflux testing. Initial empiric trial of Proton pump inhibitors (PPI) twice daily for 2-3 months is convenient, but risks overtreatment and delayed diagnosis if patient complaints are not from LPR. Dietary modifications, H2-antagonists, alginates, and fundoplication are other possible LPR treatments. If objective diagnosis is desired or patients' symptoms are refractory to empiric treatment, pH testing with/without impedance should be considered. Additionally, evaluation for non-reflux etiologies of complaints should be performed, including laryngoscopy or videostroboscopy.

Achalasia is the prototypical obstructive motor disorder diagnosed using HRM, but non-achalasia motor disorders are often identified in symptomatic patients. The clinical relevance of these disorders are assessed using ancillary HRM maneuvers (multiple rapid swallows, rapid drink challenge, solid swallows) that augment the standard supine HRM evaluation by challenging peristaltic function. Finding obstructive motor physiology in non-achalasia motor disorders may raise the option of invasive management akin to achalasia. Certain non-achalasia disorders, particularly hypermotility disorders, may manifest as epiphenomena seen with esophageal hypersensitivity. Symptomatic management is offered for superimposed reflux disease, psychological disorders, functional esophageal disorders, and behavioral disorders.

The gastrointestinal tract is the second largest organ system in the body and is often affected by connective tissue disorders. Scleroderma is the classic rheumatologic disease affecting the esophagus; more than 90% of patients with scleroderma have esophageal involvement. This article highlights esophageal manifestations of scleroderma, focusing on pathogenesis, clinical presentation, diagnostic considerations, and treatment options. In addition, this article briefly reviews the esophageal manifestations of other key connective tissue disorders, including mixed connective tissue disease, myositis, Sjogren syndrome, systemic lupus erythematosus, fibromyalgia, and Ehlers-Danlos syndrome.

The aim of this review is to explore the relationship between esophageal syndromes and pulmonary diseases considering the most recent data available. Prior studies have shown a close relationship between lung diseases such as asthma, chronic obstructive pulmonary disorders (COPD), Idiopathic pulmonary fibrosis (IPF), and lung transplant rejection and esophageal dysfunction. Although the association has long been demonstrated, the exact relationship remains unclear. Clinical experience has shown a bidirectional relationship where esophageal disease may influence the outcomes of pulmonary disease and vice versa. The impact of esophageal dysfunction on pulmonary disorders may also be related to 2 different mechanisms: the reflux pathway leading to microaspiration and the reflex pathway triggering vagally mediated airway reactions. The aim of this review is to further explore these relationships and pathophysiologic mechanisms. Specifically, we discuss the proposed hypotheses for the relationship between the 2 diseases, as well as the pathophysiology and new developments in clinical management.

Therapeutic gastrointestinal endoscopy is rapidly evolving, and this evolution is quite apparent for esophageal diseases. Minimally invasive endoluminal therapy now allows outpatient treatment of many esophageal diseases that were traditionally managed surgically. In this review article, we explore the most exciting new developments. We discuss the use of peroral endoscopic myotomy for treatment of achalasia and other related diseases, as well as the modifications that have allowed its use in treatment of Zenker diverticulum. We cover endoscopic treatment of gastroesophageal reflux disease and Barrett's esophagus. Further, we explore advanced endoscopic resection techniques.

> The esophagus plays a crucial role in oral nutrition and digestive pathophysiology. In addition, diet is now considered an important primary or augmentative therapy in several esophageal disease states. This review highlights common dietary therapies used in treating diseases of the esophagus as well as the underlying data that support such practices. Specially, diet and its relationship to swallowing dysfunction, motility disorders, malignancies, and inflammatory mucosal diseases such as gastroesophageal reflux disease and eosinophilic esophagitis is explored.

GASTROENTEROLOGY
CLINICS OF NORTH AMERICA

FORTHCOMING ISSUES

March 2022
Pelvic Floor Disorders
Darren M. Brenner, *Editor*

June 2022
Medical and Surgical Management of Crohn's Disease
Sunanda V. Kane, *Editor*

September 2022
Diagnosis and Treatment of Gastrointestinal Cancers
Marta Davila and Raquel E. Davila, *Editors*

RECENT ISSUES

September 2021
Irritable Bowel Syndrome
William D. Chey, *Editor*

June 2021
Gastrointestinal Infections
M. Nedim Ince and David E. Elliot, *Editor*

March 2021
Nutritional Management of Gastrointestinal Diseases
Gerard E. Mullin and Berkeley N. Limketkai, *Editors*

SERIES OF RELATED INTEREST

Gastrointestinal Endoscopy Clinics of North America
(Available at: https://www.giendo.theclinics.com)
Clinics in Liver Disease
(Available at: https://www.liver.theclinics.com)

Preface

A Comprehensive Approach to Esophageal Symptoms and Disorders

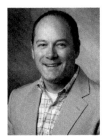

John O. Clarke, MD, AGAF, FACG, FACP, FASGE
Editor

Esophageal symptoms and disease are highly prevalent and comprise a significant burden to patients and society. Thankfully, our understanding of pathophysiology and treatments continues to expand. As we enter the 2020s, we are better able to diagnose and treat our affected patients (although much remains still to be discovered).

As I look back at prior issues of *Gastroenterology Clinics of North America*, it is striking how much advancement has occurred since the last issue dedicated specifically to diverse esophageal disorders was published in 2008. Just in the last year alone, over 3000 articles have been published on dysphagia, over 1500 articles have been published on gastroesophageal reflux, and even less prevalent conditions, such as eosinophilic esophagitis and achalasia, each have several hundred new publications. Over the past decade, we have witnessed the rise and refinement of new diagnostic modalities, including the Functional Lumen Imaging Probe and Mucosal Integrity testing, plus a revolution in the treatment in certain disciplines, such as Barrett's esophagus and early esophageal cancer. Even for areas with less drastic change, such as endoscopic dilation and nutrition, we have increased experience and understanding to better guide management decisions.

In this issue, we have assembled a diverse panel of experts from multiple disciplines to review the key esophageal symptoms and disorders that plague our patients, with the goal of providing a comprehensive approach to the esophageal landscape as it stands today. As reflux affects approximately 20% of American adults and is the main esophageal disorder seen by practicing gastroenterologists today, we have devoted several articles to various aspects of this disorder, including (a) endoscopic and surgical management, (b) the connection to obesity, (c) the relationship to pulmonary disease, and (d) how to approach laryngopharyngeal reflux. We have also focused

Gastroenterol Clin N Am 50 (2021) xiii–xiv
https://doi.org/10.1016/j.gtc.2021.08.011
0889-8553/21/© 2021 Elsevier Inc. All rights reserved.

two articles specifically on sequelae of reflux, namely Barrett's esophagus and early esophageal cancer. Other common esophageal complaints, such as dysphagia and chest pain, have also been addressed in separate articles. Emerging conditions that have had significant updates in the last decade, such as achalasia, motility disorders other than achalasia, eosinophilic esophagitis, and scleroderma (as it pertains to the esophagus), are also reviewed. Two articles focus specifically on therapeutic endoscopy implications for esophageal disease, including Bill Ravich's article reflecting on 40 years of personal experience with the technique of esophageal dilation. The final article addresses nutritional concerns in esophageal disease, an important consideration for all esophageal symptoms and disorders. I would like to personally thank all the authors for their contributions and for writing such thorough and eloquent articles in a timely fashion.

The past decade has seen significant change in our knowledge of esophageal disease, but we still have much progress to make. This issue provides a map of the esophageal landscape as it stands in December 2021.

John O. Clarke, MD, AGAF, FACG, FACP, FASGE
Division of Gastroenterology & Hepatology
Stanford University School of Medicine
Redwood City, CA 94063, USA

E-mail address:
john.clarke@stanford.edu

Achalasia
Diagnosis, Management and Surveillance

Sydney Pomenti, MD, John William Blackett, MD, MSc,
Daniela Jodorkovsky, MD*

KEYWORDS

- Achalasia • Esophageal manometry • Esophagram
- Functional luminal imaging probe • Heller myotomy • Pneumatic dilation
- Peroral endoscopic myotomy • Esophageal cancer

KEY POINTS

- Achalasia is characterized by incomplete relaxation of the lower esophageal sphincter and abnormal peristalsis.
- Symptoms include dysphagia, regurgitation, chest pain, or heartburn.
- High-resolution esophageal manometry is the gold standard for diagnosis.
- Treatments include pneumatic dilation, Heller myotomy with fundoplication, and peroral endoscopic myotomy.

INTRODUCTION

Achalasia is a rare esophageal motor disorder characterized by abnormal or absent peristalsis associated with incomplete relaxation of the lower esophageal sphincter (LES) with deglutition. The pathophysiologic mechanism is thought to be an immune-mediated degeneration of myenteric neurons in response to an unidentified antigen/infection.[1,2] Loss of inhibitory ganglion cells in the distal esophagus results in increased basal pressure of the LES, lack of normal LES relaxation, and loss of normal peristalsis.[3] The annual incidence ranges from 1.6 to 2.8 per 100,000 individuals with a prevalence of 10.8 per 100,000 individuals.[4] The prevalence does seem to be increasing based on recent studies from the United States, potentially due to increased disease awareness and improvements in technology, especially high-resolution manometry (HRM).[5]

DIAGNOSIS
Historical Cues

Solid food dysphagia in conjunction with variable degrees of dysphagia to liquids (70%–97%) is a hallmark of achalasia. The onset of dysphagia is usually gradual,

Division of Digestive and Liver Diseases, Columbia University Irving Medical Center, 630 West 168th Street, Suite 3-401, New York, NY 10032, USA
* Corresponding author.
E-mail address: dj2470@cumc.columbia.edu

Gastroenterol Clin N Am 50 (2021) 721–736
https://doi.org/10.1016/j.gtc.2021.07.001
0889-8553/21/© 2021 Elsevier Inc. All rights reserved.

with many patients having symptoms for years before diagnosis. As the disease progresses, especially as the esophagus dilates, patients develop regurgitation of undigested food or accumulated saliva (75%–91%).[6–8] Given the delay in diagnosis and years of symptoms, patients often accommodate to these symptoms using various maneuvers including drinking carbonated beverages and lifting the neck while eating and drinking.[9] Chest pain occurs in approximately half of patients; it is more common in younger patients and is less likely to be relieved by treatments but is more likely to spontaneously resolve over time.[6,8,10] Heartburn and reflux symptoms are often endorsed by patients (40%–60%); however, symptoms are thought to be caused by bacterial fermentation of retained food leading to esophageal acidification rather than gastroesophageal reflux events.[11] Some patients complain of respiratory symptoms (40%) including cough, hiccups, hoarseness, shortness of breath, and aspiration with up to 10% having bronchopulmonary complications as a result of regurgitation and aspiration.[12] Mild weight loss can by typical for achalasia; however, more profound weight loss should raise concerns for alternate diagnoses including pseudoachalasia.

The historical cues mentioned earlier should trigger a more extensive evaluation but are unable to distinguish patients with a primary motility disorder or differentiate between different motility disorders. Upper endoscopy, barium esophagram, and HRM are often used in conjunction to establish the diagnosis of achalasia.

Esophagogastroduodenoscopy

In all patients presenting with dysphagia, mechanical obstruction must be ruled out, typically by esophagogastroduodenoscopy (EGD). EGD is often the first test for evaluating new-onset dysphagia, as it combines the ability to detect most structural causes of dysphagia with the ability to obtain biopsies to identify conditions such as eosinophilic esophagitis or therapeutically treat webs, strictures, and rings with dilation. Early in achalasia, the esophagus may seem normal, and a normal examination should not exclude the diagnosis.[8] Endoscopic findings consistent with achalasia include retained saliva and dilated esophagus with retained materials. The esophageal mucosa usually seems normal but nonspecific changes including erythema, ulceration, and even esophageal candidiasis may be seen secondary to retained materials. A puckered esophagogastric junction (EGJ) or a rosette configuration on retroflexion may be seen in patients with achalasia (**Fig. 1**). The endoscopist may experience

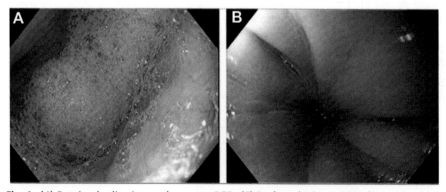

Fig. 1. (*A*) Retained saliva in esophagus on EGD. (*B*) Puckered EGJ on EGD. (*From* Vaezi MF, Pandolfino JE, Yadlapati RH, Greer KB, Kavitt RT. ACG clinical guidelines: diagnosis and management of achalasia. *Am J Gastroenterol.* 2020;115(9):1393-1411; with permission.)

resistance to intubation of the EGJ but this should be easily traversed with gentle pressure in patients with achalasia. During endoscopy, careful examination of the EGJ and the gastric cardia is critical in evaluation for obstructing lesions.

Pseudoachalasia secondary to an infiltrating neoplasm should be suspected in patients older than 60 years with new-onset symptoms, rapid weight loss, or abnormal endoscopy with increased resistance during intubation of the stomach. In these high-risk patients, endoscopic ultrasound with fine-needle aspiration of the esophagogastric junction should be considered in addition to the standard EGD to definitively rule out malignancy.[13,14]

High-Resolution Manometry

HRM incorporates up to 36 pressure sensors spaced within 1 cm on a transnasal catheter allowing for enhanced visualization and esophageal pressure topography. HRM is the current gold standard for diagnosis of achalasia.[15] The benefits of HRM over conventional manometry include improved accuracy, reproducibility, and the ability to distinguish clinically relevant subtypes of achalasia.[16–19] On HRM, achalasia is defined as incomplete relaxation of the LES characterized by an elevated integrated relaxation pressure (IRP) and no normal peristalsis. Three distinct achalasia subtypes have been established based on esophageal body topography, with differences in their responsiveness to medical and surgical therapies[15,20–23] (**Fig. 2**). All 3 subtypes of achalasia have impaired EGJ relaxation with a supine IRP greater than 15 to 22 mm Hg (depending on proprietary software).[24,25] However, the subtypes differ in their patterns of peristalsis and pressurization.[13,15]

Type I achalasia is defined by aperistalsis, with esophageal pressurization less than 30 mm Hg, type II achalasia is defined by panesophageal pressurization greater than 30 mm Hg in at least 20% of swallows with no normal peristalsis, and type III achalasia is characterized by at least 20% of swallows with premature contractions defined by a distal latency less than 4.5 seconds and no normal peristalsis.[15,20,21] Achalasia type II is the most common and increasing in prevalence, accounting for 50% to 70% of cases, whereas achalasia type I, accounting for 20% to 40% of cases, is next most common. Achalasia type III is the least common, accounting for 5% of cases.[13,26]

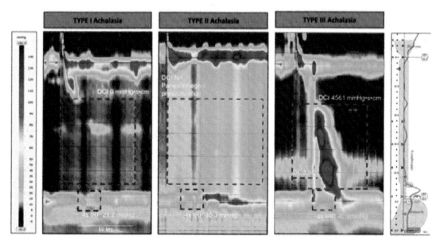

Fig. 2. Representative HRM of type I, II, and III achalasia. (*From* Yadlapati R, Kahrilas PJ, Fox MR, et al. Esophageal motility disorders on high-resolution manometry: Chicago classification version 4.0©. *Neurogastroenterol Motil*. 2021;33(1):e14058; with permission.)

Contrast Imaging

Videofluoroscopy and modified barium swallows are often used to evaluate oropharyngeal dysphagia and can also evaluate various compensatory dietary modifications, postures, and swallowing maneuvers.

In cases where endoscopy and HRM are equivocal, a barium esophagram is a complementary tool. Esophageal dilation, narrow EGJ with a "bird-beak" appearance, aperistalsis, and delayed emptying of barium suggest achalasia.[13] A timed barium esophagram is used in both diagnosis and monitoring posttherapy by measuring the barium column height at 1-, 2-, and 5-minutes after ingestion.[27,28] However, barium esophagram is not a sensitive test for diagnosis of achalasia and may be normal in approximately one-third of patients with achalasia.[8]

Functional Lumen Imaging Probe

Functional lumen imaging probe (FLIP) is a catheter that uses high-resolution impedance planimetry to measure cross-sectional area and pressure to calculate a distensibility index during controlled balloon inflation across the GEJ in a simulated 3-dimensional model.[29] Although transnasal assessment can be performed, the FLIP study is more commonly performed through the mouth during sedated EGD. FLIP has been shown to have high concordance with HRM, correlates with symptom severity, and in equivocal cases may be a useful complementary diagnostic tool.[30–32] The use of FLIP during initial endoscopy in those with high clinical suspicion for achalasia before HRM or esophagram is an area of investigation.

In addition to EGJ distensibility and diameter, the 2.0 platform captures esophageal body patterns in response to balloon inflation. The 3 main patterns that have emerged are repetitive anterograde contractions, repetitive retrograde contractions (RRCs), and absent contractility. RRCs are most noted in spastic conditions and type III achalasia.[30] The use of FLIP esophageal body patterns in the management of achalasia is still under investigation.

The authors' proposed diagnostic algorithm is pictured in **Fig. 3**.

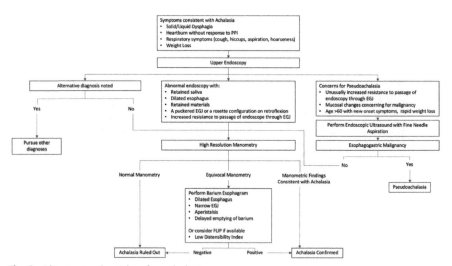

Fig. 3. Diagnostic algorithm for achalasia.

MANAGEMENT

The goals of therapy for achalasia are symptom improvement and prevention of complications, including aspiration and esophageal dilation, by improving esophageal emptying. Definitive therapies for achalasia include pneumatic dilation, surgical myotomy, and peroral endoscopic myotomy (POEM). Nondefinitive therapies include oral medications and botulinum toxin. Esophagectomy can be considered for patients who have failed other therapies.

Oral Pharmacotherapy

Oral pharmacotherapy is the least effective available treatment of achalasia. Medications that induce LES relaxation include calcium channel blockers such as nifedipine, nitrates such as isosorbide dinitrate, and phosphodiesterase inhibitors such as sildenafil.[33–37] There are few comparative studies evaluating the effectiveness of oral medications for achalasia, which are generally reserved either for patients who are not candidates for definitive therapy and have failed botulinum injection or as a bridge to more definitive therapy in symptomatic patients. Smooth muscle relaxants are limited by short duration and side effects, including headaches and hypotension.

Botulinum Injection

Botulinum toxin inhibits acetylcholine release from nerve endings, leading to decrease of muscle tone, and thus can induce LES relaxation when injected endoscopically.[38] Symptom relief occurs in approximately 80% of patients initially but only lasts for several months up to about a year.[39] The response may be better in older patients.[40] The authors inject 100U of botulinum toxin in 0.5 to 1 mL aliquots just above the GEJ. Because of the short duration of symptomatic relief, it is generally reserved for patients with a limited life expectancy or who are too sick to undergo dilation, myotomy, or POEM. Injections may lead to fibrosis and higher complication rates and worse outcomes if subsequent myotomy is performed, although this is based on observational studies[41,42]; this may be less likely to affect patients who undergo POEM after previous endoscopic injections.[43,44]

Pneumatic Dilation

Pneumatic dilation uses a rigid balloon to disrupt the LES by circumferential stretching of the muscle fibers. Standard through-the-scope balloon dilation or bougie dilation is not effective at disrupting the muscularis propria. Dilators come in 3.0, 3.5, and 4.0 cm sizes and are used sequentially if adequate symptom relief has not been achieved. Dilation typically starts at 3.0 cm and is repeated every 4 to 6 weeks as needed with sequential sizes.[13,45] The risk of perforation from pneumatic dilation is about 2%, with 1% requiring surgery.[46] Perforations are most likely to occur during the initial dilation.[47] The procedure is typically performed with fluoroscopy. The EsoFLIP hydraulic balloon does not require fluoroscopy, and small, short-term studies show symptom improvement with few complications.[48] Compared with surgical myotomy, pneumatic dilation may be more cost-effective, at least in the short-term.[49] Routine gastrografin esophagram is sometimes performed after dilation to rule out perforation but is likely unnecessary unless signs or symptoms such as chest pain, fever, and crepitus are present.[50] The efficacy of a single dilation ranges from 66% to 88% at 1 year but declines to 25% to 29% at 10 years.[46]

Surgical Myotomy

Surgical myotomy (Heller myotomy) is accomplished by division of the muscular fibers of the LES, typically done laparoscopically. The success rate of laparoscopic Heller myotomy (LHM) in randomized controlled trials (RCTs) ranges from 82% to 90% at 2 years, but one study found that the response decreased from 89% at 6 months to 57% at 6 years.[51–53] A meta-analysis of 1575 patients found that response rates are higher in type I (81%) and type II (92%) achalasia than type III achalasia (71%).[22] Gastroesophageal reflux disease (GERD) develops in approximately 30% to 50% of patients after myotomy who do not receive a fundoplication. The addition of a partial fundoplication decreases the incidence of GERD to about 10% and is now done routinely.[39,54,55]

Peroral Endoscopic Myotomy

POEM involves the endoscopic creation of a submucosal tunnel and selective myotomy of the esophagus and proximal stomach. The typical length of myotomy is 8 to 12 cm.[56] A longer myotomy may be helpful in patients with type III achalasia in order to treat the entire spastic segment of esophagus as determined by manometry. Because of ability to tailor and lengthen the myotomy, POEM may be especially effective for type III achalasia.[57] POEM should be avoided in patients who cannot tolerate general anesthesia, have coagulopathy or portal hypertension, or prior radiation, ablation, or mucosal resection in the operative field, due to risk of perforation or uncontrolled bleeding.[56] Routine esophagram after POEM is often performed but seems to have limited benefit and occasionally misses serious adverse events.[58] The success rate of POEM is at or greater than 90% in most studies.[59–61] GERD develops after POEM in up to 58% of patients, and erosive esophagitis is also more likely to occur after POEM than LHM, due to inability to add fundoplication with POEM at the time of the initial procedure.[62] POEM should therefore be avoided in patients with esophagitis or Barrett's esophagus unless planned to combine with endoscopic or surgical fundoplication.

Comparison of Treatment Modalities

Several landmark RCTs have been performed comparing the definitive treatment modalities (**Table 1**). Most investigative studies use the Eckardt score to follow symptoms and define treatment success. Each of the 4 components are scored on a 0- to 3-point scale (0: none, 1: occasionally, 2: daily, 3: each meal, for a total score out of 12).[63] A total score of 3 or more after treatment is considered suboptimal.[13] Although the Eckardt score is the current standard, the variance in patient responses mostly depends on the dysphagia symptom alone (which accounts for 50% of the variance), whereas chest pain and weight loss account for 10% of the variance each.[64] Thus, the Eckardt score alone is not sufficient to define treatment success and failure, and other methods of symptom surveillance are needed.

In a 2011 RCT, pneumatic dilation (n = 95) versus LHM with Dor fundoplication (n = 106) found no significant difference in therapeutic success, defined as Eckhardt score less than or equal to 3 at 2 years (86% in pneumatic dilation vs 90% in LHM).[52] At 2-year follow-up, there were also no significant differences in pressure at the LES on manometry, esophageal emptying on timed barium esophagram, or rates of abnormal acid exposure. One caveat to this RCT is that sequential dilation was allowed, and all the patients in the pneumatic dilation arm underwent at least 2 dilations.

More recently, a 2019 RCT comparing POEM (n = 67) versus pneumatic dilation (n = 66) found that POEM had significantly higher treatment success at 2 years,

Table 1
Overview of randomized controlled trials for achalasia interventions

Author, Year	Comparison	Location	Inclusion Criteria	N per Group	Primary Outcome	Secondary Outcome
Boeckxstaens,[52] 2011	LHM with Dor fundoplication vs PD	14 hospitals in 5 European countries	Achalasia, 18–75 y of age, Eckhardt score >3	95 PD, 106 LHM	Treatment success (Eckhardt score ≤3 at 2 y) occurred in 86% of PD and 90% of LHM patients (P = .46)	At 2-y follow-up, no significant difference in LES pressure, esophageal emptying on barium esophagram, quality of life, or esophageal acid exposure
Ponds,[65] 2019	POEM vs PD	6 hospitals in Netherlands, Germany, Italy, Hong Kong, and United States	Newly diagnosed achalasia, 18–80 y of age, Eckhardt score >3, ASA classification I–II	64 POEM, 66 PD	Treatment success (Eckhardt score ≤3 at 2 y) occurred in 92% of POEM and 54% of PD patients (P < .001).	At 2-y follow-up, no significant difference in median IRP or esophageal emptying on barium esophagram. Reflux esophagitis was more common in POEM than PD (41% vs 7%).
Werner,[53] 2019	POEM vs LHM with Dor fundoplication	8 hospitals in 6 European countries	Achalasia, ≥18 y of age, Eckhardt score >3	112 POEM, 109 LHM	Treatment success (Eckhardt score ≤3 at 2 y) occurred in 83.0% of POEM and 81.7% of LHM patients (P = .007 for noninferiority)	At 2-y follow-up, no difference in IRP, Gastrointestinal Quality of Life Index, or serious adverse events. Reflux esophagitis was more common after POEM (44% vs 29% after LHM at 2 y)

defined as Eckhardt score less than or equal to 3 and absence of severe complications or retreatment (92% for POEM vs 54% for pneumatic dilation).[65] However, the lower efficacy rate of pneumatic dilation (54%) compared with historical data was questioned. Reflux esophagitis also occurred more often in the POEM group than the pneumatic dilation group (41% vs 7%). Another 2019 RCT compared POEM (n = 112) versus LHM with Dor fundoplication (n = 109). Clinical success, defined as Eckhardt score less than or equal to 3 at 2-year follow-up without the need for additional treatments, occurred in 83.0% of POEM patients and 81.7% of LHM patients.[53] There were also no differences in the LES IRP or Gastrointestinal Quality of Life Index at 2-year follow-up between groups. Reflux esophagitis was found more often in the POEM group on endoscopy at 2-year follow-up, at 44% compared with 29% in the LHM group.

A 2018 meta-analysis and systematic review compared 53 studies of LHM (5834 patients) and 21 studies of POEM (1958) for the treatment of achalasia.[66] POEM had a slightly higher probability of improved dysphagia at both 1 year (93.5% for POEM vs 91.0% for LHM, $P = .01$) and 2-year follow-up (92.7% for POEM vs 90.0% for LHM, $P = .01$). However, POEM patients had significantly higher odds of developing GERD symptoms (odds ratio 1.69), erosive esophagitis (odds ratio 9.31), and positive pH testing (odds ratio 4.30). Mean length of stay was also 1.03 days longer in POEM versus LHM.

A 2019 meta-analysis of 20 studies of 1575 patients with achalasia compared the results of botulinum toxin, pneumatic dilatation, LHM, and POEM, stratified by subtype.[22] For type I achalasia, the pooled success rate was 18% with botulinum toxin, 61% for pneumatic dilation, 81% for LHM, and 95% for POEM. For type II achalasia, the success rate was 59% with botulinum toxin, 84% for pneumatic dilation, 92% for LHM, and 97% for POEM. For type III achalasia, the success rate was 21% for botulinum toxin, 31% for pneumatic dilation, 71% for LHM, and 93% for POEM. Type II achalasia had the highest success rates for all treatment types. POEM was superior to LHM for type I achalasia (odds ratio [OR] 2.97, 95% confidence interval [CI] 1.09–8.03, $P = .032$) and type III achalasia (OR 3.51, 95% CI 1.39–8.77, $P = .007$) but not type II achalasia (OR 1.31, 95% CI 0.48–3.55, $P = .591$). The increased risk of GERD is a significant limitation of POEM compared with LHM. A meta-analysis of 1542 patients who underwent POEM and 2581 who underwent LHM with Dor fundoplication found that POEM was associated with a significantly higher rate of posttreatment GERD, at 39.0% versus 16.8%.[67]

Esophagectomy

Approximately 10% to 15% of treated patients will progress to megaesophagus or end-stage achalasia and up to 5% require esophagectomy.[68–71] Esophagectomy carries a significant risk of respiratory complications; however, it is safe and effective in experienced centers.[72]

Therapeutic Targets

During or immediately following treatment, objective testing to confirm success with either HRM, timed barium esophagram, and more recently FLIP has been used. A postdilation LES resting pressure of less than 10 to 15 mm Hg is thought to be a predictor of long-term response.[73,74] Similarly, a greater than 50% improvement over baseline in barium height after timed barium esophagram or complete esophageal emptying at 1-minute postingestion also seems to predict a favorable outcome.[75,76] Intraoperative FLIP during POEM or LHM may be used to target a goal distensibility index (DI). A DI of 4.5 to 8.5 mm²/mm Hg may be ideal to improve symptom scores without increased reflux, and FLIP may be most predictive of postoperative treatment response.[77–79]

SURVEILLANCE

Achalasia is a chronic disease that requires life-long management and follow-up. The natural history of achalasia without treatment is progressive dilation of the esophagus, in some cases resulting in megaesophagus (esophageal diameter >6 cm), potential Barrett's esophagus, and esophageal cancer.[69] Because there is no cure for achalasia, providers must remain vigilant for recurrent symptoms or complications.

There are no clear surveillance guidelines for the long-term management of achalasia, and much is left to the discretion and judgment of individual providers. The American Society for Gastrointestinal Endoscopy guidelines suggest there is insufficient evidence to support routine surveillance. Postprocedure management options include monitoring symptoms, assessing for symptom recurrence, assessing esophageal acid exposure, and esophageal cancer screening in high-risk groups.[80,81]

Surveillance of Symptoms

For any significant change in signs or symptoms following treatment, the authors' initial first study is typically upper endoscopy to rule out esophagitis, stricture, or cancer. Otherwise, their approach is commonly a variety of testing that provide complementary and corroborative information.

Timed barium esophagram is a better predictor for treatment success than patient reported symptoms by assessing for bolus retention.[75] HRM may look for return of peristalsis, ongoing spasticity, and assess completeness of myotomy; however, esophageal stasis on timed barium esophagogram (TBE) has been shown to be a better predictor of symptom recurrence than LES pressure on manometry.[82] Some experts have suggested monitoring TBE annually after treatment over HRM to assess esophageal emptying and diameter.[13,45] However, provocative maneuvers during HRM as the rapid drink challenge may increase the utility of HRM in postachalasia treatment symptom recurrence.[83] Further, impedance sensors capturing the impedance bolus height may approximate a TBE measure of bolus stasis.[84] Finally, as stated earlier, metrics obtained during FLIP evaluation can be predictive of symptom recurrence and assess adequacy of myotomy.[79]

Surveillance of Reflux

Postintervention reflux can occur after treatment, with rates of reflux higher in POEM than Heller myotomy combined with fundoplication. A study of 36 patients who underwent POEM for achalasia and then received EGD with wireless pH testing found esophagitis in 13% and an abnormal esophageal acid exposure in 41.7% of patients. It was often asymptomatic, as only 13% had positive symptom correlation.[85] A study of 64 achalasia patients who had surgical myotomy plus fundoplication found that in those with 7- to 10-year follow-up, the prevalence of abnormal pH testing was 15%, compared with 28% in those with 10- to 20-year follow-up, and 53% in those greater than 20-year follow-up.[86] It is unclear which modality is best to evaluate acid exposure in the absence of esophagitis or if traditional pH metrics apply to achalasia patients.

Cancer Surveillance

The association of achalasia with esophageal cancer has been well established, with squamous cell carcinoma far more common than adenocarcinoma.[87–90] A 2017 meta-analysis of 11,978 achalasia patients found that the incidence of esophageal squamous cell carcinoma was 312 cases per 100,000 patient-years, compared with 21 cases per 100,000 patient-years for esophageal adenocarcinoma.[91]

The mechanisms of esophageal cancer in achalasia differs by subtype. Squamous cell carcinoma is thought to occur due to poor clearance of esophageal contents, leading to retention of toxic food contents and nitrosamine production from bacterial overgrowth, leading to chronic inflammation.[81] Although the relative risk of cancer is much higher in achalasia than the general population, the absolute risk remains low. The annual incidence of esophageal cancer ranges from 0.14% to 0.34% and the prevalence is about 1% to 3%.[87,91–96] The risk of squamous cell cancer remains significantly elevated even after treatment with myotomy in men, although not in women, in whom there is a much lower baseline risk.[89] Adenocarcinoma is thought to be mediated by increased gastroesophageal reflux and esophagitis progressing to Barrett's esophagus postdilation or myotomy.[86,93,97] However, in a Swedish cohort study of 2896 achalasia patients, the risk of esophageal cancer was not significantly different in treated versus untreated achalasia, suggesting that iatrogenic reflux is unlikely to be the only cause.[92]

Although it is clearly established that the risk of esophageal cancer is increased in achalasia, the benefits of screening are unclear. There is no consensus among achalasia experts on whether to screen achalasia patients, when to start screening, or what the appropriate screening interval should be.[81,98] The 2020 ACG guidelines note that "there are limited data to support routine screening for cancer in patients with achalasia" but they also note that "many experts are in favor of some form of endoscopic or radiographic surveillance in patients with achalasia at an interval of every 3 years if the disease has been present for more than 10 to 15 years."[13] It has been estimated that annual surveillance would require 406 endoscopies in men and 2220 in women to detect one case of esophageal cancer.[87] There are no studies evaluating the cost-effectiveness of esophageal cancer screening in achalasia.

Given these limitations, the authors' approach to postintervention surveillance in achalasia is shown in the algorithm in **Fig. 4**. For patients with well-controlled symptoms, the authors consider an upper endoscopy at 3-year intervals if there are multiple risk factors for cancer (Barrett's esophagus, family history, tobacco or daily alcohol consumption, male sex, achalasia diagnosis >10 years, esophagitis or positive pH test) (see **Fig. 4**).

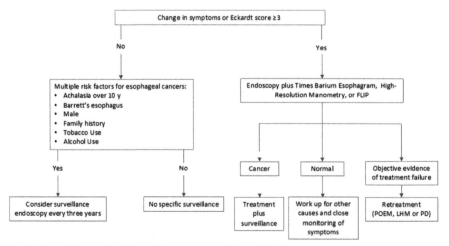

Fig. 4. Surveillance algorithm after treatment for achalasia.

CLINICS CARE POINTS

- All patients with symptoms concerning for achalasia including dysphagia, regurgitation, chest pain, and heart burn should first undergo EGD followed by HRM.
- Achalasia is defined by impaired EGJ relaxation on HRM and the subtypes are defined by their patterns of peristalsis and pressurization.
- In cases where endoscopy and HRM are equivocal, timed barium esophagram and FLIP can be used as complementary tools.
- Definitive therapies for achalasia include pneumatic dilation, surgical myotomy, and POEM, whereas botulinum injections and oral pharmacotherapy are generally reserved for patients who are not candidates for definitive therapies.
- For any significant change in signs or symptoms following treatment of achalasia, upper endoscopy should be performed evaluating for esophagitis, stricture, or cancer followed by timed barium esophagram, HRM, or FLIP.

DISCLOSURE

None.

REFERENCES

1. Hoshino M, Omura N, Yano F, et al. Immunohistochemical study of the muscularis externa of the esophagus in achalasia patients. Dis Esophagus 2013;26(1): 14–21.
2. Raymond L, Lach B, Shamji FM. Inflammatory aetiology of primary oesophageal achalasia: an immunohistochemical and ultrastructural study of Auerbach's plexus. Histopathology 1999;35(5):445–53.
3. Holloway RH, Dodds WJ, Helm JF, et al. Integrity of cholinergic innervation to the lower esophageal sphincter in achalasia. Gastroenterology 1986;90(4):924–9.
4. Sadowski DC, Ackah F, Jiang B, et al. Achalasia: incidence, prevalence and survival. A population-based study. Neurogastroenterol Motil 2010;22(9):e256–61.
5. Samo S, Carlson DA, Gregory DL, et al. Incidence and prevalence of achalasia in central Chicago, 2004-2014, since the widespread use of high-resolution manometry. Clin Gastroenterol Hepatol 2017;15(3):366–73.
6. Fisichella PM, Raz D, Palazzo F, et al. Clinical, radiological, and manometric profile in 145 patients with untreated achalasia. World J Surg 2008;32(9):1974–9.
7. Tsuboi K, Hoshino M, Srinivasan A, et al. Insights gained from symptom evaluation of esophageal motility disorders: a review of 4,215 patients. Digestion 2012; 85(3):236–42.
8. Howard PJ, Maher L, Pryde A, et al. Five year prospective study of the incidence, clinical features, and diagnosis of achalasia in Edinburgh. Gut 1992;33(8): 1011–5.
9. Vaezi MF, Richter JE. Diagnosis and management of achalasia. American College of Gastroenterology Practice Parameter Committee. Am J Gastroenterol 1999; 94(12):3406–12.
10. Eckardt VF, Stauf B, Bernhard G. Chest pain in achalasia: patient characteristics and clinical course. Gastroenterology 1999;116(6):1300–4.
11. Smart HL, Foster PN, Evans DF, et al. Twenty four hour oesophageal acidity in achalasia before and after pneumatic dilatation. Gut 1987;28(7):883–7.

12. Sinan H, Tatum RP, Soares RV, et al. Prevalence of respiratory symptoms in patients with achalasia. Dis Esophagus 2011;24(4):224–8.

13. Vaezi MF, Pandolfino JE, Yadlapati RH, et al. ACG clinical guidelines: diagnosis and management of achalasia. Am J Gastroenterol 2020;115(9):1393–411.

14. Kahrilas PJ, Kishk SM, Helm JF, et al. Comparison of pseudoachalasia and achalasia. Am J Med 1987;82(3):439–46.

15. Yadlapati R, Kahrilas PJ, Fox MR, et al. Esophageal motility disorders on high-resolution manometry: Chicago classification version 4.0©. Neurogastroenterol Motil 2021;33(1):e14058.

16. Pandolfino JE, Ghosh SK, Rice J, et al. Classifying esophageal motility by pressure topography characteristics: a study of 400 patients and 75 controls. Am J Gastroenterol 2008;103(1):27–37.

17. Bogte A, Bredenoord AJ, Oors J, et al. Reproducibility of esophageal high-resolution manometry. Neurogastroenterol Motil 2011;23(7):e271–6.

18. Fox M, Hebbard G, Janiak P, et al. High-resolution manometry predicts the success of oesophageal bolus transport and identifies clinically important abnormalities not detected by conventional manometry. Neurogastroenterol Motil 2004; 16(5):533–42.

19. Roman S, Huot L, Zerbib F, et al. High-resolution manometry improves the diagnosis of esophageal motility disorders in patients with dysphagia: a randomized multicenter study. Am J Gastroenterol 2016;111(3):372–80.

20. Pandolfino JE, Kwiatek MA, Nealis T, et al. Achalasia: a new clinically relevant classification by high-resolution manometry. Gastroenterology 2008;135(5): 1526–33.

21. Kahrilas PJ, Bredenoord AJ, Fox M, et al. The Chicago Classification of esophageal motility disorders, v3.0. Neurogastroenterol Motil 2015;27(2):160–74.

22. Andolfi C, Fisichella PM. Meta-analysis of clinical outcome after treatment for achalasia based on manometric subtypes. Br J Surg 2019;106(4):332–41.

23. Ou YH, Nie XM, Li LF, et al. High-resolution manometric subtypes as a predictive factor for the treatment of achalasia: a meta-analysis and systematic review. J Dig Dis 2016;17(4):222–35.

24. Ghosh SK, Pandolfino JE, Rice J, et al. Impaired deglutitive EGJ relaxation in clinical esophageal manometry: a quantitative analysis of 400 patients and 75 controls. Am J Physiol Gastrointest Liver Physiol 2007;293(4):G878–85.

25. Herregods TVK, Roman S, Kahrilas PJ, et al. Normative values in esophageal high-resolution manometry. Neurogastroenterol Motil 2015;27(2):175–87.

26. Zhou MJ, Kamal A, Freedberg DE, et al. Type II achalasia is increasing in prevalence. Dig Dis Sci 2020. https://doi.org/10.1007/s10620-020-06668-7.

27. de Oliveira JM, Birgisson S, Doinoff C, et al. Timed barium swallow: a simple technique for evaluating esophageal emptying in patients with achalasia. AJR Am J Roentgenol 1997;169(2):473–9.

28. Neyaz Z, Gupta M, Ghoshal UC. How to perform and interpret timed barium esophagogram. J Neurogastroenterol Motil 2013;19(2):251–6.

29. Mearin F, Malagelada JR. Complete lower esophageal sphincter relaxation observed in some achalasia patients is functionally inadequate. Am J Physiol Gastrointest Liver Physiol 2000;278(3):G376–83.

30. Carlson DA, Kahrilas PJ, Lin Z, et al. Evaluation of esophageal motility utilizing the functional lumen imaging probe. Am J Gastroenterol 2016;111(12):1726–35.

31. Pandolfino JE, de Ruigh A, Nicodème F, et al. Distensibility of the esophagogastric junction assessed with the functional lumen imaging probe (FLIP™) in achalasia patients. Neurogastroenterol Motil 2013;25(6):496–501.

32. Ponds FA, Bredenoord AJ, Kessing BF, et al. Esophagogastric junction distensibility identifies achalasia subgroup with manometrically normal esophagogastric junction relaxation. Neurogastroenterol Motil 2017;29(1). https://doi.org/10.1111/nmo.12908.

33. Coccia G, Bortolotti M, Michetti P, et al. Prospective clinical and manometric study comparing pneumatic dilatation and sublingual nifedipine in the treatment of oesophageal achalasia. Gut 1991;32(6):604–6.

34. Traube M, Dubovik S, Lange RC, et al. The role of nifedipine therapy in achalasia: results of a randomized, double-blind, placebo-controlled study. Am J Gastroenterol 1989;84(10):1259–62.

35. Gelfond M, Rozen P, Gilat T. Isosorbide dinitrate and nifedipine treatment of achalasia: a clinical, manometric and radionuclide evaluation. Gastroenterology 1982; 83(5):963–9.

36. Wen ZH, Gardener E, Wang YP. Nitrates for achalasia. Cochrane Database Syst Rev 2004;(1):CD002299.

37. Eherer AJ, Schwetz I, Hammer HF, et al. Effect of sildenafil on oesophageal motor function in healthy subjects and patients with oesophageal motor disorders. Gut 2002;50(6):758–64.

38. Pasricha PJ, Ravich WJ, Hendrix TR, et al. Intrasphincteric botulinum toxin for the treatment of achalasia. N Engl J Med 1995;332(12):774–8.

39. Campos GM, Vittinghoff E, Rabl C, et al. Endoscopic and surgical treatments for achalasia: a systematic review and meta-analysis. Ann Surg 2009;249(1):45–57.

40. Pasricha PJ, Rai R, Ravich WJ, et al. Botulinum toxin for achalasia: long-term outcome and predictors of response. Gastroenterology 1996;110(5):1410–5.

41. Patti MG, Feo CV, Arcerito M, et al. Effects of previous treatment on results of laparoscopic Heller myotomy for achalasia. Dig Dis Sci 1999;44(11):2270–6.

42. Smith CD, Stival A, Howell DL, et al. Endoscopic therapy for achalasia before Heller myotomy results in worse outcomes than heller myotomy alone. Ann Surg 2006;243(5):579–84 [Discussion 584].

43. Orenstein SB, Raigani S, Wu YV, et al. Peroral endoscopic myotomy (POEM) leads to similar results in patients with and without prior endoscopic or surgical therapy. Surg Endosc 2015;29(5):1064–70.

44. Jones EL, Meara MP, Pittman MR, et al. Prior treatment does not influence the performance or early outcome of per-oral endoscopic myotomy for achalasia. Surg Endosc 2016;30(4):1282–6.

45. Vaezi MF, Pandolfino JE, Vela MF. ACG clinical guideline: diagnosis and management of achalasia. Am J Gastroenterol 2013;108(8):1238–49 [quiz 1250].

46. Katzka DA, Castell DO. Review article: an analysis of the efficacy, perforation rates and methods used in pneumatic dilation for achalasia. Aliment Pharmacol Ther 2011;34(8):832–9.

47. van Hoeij FB, Prins LI, Smout AJPM, et al. Efficacy and safety of pneumatic dilation in achalasia: a systematic review and meta-analysis. Neurogastroenterol Motil 2019;31(7):e13548.

48. Schnurre L, Murray FR, Schindler V, et al. Short-term outcome after singular hydraulic EsoFLIP dilation in patients with achalasia: a feasibility study. Neurogastroenterol Motil 2020;32(9):e13864.

49. Kostic S, Johnsson E, Kjellin A, et al. Health economic evaluation of therapeutic strategies in patients with idiopathic achalasia: results of a randomized trial comparing pneumatic dilatation with laparoscopic cardiomyotomy. Surg Endosc 2007;21(7):1184–9.

50. Zori AG, Kirtane TS, Gupte AR, et al. Utility of clinical suspicion and endoscopic re-examination for detection of esophagogastric perforation after pneumatic dilation for achalasia. Endoscopy 2016;48(2):128–33.

51. Vela MF, Richter JE, Khandwala F, et al. The long-term efficacy of pneumatic dilatation and Heller myotomy for the treatment of achalasia. Clin Gastroenterol Hepatol 2006;4(5):580–7.

52. Boeckxstaens GE, Annese V, des Varannes SB, et al. Pneumatic dilation versus laparoscopic Heller's myotomy for idiopathic achalasia. N Engl J Med 2011; 364(19):1807–16.

53. Werner YB, Hakanson B, Martinek J, et al. Endoscopic or surgical myotomy in patients with idiopathic achalasia. N Engl J Med 2019;381(23):2219–29.

54. Richards WO, Torquati A, Holzman MD, et al. Heller myotomy versus Heller myotomy with Dor fundoplication for achalasia: a prospective randomized double-blind clinical trial. Ann Surg 2004;240(3):405–12 [Discussion 412].

55. Kummerow Broman K, Phillips SE, Faqih A, et al. Heller myotomy versus Heller myotomy with Dor fundoplication for achalasia: long-term symptomatic follow-up of a prospective randomized controlled trial. Surg Endosc 2018;32(4): 1668–74.

56. Grimes KL, Inoue H. Per oral endoscopic myotomy for achalasia: a detailed description of the technique and review of the literature. Thorac Surg Clin 2016;26(2):147–62.

57. Kumbhari V, Tieu AH, Onimaru M, et al. Peroral endoscopic myotomy (POEM) vs laparoscopic Heller myotomy (LHM) for the treatment of Type III achalasia in 75 patients: a multicenter comparative study. Endosc Int Open 2015;3(3):E195–201.

58. Reddy CA, Tavakkoli A, Abdul-Hussein M, et al. Clinical impact of routine esophagram after peroral endoscopic myotomy. Gastrointest Endosc 2021;93(1):102–6.

59. von Renteln D, Inoue H, Minami H, et al. Peroral endoscopic myotomy for the treatment of achalasia: a prospective single center study. Am J Gastroenterol 2012;107(3):411–7.

60. Inoue H, Kudo S-E. [Per-oral endoscopic myotomy (POEM) for 43 consecutive cases of esophageal achalasia]. Nippon Rinsho 2010;68(9):1749–52.

61. Inoue H, Sato H, Ikeda H, et al. Per-oral endoscopic myotomy: a series of 500 patients. J Am Coll Surg 2015;221(2):256–64.

62. Kumbhari V, Familiari P, Bjerregaard NC, et al. Gastroesophageal reflux after peroral endoscopic myotomy: a multicenter case-control study. Endoscopy 2017;49(7):634–42.

63. Eckardt AJ, Eckardt VF. Treatment and surveillance strategies in achalasia: an update. Nat Rev Gastroenterol Hepatol 2011;8(6):311–9.

64. Taft TH, Carlson DA, Triggs J, et al. Evaluating the reliability and construct validity of the Eckardt symptom score as a measure of achalasia severity. Neurogastroenterol Motil 2018;30(6):e13287.

65. Ponds FA, Fockens P, Lei A, et al. Effect of peroral endoscopic myotomy vs pneumatic dilation on symptom severity and treatment outcomes among treatment-naive patients with achalasia: a randomized clinical trial. JAMA 2019;322(2): 134–44.

66. Schlottmann F, Luckett DJ, Fine J, et al. Laparoscopic heller myotomy versus peroral endoscopic myotomy (POEM) for achalasia: a systematic review and meta-analysis. Ann Surg 2018;267(3):451–60.

67. Repici A, Fuccio L, Maselli R, et al. GERD after per-oral endoscopic myotomy as compared with Heller's myotomy with fundoplication: a systematic review with meta-analysis. Gastrointest Endosc 2018;87(4):934–43.e18.

68. Devaney EJ, Lannettoni MD, Orringer MB, et al. Esophagectomy for achalasia: patient selection and clinical experience. Ann Thorac Surg 2001;72(3):854–8.
69. Eckardt VF, Hoischen T, Bernhard G. Life expectancy, complications, and causes of death in patients with achalasia: results of a 33-year follow-up investigation. Eur J Gastroenterol Hepatol 2008;20(10):956–60.
70. Orringer MB, Stirling MC. Esophageal resection for achalasia: indications and results. Ann Thorac Surg 1989;47(3):340–5.
71. Vela MF, Richter JE, Wachsberger D, et al. Complexities of managing achalasia at a tertiary referral center: use of pneumatic dilatation, Heller myotomy, and botulinum toxin injection. Am J Gastroenterol 2004;99(6):1029–36.
72. Aiolfi A, Asti E, Bonitta G, et al. Esophagectomy for end-stage achalasia: systematic review and meta-analysis. World J Surg 2018;42(5):1469–76.
73. Eckardt VF, Aignherr C, Bernhard G. Predictors of outcome in patients with achalasia treated by pneumatic dilation. Gastroenterology 1992;103(6):1732–8.
74. Hulselmans M, Vanuytsel T, Degreef T, et al. Long-term outcome of pneumatic dilation in the treatment of achalasia. Clin Gastroenterol Hepatol 2010;8(1):30–5.
75. Vaezi MF, Baker ME, Achkar E, et al. Timed barium oesophagram: better predictor of long term success after pneumatic dilation in achalasia than symptom assessment. Gut 2002;50(6):765–70.
76. Oezcelik A, Hagen JA, Halls JM, et al. An improved method of assessing esophageal emptying using the timed barium study following surgical myotomy for achalasia. J Gastrointest Surg 2009;13(1):14–8.
77. Su B, Callahan ZM, Novak S, et al. Using impedance planimetry (endoflip) to evaluate myotomy and predict outcomes after surgery for achalasia. J Gastrointest Surg 2020;24(4):964–71.
78. Chang J, Yoo IK, Günay S, et al. Clinical usefulness of esophagogastric junction distensibility measurement in patients with achalasia before and after peroral endoscopic myotomy. Turk J Gastroenterol 2020;31(5):362–7.
79. Teitelbaum EN, Soper NJ, Pandolfino JE, et al. Esophagogastric junction distensibility measurements during Heller myotomy and POEM for achalasia predict postoperative symptomatic outcomes. Surg Endosc 2015;29(3):522–8.
80. Khashab MA, Vela MF, Thosani N, et al. ASGE guideline on the management of achalasia. Gastrointest Endosc 2020;91(2):213–27.e6.
81. Eckardt AJ, Eckardt VF. Editorial: cancer surveillance in achalasia: better late than never? Am J Gastroenterol 2010;105(10):2150–2.
82. Rohof WO, Lei A, Boeckxstaens GE. Esophageal stasis on a timed barium esophagogram predicts recurrent symptoms in patients with long-standing achalasia. Am J Gastroenterol 2013;108(1):49–55.
83. Ponds FA, Oors JM, Smout AJPM, et al. Rapid drinking challenge during high-resolution manometry is complementary to timed barium esophagogram for diagnosis and follow-up of achalasia. Neurogastroenterol Motil 2018;30(11):e13404.
84. Cho YK, Lipowska AM, Nicodème F, et al. Assessing bolus retention in achalasia using high-resolution manometry with impedance: a comparator study with timed barium esophagram. Am J Gastroenterol 2014;109(6):829–35.
85. Arevalo G, Sippey M, Martin-Del-Campo LA, et al. Post-POEM reflux: who's at risk? Surg Endosc 2020;34(7):3163–8.
86. Csendes A, Braghetto I, Burdiles P, et al. Very late results of esophagomyotomy for patients with achalasia: clinical, endoscopic, histologic, manometric, and acid reflux studies in 67 patients for a mean follow-up of 190 months. Ann Surg 2006; 243(2):196–203.

87. Sandler RS, Nyrén O, Ekbom A, et al. The risk of esophageal cancer in patients with achalasia. A population-based study. JAMA 1995;274(17):1359–62.
88. Streitz JM, Ellis FH, Gibb SP, et al. Achalasia and squamous cell carcinoma of the esophagus: analysis of 241 patients. Ann Thorac Surg 1995;59(6):1604–9.
89. Zaninotto G, Rizzetto C, Zambon P, et al. Long-term outcome and risk of oesophageal cancer after surgery for achalasia. Br J Surg 2008;95(12):1488–94.
90. Gillies CL, Farrukh A, Abrams KR, et al. Risk of esophageal cancer in achalasia cardia: a meta-analysis. JGH Open 2019;3(3):196–200.
91. Tustumi F, Bernardo WM, da Rocha JRM, et al. Esophageal achalasia: a risk factor for carcinoma. A systematic review and meta-analysis. Dis Esophagus 2017; 30(10):1–8.
92. Zendehdel K, Nyrén O, Edberg A, et al. Risk of esophageal adenocarcinoma in achalasia patients, a retrospective cohort study in Sweden. Am J Gastroenterol 2011;106(1):57–61.
93. Leeuwenburgh I, Scholten P, Alderliesten J, et al. Long-term esophageal cancer risk in patients with primary achalasia: a prospective study. Am J Gastroenterol 2010;105(10):2144–9.
94. Markar SR, Wiggins T, MacKenzie H, et al. Incidence and risk factors for esophageal cancer following achalasia treatment: national population-based case-control study. Dis Esophagus 2019;32(5):doy106.
95. Harvey PR, Thomas T, Chandan JS, et al. Incidence, morbidity and mortality of patients with achalasia in England: findings from a study of nationwide hospital and primary care data. Gut 2019;68(5):790–5.
96. Zagari RM, Marasco G, Tassi V, et al. Risk of squamous cell carcinoma and adenocarcinoma of the esophagus in patients with achalasia: a long-term prospective cohort study in Italy. Am J Gastroenterol 2020. https://doi.org/10.14309/ajg.0000000000000955.
97. Leeuwenburgh I, Van Dekken H, Scholten P, et al. Oesophagitis is common in patients with achalasia after pneumatic dilatation. Aliment Pharmacol Ther 2006; 23(8):1197–203.
98. Ravi K, Geno DM, Katzka DA. Esophageal cancer screening in achalasia: is there a consensus? Dis Esophagus 2015;28(3):299–304.

The Art of Endoscopic Dilation
Lessons Learned Over 4 Decades of Practice

William J. Ravich, MD

KEYWORDS

- Esophageal dilation • Esophageal stenosis • Esophageal stricture

KEY POINTS

- The adage that solid food dysphagia is a stenosis until proven otherwise may require empirical dilation to prove, or disprove, the presence of a stenosis.
- The endoscopist should be familiar with the interpretation of barium esophagrams and should review the studies performed on the patient before endoscopic dilation.
- The Rule of Threes does not apply to all situations equally.
- Inflammatory strictures represent a combination of edema and scarring. Control of inflammation is essential to slow the rate of restenosis.
- Pharyngoesophageal segment (PES) stenosis is an underappreciated cause of dysphagia and can be easily missed endoscopically.

DEFINITIONS

Art (noun): "The principles or methods governing any craft or branch of learning."[1]
Lesson (noun): "A useful piece of practical wisdom acquired by experience or study."[1]
Stricture (noun): "An abnormal contraction of any passage or duct of the body."[1]

CLASSIFICATION OF ESOPHAGEAL STENOTIC LESIONS

If a stricture is an abnormal contraction of any passage or duct of the body, any pathologic stenotic lesion of the esophagus would qualify as an esophageal stricture. Esophageal stenosis can be classified in different ways (**Box 1**). The various categories have different implications for the role and approach to dilation.

Mural Strictures

Mural stenotic lesions might be considered "true strictures". It is important to appreciate that mural strictures represent a variable combination of active inflammation and

Section of Digestive Diseases, Yale School of Medicine, 40 Temple St., Suite !A, New Haven, CT 06510, USA
E-mail address: william.ravich@yale.edu

Gastroenterol Clin N Am 50 (2021) 737–750
https://doi.org/10.1016/j.gtc.2021.07.002
0889-8553/21/© 2021 Elsevier Inc. All rights reserved.

> **Box 1**
> **Esophageal stenotic lesions**
>
> Mucosal webs
> - Esophageal webs
> - Schatzki rings
>
> Mural strictures
> - Pill-induced esophagitis-related strictures
> - Atypical esophagitis-related strictures (EoE, lymphocytic esophagitis, lichen planus, cicatricial pemphigoid)
> - Radiation-induced and caustic injury-induced strictures
> - Peptic strictures
> - Anastomotic strictures
>
> Extrinsic or intramural compression
> - Intramural tumors
> - Duplications
> - Vascular compression (dysphagia lusoria, tortuous aorta, aortic aneurysm, enlarged left atrium)
> - Mediastinal masses
>
> Sphincteric dysfunction
> - PES dysfunction
> - Esophageal A-ring
> - EGJOO
> - Achalasia
>
> EGJOO, esophagogastric junction outflow obstruction; EoE, eosinophilic esophagitis; PES, pharyngoesophageal segment.

mature fibrosis. Active inflammation causes edema with little fibrosis and can, with control of the inflammatory process, resolve without luminal compromise. Over time, however, inflammation often leads to fibrosis. Even if the inflammatory process is controlled, fibrosis remains and may continue to evolve at the expense of the lumen.

Mucosal Webs

Mucosal webs are thin membranes that protrude into the esophageal lumen, producing a shelflike stenosis. Mucosal webs can be seen anywhere in the esophagus, but are most often found in the pharyngoesophageal (PE) segment and cervical esophagus or at the esophagogastric (EG) junction. Those in the proximal esophagus tend to be asymmetric, indenting the lumen from one direction, whereas those at the EG junction (the Schatzki ring) are typically circumferential and relatively symmetric. Often assumed to be part of the Plummer-Vinson syndrome, in my experience proximal esophageal webs are rarely associated with iron deficiency, a sine qua non for that syndrome. Esophageal webs in the esophageal body can be seen in various inflammatory conditions of the esophagus, such as eosinophilic esophagitis (EoE), lymphocytic esophagitis, and esophagitis associated with mucous membrane diseases, but are uncommon in reflux esophagitis. Isolated esophageal webs of the esophagus may be congenital in origin, but I have seen midesophageal webs after what, on the basis of their history, seems to have been associated with an acute episode of pill-induced esophagitis.

Esophageal Compression

The esophageal lumen can be compromised by intramural or extrinsic conditions. Benign or malignant tumors or duplication cysts are examples of intrinsic lesions; these need to grow to considerable size before they cause dysphagia. Extrinsic lesions might include pathologic conditions affecting mediastinal structures. These conditions can include mediastinal or pulmonary tumors, and also aberrant blood vessels (dysphagia lusoria), enlarged left atrium, tortuous aortas, or aortic aneurysms. Compressive lesions cannot be effectively treated by dilation because the noninvolved wall of the esophagus remains elastic and is simply stretched during passage of the dilator, only to recoil back to its original position when the dilator is removed.

Sphincteric Dysfunction

Sphincteric dysfunction may affect the upper esophageal sphincter (UES) or lower esophageal sphincter (LES). The most common LES motor abnormality that can cause dysphagia is achalasia. Although the term "achalasia" specifically relates to the failure of the EG junction to relax, the condition involves severe dysfunction of the smooth muscle segment of the esophagus as well as the LES. A recently described entity called EG junction outlet obstruction (EGJOO) involves dysfunction that is limited to the LES. Although treatment overlaps with that of achalasia, the pathogenesis of EGJOO is not necessarily related to that of achalasia from a pathophysiologic stand-point, and assumptions that EGJOO might represent an early phase of achalasia may be incorrect. Esophageal A-rings are thick muscle rings that are localized a few cen-timeters above the squamocolumnar junction. Although assumed to be rare, they are often missed in the interpretation of barium esophagram and on endoscopy. Similarly, I believe that endoscopists fail to appreciate the frequency with which dysfunction of the PE segment produces dysphagia.

TOOLS OF THE TRADE
Types of Dilators

There are essentially 3 types of dilators currently used for dilation of benign esopha-geal stenosis: nonguided serial dilators, guided serial dilators, and standard balloon dilators.[2] Serial dilators are referred to as bougies. The term bougie, French for wax candle, apparently dates to the eighteenth century; named after the Algerian town of Bujayah, which specialized in wax candle production, early dilators were made from tightly wound cylinders of wax-impregnated linen. Bougies apply pressure along the principles of a wedge, gradually forcing the stricture open incrementally by the passage of successive dilators of gradually increasing diameter. Balloon dilators, on the other hand, are typically placed across the stricture segment and inflated with liquid. Studies have not demonstrated significant differences in the efficacy of bougies and balloon for most strictures.[3]

Nonguided Serial Dilators

There are 2 basic types of nonguided dilators: Maloney and Hurst dilators (**Fig. 1**). Both are composed of rubber or silicone outer sheaths with a core filled with a pliable metal (previously mercury, now tungsten). Nonguided dilators are best suited for mildly to moderately stenotic lesions that are tapered or weblike in nature and that offer limited resistance to the passage of dilators. These dilators are ineffective with very fibrotic strictures where they tend to snake up above the stricture. Nonguided bougie dilators have been associated with a higher rate of complications.[4] However, these dilators have a long history of safety when properly used, and the influence of user experience and inappropriate choice of dilators may have been factors. These dilators are best avoided with long strictures or fibrotic strictures, with those that are tortuous, or with those that have a proximal shelf or pulsion diverticulum. I believe they should

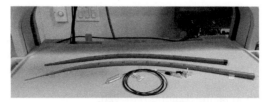

Fig. 1. Available dilators for dilation of fixed esophageal stenotic lesions (all shown with 18 mm (54F) external diameter. (*Top*) Nonguided serial dilator. The dilators would be available as a set of gradually increasing maximum diameter; they are constructed of a natural or synthetic rubber with a flexible metal core (formerly mercury, but now typically tungsten). In a Maloney-type dilator (shown), the tip of the dilator is tapered, whereas in a Hurst-type dilator the end would be shorter with a rounded tip. (*Middle*) Guidewire-directed serial dilator. As with the guided dilators, the dilators would be available as a set of gradually increasing maximum diameter. A guidewire is seen protruding from a channel that runs through the center of the polyvinyl dilator. The tapered end in available sets may be of varying lengths. To be effective, the end of the guidewire must be far enough beyond the stenosis to permit the widest part of the dilator to pass beyond the distal end of the stenosis. (*Bottom*) A balloon dilator. Most currently available balloon dilators used for fixed stenotic lesions are "controlled radial expansion" balloons, which achieve up to 3 diameters of distention, depending on the amount of pressure applied by a syringe attached to a pressure gauge. Unlike the serial dilators, which dilate by means of axial pressure along the principle of the wedge, balloon dilators, when positioned across the stenotic segment, apply pressure radially. Although initially proposed to be safer than serial dilators, the efficacy and safety of serial and balloon dilators have not been proven to be significantly different.

also be avoided when the dilation is performed with the patient undergoing deep sedation, during which the patient will be unable to react to a dilator inadvertently entering the airway.

Guided Serial Dilators

Currently available guided serial dilators are made of polyvinyl. These dilators have tapered tips with a central channel through which a previously placed guidewire is passed in a retrograde manner. The guidewire, secured in the hand of the endoscopist or an endoscopy assistant, "guides" the dilator through the stricture. Guidewires have radio-opaque markers and can be used with or without fluoroscopic imaging. The guidewire is usually introduced endoscopically, with the guidewire tip positioned well beyond the stricture, ideally in the gastric antrum. The guidewire keeps the dilator within the stricture lumen, so that even strictures that are irregular and tortuous can be dilated. Dilators of gradually increasing size are sequentially passed over the guidewire and through the stenotic segment. The key to their use is that the guidewire remains beyond the stricture. With successive passage and withdrawal of the dilators, the guidewire may become displaced, either curling in the stomach or, worse, inadvertently withdrawn into the strictured segment. The need for fluoroscopic guidance is controversial, but it does permit monitoring of the position of the guidewire. An essential part of training involves learning how to effectively keep the guidewire in place during successive passage and withdrawal of the dilators, and experience performing dilation under fluoroscopic guidance is an important part of the learning process.

Balloon Dilators

In the early 1980s, small-diameter balloon dilators, made of thermoplastic polymers, that could be passed through the accessory channel of an endoscope were introduced for use for the dilation of fixed esophageal strictures and are now routinely available in most, if not all, endoscopy facilities. Current balloon dilators can be distended in increments, usually to 3 successive sizes, based on the amount of pressure applied. Referred to as controlled radial expansion, the process simulates the effect of sequential dilation with bougie dilators. The balloons can be inflated with water, saline, or (for visualization under fluoroscopy) radio-opaque contrast. Although originally proposed as safer than bougies because they dilated by means of purely radial pressure, thereby avoiding the shearing effect of bougies,[5] the limited information available suggests that any safety advantages may be small.[3]

Other Critical Equipment

Aside from the standard adult gastroscope, with which most endoscopies are performed, an ultrathin pediatric scope can be critical for passage of tight strictures and also may be the difference between success or failure in passing guidewires for performing guided bougie dilations. Access to fluoroscopic equipment is essential for some guided bougie dilations and may be helpful even when not essential. For the trainee, a period of training in bougie dilation using fluoroscopic guidance can be particularly important in learning proper technique. Guidewires for guided bougie dilators come in various forms. I avoid the type with spring tips due to concern that resistance encountered when the dilator reaches the spring might be misinterpreted as resistance from the stricture. The guidewire used for esophageal dilation should be about 250 cm long, long enough to allow the complete withdrawal of the scope, so that the wire can be secured at the patient's mouth with the tip of the wire in the antrum. A thorough description of dilator characteristics can be found in a 2007 American Society for Gastrointestinal Endoscopy Technology Status Assessment.[6]

TRICKS OF THE TRADE
A Stricture till Proven Otherwise

A common wisdom is that solid food dysphagia is a stricture until proven otherwise; this begs the question of what is required to prove the negative. In general, I favor performing contrast radiography as the first step in the evaluation of dysphagia. The barium esophagram, by an experienced and interested radiologist, provides information about both motor function and structure, therefore providing a broader net for the evaluation of dysphagia than endoscopy. When a stricture is found, it provides a roadmap for the endoscopist and information about what the best approach to dilation might be. When negative, it narrows the possibilities that remain.

Review Your Patient's Barium Studies

Unfortunately, the quality of contrast radiology has deteriorated because other imaging technologies have been proved to be more attractive to newly minted radiologists. The radiologist may miss a finding, or the quality of the study may leave some segments inadequately examined. If the initial contrast study with liquid barium gives negative result, the study in a patient with pure solid food dysphagia is not complete until a radio-opaque tablet or barium-coated food bolus is swallowed and passes without difficulty. The gastroenterologist who reviews his or her patient's barium study serves as a double-check on the quality of the study and can question findings that might have been unappreciated by the radiologist. If I have a question, I am never shy about calling the radiologist to review the study together.

In a Patient with Pure Solid Food Dysphagia, Consider Dilation Even if No Stenotic Lesion is Seen

Endoscopy, for all its advantages, is not particularly good at detecting subtle stenotic lesions. There are regions where clinically significant stenosis can be easily missed, particularly the PE segment, which virtually never distends well during routine endoscopy, or the EG junction, which is often approached at an angle and may be difficult to distend with air. Even in the tubular esophagus, decreased distensibility can go unappreciated. The old adage that if the scope passes through it, there is no significant stenosis was not true when I entered gastroenterology when the typical scope diameter was 13 to 14 mm; it is certainly not true today when the typical adult gastroscope is 9 to 10 mm. When uncertain, I have a low threshold for performing dilation in a patient with pure solid food dysphagia. In this situation when no explanation is found, I will pass an 18- to 20-mm balloon dilator in the stomach and drag it back, fully distended to 20 mm, through the EG junction and the rest of the esophagus and, when symptoms are compatible with a pharyngeal stenosis, through the PE segment as well. In the normal esophagus, the balloon will pass with little or no resistance. If resistance is recognized, a stricture can often be appreciated, splayed out on the balloon (**Fig. 2**). If the balloon comes out without resistance, then I can be confident that no clinically significant stenosis is present. What I do once a stricture is recognized by this method is discussed in the section on "Stenosis-Specific Approach to Dilation."

Schatzki's Legacy and the Goal of Dilation

The usual target diameter for dilation is largely based on the work of Richard Schatzki. Schatzki, a radiologist, described the correlation between luminal diameter and symptoms in patients with the eponymously named Schatzki ring. The term *ring* is frequently used for a variety of abnormalities in the esophagus. Some are thin mucosal weblike structures. Others are thickening due to fibrosis or muscular dysfunction. The Schatzki ring is an example of a mucosal web, and its treatment is based on this interpretation. He stated that if the ring was 12 mm or less, everyone was symptomatic, and when it was 20 mm or more, recurrent dysphagia was rare.[7] His studies are often misquoted with figures of 10 and 12 for diameter at which everyone is symptomatic and 18 and 20 as the diameter at which no one is symptomatic. These are at best approximations

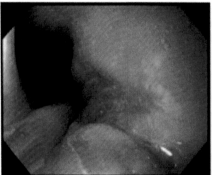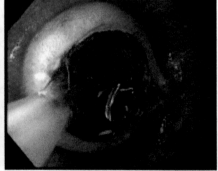

Fig. 2. Schatzki ring in patient with solid-food dysphagia. On initial intubation, there was no evidence of a ring and nothing to suggest the presence of stenotic lesion at the EG junction, even with use of air insufflation. A Schatzki ring became obvious when a fully inflated 20-mm balloon dilator was withdrawn across the EG junction. (*Courtesy of* Jill Deutsch, MD, Yale School of Medicine, New Haven, CT.)

of what he actually recorded. A few caveats are warranted. First, Schatzki's observations were radiographic and there may have been effect of magnification in the radiographic images. Second, the numbers provided may seem more precise than they really are. Third, at least in theory patients with Schatzki ring do not have significant abnormalities of esophageal motility. Normal esophageal motility cannot be assumed in patients with esophageal inflammation or long esophageal strictures, where the propulsive force to push the swallowed bolus through the stenotic segment may be diminished. Nonetheless, by tradition, 18-20 is the usual target for dilation and the maximum diameter of the dilators generally available for most dilator systems manufactured for use in benign stenosis.

The "Rule of Three"

The Rule of Three warns that you should dilate only by 3 increments of dilator diameter at one session.[8] Often attributed to Worth Boyce, a legendary esophagologist, he in turn credited the rule to another famous gastroenterologist, Eddy Palmer.[9] There are several limitations to its application. In early descriptions, it often failed to mention the starting point. Later formulations mentioned the presence of moderate or greater resistance as the point at which the count starts, but the consistency with which endoscopists interpret the amount of resistance is open to question. The endoscopic assessment of the initial diameter of a stenosis is highly subjective. In addition, the increments between dilators in various dilator systems and between different endoscopy facilities vary. Nonguided bougies are available in 2F increments [1F = 1/ 3.14 mm]. Some guided bougies are available in 3F increments. At Johns Hopkins where I spent much of my career, we had nonguided bougies in 4F increments. It was only after I became director of GI endoscopy and was responsible for purchasing equipment that I realize that my 3 dilators permitted under the "Rule of Three" was twice as aggressive as Boyce might have intended. Absolute adherence would dictate limiting dilations to as little as 1 mm per session and require 8 separate sessions to dilate a 10-mm stricture to 18 mm. Finally, the entire concept of using resistance as a measure of how far to dilate does not translate easily to balloon dilators, where the tactile sense of resistance is often in the hands of an assistant and is of uncertain reliability. I tend to use the Rule of Three more as a caution than as a strict rule, a practice supported by a study of endoscopic practice that did not show an increased risk of perforation when the rule was not adhered to strictly.[10] In nonulcerated refluxinduced stricture, I do not adhere to it rigidly, as long as the successive dilators do not meet with a significant increase in resistance. Once progressive resistance is appreciated I will go up to 1 or 2 additional dilator diameters, depending on the severity of resistance encountered, and then call it a day, deferring further dilation to another day. With balloon dilators, I estimate the diameter of the stricture, pick a graded balloon dilator with its lowest diameter just a bit above that diameter, and use the observed effect to decide on whether to stop at the point of full balloon distention or go on to the next balloon catheter in the series to continue dilation.

Refractory Strictures

Some strictures prove refractory to dilation. If inflammation is present, the cause of inflammation must be determined and effective treatment instituted. Often patience is all that is required. I have had patients referred to me for refractory strictures who simply needed a few more sessions and perhaps a slightly more aggressive dilation to achieve sustained results. Intralesional steroids have been helpful in some patients.[11] I have found steroid injections to be most helpful in short strictures of any type. I have had limited experience with stents for benign esophageal strictures and

I am concerned that they may propagate inflammation and are associated with a high rate of displacement and other complications.[12] I consider it only when my hand is forced. Finally, incisional therapy has been advocated for webs, sometimes simply biopsying multiple times around the circumference of the web. Although appealing, I am unconvinced that incisional therapy yields better results than dilation.[13] For longer, fibrotic strictures, improvement in equipment and technique may be required to make incisional therapy practical.

STENOSIS-SPECIFIC APPROACH TO DILATION
Rings and Webs

The Schatzki ring is the most commonly diagnosed and most commonly missed cause of solid food dysphagia in gastroenterologic practice. When using a nonguided bougie, I typically take a 32F dilator, not for the purpose of initiating dilation, but to permit the patient to get used to the experience of the dilator passing. I then take a 56F or 60F dilator (in general 56F for women and 60F for men) and pass it down smoothly but relatively quickly to its full length. If the patient demonstrates discomfort during dilator passage, I will either withdraw or, if the proximal esophagus has been intubated, maintain the dilator position until the patient can receive additional sedation and relaxes. I use nonguided bougies only in a patient under conscious sedation due to concern of a greater risk of unappreciated airway penetration with deep sedation. With deep sedation, if I use a guided bougie dilator, I skip the smaller-diameter dilator and go directly to the larger-diameter dilator.

I must admit to a preference for using balloon dilators in webs and mucosal rings I do not have and have never had a financial relationship with an endoscopic balloon manufacturer; my inclination toward using balloons comes entirely from personal endoscopic experience. The balloon allows me to adjust my technique if necessary and assess the effect of dilation immediately after dilation is completed and before any bleeding obscures the field. My approach is to position a multistage 18- to 20-mm balloon in the stomach, inflate it to 20 mm with water, and maintain the proximal end of the balloon a few centimeters beyond the endoscope by grabbing the catheter with my fifth finger as it comes out of the accessory channel. Then by withdrawing the balloon and scope as a single unit, I keep the balloon in sight of the scope. Even if the ring is not appreciated during initial intubation, the maneuver will reveal a clinically significant ring if it is present (see **Fig. 2**). If I am able to pull the fully inflated balloon through the ring segment without excessive resistance, a matter of feel based on experience, I will rupture the ring by continuing to withdraw the scope. If I do encounter substantial resistance, I will deflate the balloon, reposition it across the EG junction, and ask my endoscopic assistant to blow the balloon up as quickly as possible. Success will usually be confirmed by modest bleeding and a recognizable mucosal tear. If not observed, I will repeat the original retrograde pull-through, which will usually be possible without undue resistance, to complete the job. Proximal esophageal webs, with the exception of those associated with eosinophilic and other atypical esophagitis, are handled in a similar manner with the exception that the balloon can be blown up in the tubular esophagus rather than in the stomach.

Pill-Induced Esophageal Strictures

Pill-induced esophagitis is a condition in which a medication swallowed in pill form is retained in the esophagus and causes a direct caustic injury. Although pill-induced esophagitis has been attributed to a large number of medications, the most common are nonsteroidal inflammatory drugs, tetracycline, iron, potassium, quinidine, alendronates, and clindamycin. The patient often recognizes the association of the onset of pain with pill ingestion, but fails to realize its significance. Once symptoms begin, they are likely to recur with each subsequent ingestion of the same medication, presumably a result of esophageal edema and spasm, making it more likely for the same medication to be retained perpetuating the downward cycle. Pill-induced esophagitis may cause deep ulceration, fistulization, as well as stricture formation. The condition is a somewhat unique model for an esophagitis-related stricture in which the cause, once recognized, can be completely removed. My experience with this condition is that the stricture develops rapidly after the onset of symptoms. Once the drug-induced cause is recognized and the drug is suspended, the ulcers heal over a period of weeks, but the fibrosis may continue and require periodic dilations. Over time, the frequency with symptom recurrence decreases and eventually, perhaps in a year or more, ceases altogether. Bougies or balloon dilators work equally well, but I again prefer to use balloon dilators, which permit me to see my work in progress, gauge how much I can dilate, and when to stop if excessive bleeding or a tear develops. I tend to follow more or less the Rule of Three with the proviso that if only modest resistance is detected with bougies or no appreciable split or significant looking bleeding is seen, I may extend the dilation further. My ultimate target for dilation is 18 mm, but I aim to reach this target in incremental steps of successive dilation sessions. There is a suggestion in the literature that pill-induced esophagitis may be more common in patients with a history of swallowing problems, implying that an underlying swallowing disorder may predispose to pill retention. All patients with dysphagia, and particularly those with a known stenotic lesion of any type, should be educated about the medications that have been implicated in producing pill-induced esophagitis. If a patient must take one of the medications implicated in causing this condition, options include taking it as a suspension or in crushed form or taking the smallest size pill or capsule available with ample amounts of water and for the shortest time possible. Enteric-coated formulations are not solutions to this problem, because they tend to be larger than uncoated pills, can swell when exposed to saliva, and may be more likely to adhere to the esophageal mucosa.

Reflux-Induced Strictures

An untreated or inadequately treated reflux-induced stricture represents a form of stricture characterized by the simultaneous effect of active inflammation and fibrosis. Because of the edema from active inflammation, symptoms may initially improve with effective reflux treatment alone, only to recur and progress as the lumen continues to narrow as a result of fibrosis. In patients with strictures without frequent obstructive symptoms, dilation can be deferred until the effect of medical treatment of reflux disease is determined. If the patient does have obstructive symptoms or if the patient has a history of food impaction, I do not hesitate to perform a dilation at the time of the initial endoscopy, even if severe inflammation or frank ulceration is present, to provide immediate symptomatic relief and to bide time to allow medical management to work. A diagnosis of food impaction does not require the patient to have gone to an emergency department because of dysphagia. Prolonged episodes of solid food dysphagia with an inability to swallow liquids or the patient's own saliva represents food impaction, even if the symptoms clear spontaneously or with self-induced regurgitation. Like for Schatzki rings, nonguided or guided bougies can be used, with guided bougies preferred for procedures performed under deep sedation. And as with Schatzki ring, I have a preference for using balloon dilators. However, serial dilation rather than abrupt dilation should be performed. My ultimate goal is to pass an 18-mm dilator. Treatment of a reflux-induced esophageal stricture does not end with effective dilation. The stricture will recur more quickly and require dilation more often than if the reflux-induced mucosal injury is not effectively controlled.[14] Histamine receptor 2 antagonists alone will prove insufficient, and proton pump inhibitors, often in twice a day dosing, will be required.[15] I tend to treat reflux aggressively and worry about fine-tuning treatment after control of inflammation is endoscopically confirmed. Although a continuous pH study might be used to confirm adequate therapeutic response, a follow-up endoscopy should be performed in 3 months to confirm control of active inflammation. At a minimum, erosions or ulcers should have resolved. Any attempt to decrease the level of acid suppression should be followed by another endoscopy to confirm adequate control of inflammation.

Eosinophilic Esophagitis-Induced Strictures

EoE in the adult typically presents as dysphagia for solids, and the dysphagia is usually due to esophageal strictures. Strictures can vary in appearance. The stricture may be weblike or fibrotic looking. There may be multiple strictures. Long strictures that severely narrow most if not all of the esophagus ("small-caliber esophagus") can occur. The strictures may be punctuated by a series of thick indentations that look like tracheal rings (referred to as trachealization). The rings may be so impressive that the lack of distensibility of the underlying esophageal wall may not be appreciated. The tendency to develop deep mucosal tears during esophageal dilation was recognized early on, resulting in a tendency among gastroenterologists to avoid dilation in this condition altogether. Dysphagia can be severe and esophageal dilation unavoidable. The key is to perform dilation with caution. With EoE, I stick closely to the Rule of Three because overenthusiastic dilation will lead to complications. Many authorities prefer guided serial dilators for this condition. However, my experience is that once a mucosal tear develops and the wall integrity is breached, the perception of resistance upon which the application of the rule depends may no longer be reliable. Unless the lumen is so compromised that an adult endoscope cannot pass, I will pass the endoscope to the distal end of the stricture; choose a controlled radial expansion balloon dilator, selecting the balloon diameter according to my goal for dilation during that session; inflate the balloon to the lowest increment; hold it for 15 to 30 seconds; deflate it; and visually determine the mucosal integrity. If no split has occurred, I will repeat the dilation to the next balloon increment. If there is again no evidence of a mucosal tear, I will go to the final increment. I then withdraw the scope to the next segment of the esophagus and repeat the process. If a split is noted at any point, I will suspend attempt to dilate further at that level, but I am willing to withdrawn a balloon length and repeat the sequence within the next segment. Depending on the length of the stenotic segment, the session may require 3 or 4 series of segmental dilations. Further dilation is deferred to anther endoscopy session unless I conclude that I underestimated the original luminal diameter. Above all, it is essentially not to be greedy; if in doubt, stop. In patients with a small-caliber esophagus, serial dilation with a guided bougie dilator is usually unavoidable. If an ultrathin pediatric endoscope will pass, I will examine the length of the stricture and then place a guidewire in the stomach. If even the ultrathin scope is unable to pass, I will pass the guidewire carefully under fluoroscopic control. Although chest pain after dilation in EoE is common, with appropriate caution the rate of clinically significant perforations is not increased.[16] However, the critical phrase here is appropriate caution. Once the diagnosis is recognized, therapeutic interventions should be initiated in parallel with dilation with a goal to minimize the rate of restenosis and the need for repeat dilation. The susceptibility to mucosal tears seen in EoE can occur in less common conditions such as lymphocytic esophagitis or in certain mucous membrane disorders that can affect the esophagus, such as pemphigoid and lichen planus, conditions that I generally approach in a similar manner.

Radiation- and Caustic Ingestion-Induced Strictures

Among the most difficult strictures to dilate are radiation-induced strictures. Once established, they may be long and very fibrotic. Except when the strictures are short, balloon dilators and nonguided serial dilators are too compliant to effective dilate. If observed under fluoroscopy, the balloon dilators simply do not achieve the anticipated diameter and the nonguided dilators tend to curl up above the stricture. Serial guided bougies are almost mandatory and even they may curl or arch above the stricture rather than effectively expand the lumen. Here is the one situation in which the old Eder-Peustow dilators (no longer commercially available), composed of metal olives of increasing size and articulated metal rods that serve to push the olives through the stricture, might prove helpful (see **Fig. 1**). With a short radiation stricture, intralesional steroids (generally using triamcinolone injected via sclerotherapy catheter) might be considered, but the fibrosis is often so dense that it may be difficult to inject the thick suspension into the esophageal wall. In general, as time lapses, the acute mucosal inflammatory response resolves. If inflammation persists, the possibility of an interposed reflux esophagitis as a consequence of the effect of fibrosis on LES function and esophageal clearance should be considered. In this situation, aggressive reflux therapy might make subsequent dilation more effective.

Anastomotic Strictures

Like a pill-induced stricture, an anastomotic stricture after esophageal resection represents a cause of stricture in which the acute inflammatory response from surgery recedes, leaving a fibrotic stricture. The presence of persistent inflammation should raise the possibility of superimposed reflux esophagitis, a common sequela of surgery in which the LES has been removed. Reflux, if present or considered likely, should be either confirmed or treated aggressively. In apparently refractory anastomotic strictures, patience is a virtue. Most patients referred to me for this diagnosis just need more time and a few more dilations. On occasion, in patients requiring frequent dilations, an intralesional steroid injection may be helpful. Although stents or incisional therapy can be considered, I have not been impressed that either is particularly effective in this situation.

Esophageal A-Rings

Esophageal A-rings are a thick circumferential ring, located a few centimeters above the EG junction. Under fluoroscopic examination, it can appear to contract and relax intermittently; it is assumed to represent a muscular contraction at the proximal end of the phrenic ampulla, but unlike spasm, the location is quite consistent and it can occur without evidence of spasm elsewhere in the esophagus. Generally assumed to be a rare condition, in my experience it can be appreciated fairly often on radiographic studies, especially if performed using video, as well as during endoscopy if the endoscopist is patient and willing to spend a little extra time looking for it. The endoscopist can observe the squamocolumnar (SC) junction a few centimeters beyond the ring as it opens and closes and on occasion an obvious Schatzki's ring can be seen through the lumen of the muscular ring. Rather than rare, it is probably more accurate to say that it is an uncommon cause of dysphagia. It is possible that this finding accounts for at least some patients with EGJOO described manometrically. The withdrawal technique with a fully inflated 20-mm balloon (described previously) can often bring out the ring as it resists balloon passage. Brusque dilation by continuing the balloon withdrawal or rapid inflation with the balloon placed across the constricting segment in a manner similar to that described for the Schatzki ring, can be effective, but not as reliably as with a Schatzki ring. Alternative approaches might include botulinum toxin injection or large-diameter balloon dilation, if the ring is thought to represent the cause of symptoms.

Pharyngoesophageal segment stenosis

PE segment stenosis is the most underappreciated condition. Often referred to as a hypopharyngeal, or cricopharyngeal, bar when seen during a barium study, because of its appearance on lateral views of the neck during barium esophagrams, it represents incomplete opening or, in some cases, premature closure of the PE segment during bolus transit. The pathophysiology of the bar and its relationship to the UES and the cricopharyngeus are outside the scope of this presentation. The bar is a common finding on contrast radiography, but frequently missed on endoscopy. The bar may represent a secondary effect of inadequate bolus propulsion from the pharynx, inadequate hyoid elevation, or a reaction to increased downstream pressure from esophageal dysfunction or obstructive lesions. It may be difficult to determine whether it is a cause of symptoms or simply an incidental finding. As a rule of thumb, hypopharyngeal bars that narrow the lumen by less than 50% are unlikely to cause symptoms. I have found that the bar rarely causes difficulty with passing the standard endoscope into the esophagus. If the endoscopist is unable to intubate the PE segment, it should be considered a stricture, not a muscular disorder. There is often a distinct sense of traction on the scope during withdrawal, something that the average endoscopist may not notice. Further evidence that the PE segment might be the cause of symptoms comes if a 20-mm balloon dilator is passed through the scope into the esophagus, inflated, and then an attempt is made to pull it through the PE segment in a retrograde manner. An attempt to withdraw the balloon and scope as a unit will meet marked resistance to balloon passage and the cricopharyngeus will be pulled up like a stiff rubber band. On the assumption that the condition represented muscular dysfunction, I used to dilate the PE segment by forcefully pulling the balloon through the PE segment. However, I have become more cautious with age, preferring to deflate the balloon, withdraw it across the PE segment, and inflate it rapidly. Confirmation of a therapeutic effect is often recognized by the presence of a mucosal tear through the PE segment, a finding that simply does occur in a normally elastic PE segment. A guided or nonguided bougie could be used for the same purpose; however, you would have to go to a large-size (56F–60F) bougie to have the same effect, but it may not provide as much information about resistance and effect.

KNOWN UNKNOWNS

There are many unknowns concerning the practice of esophageal dilation. How to determine "moderate resistance" and how does the wish to proceed with further dilation, dictate the thought? How much pressure is too much pressure? How long should you maintain dilating pressure with balloon dilators? If a series of dilation sessions are required, is there a minimum and maximum interval at which the sessions should occur for maximizing effect and minimizing risk? What is the role that dysmotility above a stricture plays in the severity of symptoms and would there be any value to dilating more than suggested in Schatzki's original studies on the Schatzki ring? How much do differences between users in the choice or application of devices affect the benefit or safety of different approaches to dilation. In many cases there are simply no studies at all that address these issues. Where studies exist, they are often few and flawed in design. In their absence, personal experience is likely to remain as good a guide as any. It is hoped that in the future, opinion can be replaced by facts.

CLINICS CARE POINTS

- Both barium radiography and endoscopy can miss clinically significant strictures.
- In patients with solid food dysphagia, when in doubt, dilate.
- Learn how to interpret barium studies and review those performed on your patient's before performing endoscopy on them.

DISCLOSURE

The author owns stock in Johnson & Johnson.

REFERENCES

1. The Random House Dictionary of the English Language. 2nd edition. New York: Random House, Inc.; 1987. Unabridged. (Stuart Berg Flexner, Editor in Chief; Leonore Crary Houch, Managing Editor).
2. Siddiqui UD, Banerjee S, Barth B, et al. ASGE Technology Committee: Tools for endoscopic stricture dilation. Gastrointest Endosc 2013;78:391–404.
3. Cox JG, Winter RK, Mslin SC, et al. Balloon or bougie for dilatation of benign esophageal stricture? Dig Dis Sci 1994;39. 776–81.
4. Hernandez LV, Jacobson JW, Harris MS. Comparison among the perforation rates of Maloney, balloon, and savary dilation of esophageal strictures. Gastrointest Endosc 2000;51:460–2.
5. Abele JE. The physics of esophageal dilatation. Hepatogastroenterology 1992; 38:486–9.
6. Carr-Locke DL, Branch MS, Byrne WJ, et al. ASGE technology assessment status evaluation: guidewires in GI endoscopy. Gastrointest Endosc 2007;47: 579–83.
7. Schatzki R. The lower esophageal ring: long term follow-up of symptomatic and asymptomatic rings. Am J Roentgenol Radium Ther Nucl Med 1963;90:805–10.
8. Boyce HW. Dilation of difficult benign esophageal strictures. Am J Gastroenterol 2005;100:744–5.
9. Richter JE. Rule of three for esophageal dilation: like the tortoise versus the rabbit, low and slow is our friend and our patients' win. Gastrointest Endosc 2017; 85(2):338–9.
10. Grooteman KV, Wong K, Song LM, et al. Non-adherence to the rule of 3 does not increase the risk of adverse events in esophageal dilation. Gastrointest Endosc 2017;85:332–7.e1.
11. Ramage JI, Rumalla A, Baron TH, et al. A prospective, randomized, double-blind, placebo-controlled trial of endoscopic steroid injection therapy for recalcitrant esophageal peptic strictures. Am J Gastroenterol 2005;100:2419–25.
12. Sharma P, Kozarek R. Practice Parameters Committee of American College of Gastroenterology: Role of esophageal stents in benign and malignant diseases. Am J Gastroenterol 2010;105:258–73.
13. Hordijk ML, van Hooft JE, Hansen BE, et al. A randomized comparison of electrocautery incision with Savary bougienage for relief of anastomotic gastroesophageal strictures. Gastrointest Endosc 2009;70:849–55.

14. Ruigómez A, García Rodríguez LA, Wallander MA, et al. Esophageal stricture: incidence, treatment patterns, and recurrence rate. Am J Gastroenterol 2006; 101(12):2685–92.
15. Smith PM, Kerr GD, Cockel R, et al. A comparison of omeprazole and ranitidine in the prevention of recurrence of benign esophageal stricture. Restore Investigator Group. Gastroenterology 1994;107:1312–8.
16. Jacobs JW, Spechler SJ. A systematic review of the risk of perforation during esophageal dilation for patients with eosinophilic esophagitis. Dig Dis Sci 2010; 55:1512–5.

Barrett's Esophagus
Diagnosis, Management, and Key Updates

Karen Chang, DO[a], Christian S. Jackson, MD[b],
Kenneth J. Vega, MD[c],*

KEYWORDS

- Barrett's esophagus • Dysplasia • Management • Screening • Surveillance
- Ablation • Artificial intelligence • Biomarkers

KEY POINTS

- Barrett's esophagus (BE) is accepted as the single precursor lesion for development of esophageal adenocarcinoma (EAC).
- BE screening/surveillance has not provided the anticipated EAC reduction benefit to date.
- Noninvasive cell sampling devices or biomarkers are increasingly available or under study to screen for BE among those with and without known risk factors.
- Implementation of artificial intelligence platforms to aid the endoscopist during screening and surveillance will likely become routine, minimizing missed lesions during endoscopy.
- BE with low-grade dysplasia can be managed with removal of visible lesions combined with endoscopic eradication therapy or surveillance per recent guidelines.

INTRODUCTION

Barrett's esophagus (BE) is a metaplastic columnar epithelial change that results from chronic esophageal mucosal injury to the normal squamous esophageal mucosa.[1] BE prevalence has been observed to vary from 1% to 2% in general populations as well as in those undergoing endoscopy, with higher frequency found in patients with gastroesophageal reflux disease (GERD).[2–6] Therefore, in the United States, approximately 3 to 6 million individuals are estimated to have BE with the overwhelming majority clinically unaware of its presence.

BE is also accepted as the single precursor lesion for the development of esophageal adenocarcinoma (EAC). This occurs through a succession of changes due to

Author contributions: All authors planned the review and assessed all data included. All authors wrote the review and revised it for intellectual content. All authors approved the final submitted version. K.J. Vega is the review guarantor.
[a] Department of Internal Medicine, University of California, Riverside School of Medicine, 900 University Avenue, Riverside, CA 92521, USA; [b] Section of Gastroenterology, Loma Linda VA Healthcare System, 11201 Benton Street, 2A-38, Loma Linda, CA 92357, USA; [c] Division of Gastroenterology & Hepatology, Augusta University-Medical College of Georgia, 1120 15th Street, AD-2226, Augusta, GA 30912, USA
* Corresponding author.
E-mail address: kvega@augusta.edu

gastro.theclinics.com

continued injury from nondysplastic BE (NDBE) to BE with low-grade dysplasia (LGD) and BE with high-grade dysplasia (HGD) before cancer development. NDBE progression risk to EAC ranges from 0.2% to 0.5% per patient year.[7–11] LGD progresses at a rate between 0.6% and 13.4% per patient year to EAC.[6,7,12–15] Finally, progression from HGD to EAC occurs at between 5% and 8% per year.[16,17]

Unfortunately, BE screening/surveillance to prevent EAC has not provided the anticipated cancer reduction benefit despite guidelines advocating for early BE detection and improvements in endoscopic management after BE discovery. This is due to the majority of newly diagnosed EAC cases not having known BE prior.[18] Therefore, improvement in early diagnosis/screening and maximizing management before cancer development is of greatest importance among all those with BE.

DEFINITION AND EPIDEMIOLOGY OF BARRETT'S ESOPHAGUS

BE is defined as columnar-type epithelium at least 1 cm proximal from the gastroesophageal junction (GEJ) detected at endoscopy with biopsy confirmed presence of intestinal metaplasia.[1] Long-segment BE (LSBE) is defined as BE length $\geq$3 cm, whereas short-segment BE (SSBE) is less than 3 cm but greater than 1 cm above the GEJ.[19] Columnar epithelium less than 1 cm proximal of the GEJ should be classified as specialized intestinal metaplasia of the esophagogastric junction (SIM-EGJ) and not BE because of elevated interobserver variability along with low risk for EAC development. This is because patients with SIM-EGJ have not demonstrated a propensity for dysplasia or EAC development in large cohorts after long-term follow-up compared to those with segments greater than 1 cm.[20] Furthermore, the use of the Seattle protocol for biopsy along with Prague criteria for endoscopic description has resulted in a standard method for endoscopists to characterize and biopsy BE seen at esophagogastroduodenoscopy (EGD).[21,22] Accurate representation and biopsy of the BE segment is important as increasing BE length is associated with an increased risk of progression to dysplasia and EAC.[23]

Overall BE prevalence in the general population is not clearly known across the world as many with it are not symptomatic.[24] Within selected populations, for example, endoscopic or surgical series, data do exist on BE prevalence, but these studies have inherent bias. Only 3 studies in the literature have assessed BE prevalence in random patient samples from western nations.[2,3,25] Two of these studies are from randomly selected populations undergoing endoscopy from Sweden and Italy with BE population prevalences of 1.3% to 1.6%.[2,3] In both these investigations, SSBE was the predominant form of BE. The other general population study was performed at the Mayo Clinic comparing LSBE prevalence found in a randomly selected autopsy sample to endoscopy.[25] The prevalence of LSBE in the autopsy group was 0.38%, more than 20 times higher than expected based on their endoscopic data. Modeling to estimate the US population prevalence has also been performed.[26] Using EAC rates from the Surveillance, Epidemiology and End Results registry, the estimated US BE population prevalence was 5.6%. Interestingly, BE population prevalence in Asia ranges from 0.7% to 2.6% with most cases identified as SSBE.[27,28]

BE incidence trends are difficult to determine as well because of the presumed large number of asymptomatic individuals. However, endoscopic data have been used with the expectation that such changes seen also represent all BE cases, including those never discovered. Multiple population-based studies have reported an increase in incidence rates.[8,29–32] This was explained by an increase in endoscopy performed along with introduction of society recommendations and guidelines published for screening those with GERD.[33,34] Recent data have indicated a stabilization of BE incidence over at least the last 15 years.[35,36]

Demographics of BE in the United States are changing over time. Males and non-Hispanic whites (nHw) have been the primary groups affected with BE.[37-39] New data indicate, using an aggregate electronic medical record database, that the male-to-female BE ratio has decreased and Hispanic Americans (Hisp) diagnosed with BE have increased from 2006 to 2016.[40] The authors speculate that the change in male/female ratio may be due to an increased rate of females diagnosed with BE. No comment was provided for the observed BE increase among Hisp. Each phenomenon deserves confirmation, and assessing EAC rates in a similar fashion could serve as a potential surrogate form of validation.

RISK FACTORS AND SCREENING FOR BARRETT'S ESOPHAGUS
Risk Factors and Who to Screen?

Known BE risk factors include age greater than 50 years, male sex, Caucasian race, smoking, central obesity, chronic (>5 years) or frequent (>once weekly) GERD, as well as family hx (first degree relative) of BE or EAC.[1,41,42] Published guidelines are available from multiple national and multinational gastroenterologic societies providing criteria to identify individuals for BE screening[1,43-46] (**Table 1**). Screening criteria used in these guidelines are based primarily on the known BE risk factors mentioned previously. Overall, screening is not endorsed in the general population by all organizations but are advised in those considered high-risk.[1,43-46] Furthermore, discussion about whether to perform BE screening should occur with the patient. Items important for dialog include the potential impact of BE discovery with resulting surveillance and/or treatment if dysplasia is found. Additional factors from a physician perspective requiring consideration include anticipated patient life expectancy and impact of comorbidities on potential therapeutic interventions if dysplasia is discovered. The current guideline from the American Gastroenterological Association advises BE screening in those with multiple EAC risk factors (age>50, male, white race, chronic GERD, hiatal hernia presence, BMI elevated, and body fat distribution intraabdominally).[43] The American College of Gastroenterology guideline recommends BE screening in men with chronic (>5 years) and/or frequent (weekly or more) GERD as well as two or more risk factors from the following: 50 year old or greater, white race, central obesity, current/past smoking history, and confirmed first-degree relative with BE or EAC.[1] BE screening in women was not recommended because of low risk but could be performed if multiple risk factors exist.[1] The British Society of Gastroenterology guideline endorses BE screening in patients with chronic GERD and a minimum of 3 risk factors from the following: age 50 years or older, white race, male sex, and obesity.[44] Additionally, the requirement of 3 risk factors should be lowered in those with a family history of a first-degree relative with BE or EAC.[44] The BE screening approach from the American Society of Gastrointestinal Endoscopy endorses identification of individuals at risk for EAC.[45] At-risk populations are divided into high risk (family history of BE and EAC) or moderate risk (patients with GERD and at least 1 other risk factor for EAC including age >50 years, obesity/central adiposity, smoking history, or male gender).[45] Finally, the European Society of Gastrointestinal Endoscopy proposes that BE endoscopic should be considered only in high-risk individuals, those with long-standing GERD symptoms (ie, >5 years), and multiple risk factors (age >50 years, white race, male sex, obesity, or first-degree relative with BE or EAC).[46]

Publications evaluating BE risk factors in a screening population have evaluated only a single item such as male sex, GERD, abdominal obesity, and smoking.[36,47-49]

Table 1
Society BE definitions, guidelines for screening, surveillance, and management

Society	BE Definition	Screening	NDBE Surveillance	LGD Management	HGD Management	EAC T1a Management
ACG	≥1 cm CE that replaces squamous epithelium with presence of IM	Males with chronic ≥5 y or freq (≥once weekly) GERD AND ≥2 risk factors: age ≥50 y, Caucasian race, central obesity, past/current smoking, BE or EAC family history	Repeat endoscopy every 3–5 y	• Repeat biopsy every 12 mo OR • EET	• EET unless there is a life-limiting comorbidity • Endoscopic ablative therapy of remaining BE	• EET • Endoscopic ablative therapy of remaining BE
AGA	CE proximal to the GEJ with presence of IM	Recommended in Individuals with multiple risk factors (weak evidence)	Repeat endoscopy every 3–5 y	Repeat biopsy after 3–6 mo while on optimal acid-suppressive therapy Surveillance every 6–12 mo EET is reasonable	• EET • Flat HGD should be re-evaluated in 6–8 wk to look for a visible lesion	EET is reasonable if: • <500 nm invasion into submucosa • Good to moderate differentiation • No lymphatic invasion
ASGE	CE proximal to the GEJ with presence of IM	High risk: family hx of BE or EAC, screening recommended Moderate risk: presence of GERD + at least 1 other risk factor, may benefit from screening Low risk: no screening	Repeat endoscopy every 3–5 y	EET vs surveillance should be a shared decision with the patient	• EET • Recommend against esophagectomy	• EET • Recommend against esophagectomy

ESGE	≥1 cm CE that replaces squamous epithelium with presence of IM	Can be considered in patients with chronic GERD (≥5 y) AND multiple risk factors	For BE <1 cm, no further surveillance. For BE ≥1 cm, <3 cm, surveillance every 5 y. For BE ≥3 cm and <10 cm, surveillance every 3 y. For BE ≥10 cm, referral to BE expert center	Repeat biopsy in 6 mo: • If no dysplasia: interval increased to 1 y. After two consecutive endoscopies with negative dysplasia, move to NDBE schedule • If repeat LGD, perform EET	Repeat biopsy: • If no visible dysplasia, repeat biopsies in 3 mo • If visible lesions, perform EET	EET
BSG	CE ≥1 cm proximal to the GEJ	Chronic GERD and 3 or more risk factors or Chronic GERD and family history of BE/EAC	For BE <3 cm, surveillance every 3–5 y. For BE ≥3 cm, surveillance every 2–3 y	EET or repeat biopsy in 6 mo	EET	EET

Abbreviations: ACG, American College of Gastroenterology; AGA, American Gastroenterological Association; ASGE is American Society for Gastrointestinal Endoscopy; BE, Barrett's esophagus; BSG, British Society of Gastroenterology; CE, columnar epithelium; EAC, esophageal adenocarcinoma; EET, endoscopic eradication therapy; ESGE, European Society of Gastrointestinal Endoscopy; GEJ, gastroesophageal junction; HGD, high-grade dysplasia; IM, Intestinal metaplasia; LGD, low-grade dysplasia; NDBE, nondysplastic Barrett's esophagus.

Qumseya and associates addressed this limitation, reporting in a systemic review and meta-analysis that the highest risk for BE was in those with a family history of BE or EAC.[27] The risk increased further with the addition of GERD. Furthermore, for every other additional risk factor studied, the rate of BE increased by 1.2%. Investigators have also developed clinical prediction tools to improve selection of individuals for EGD to maximize benefit and yield of endoscopic screening for BE.[50–54] Recently, Rubinstein and colleagues[55] validated and compared multiple tools to select individuals for BE screening. All tools assessed were compared to the presence of GERD symptoms and found to differentiate BE better than symptom presence alone. Limitations of all tools assessed by Rubinstein were study performance in a population that was 85% nHw along with 3 of the tools evaluated not integrating race/ethnicity in their models.

How to Screen?

Endoscopic methods
Endoscopy with biopsy. Currently, the gold standard method for identifying BE is by EGD with biopsy using the Seattle protocol in patients with GERD and risk factors described previously.[1,21,22,43–46] This method has multiple limitations. It is well known that BE is diagnosed in those without GERD symptoms.[56,57] Also known is less than 10% of all EAC cases have a prior diagnosis of BE.[58,59] Further complicating matters, approximately 5% of the BE segment is adequately sampled with this method resulting in potential for missed dysplasia or cancer.[60,61] Moreover, adherence to the Seattle protocol is a concern based on BE length due to time, sedation, and patient factors. Investigators have found that adherence to BE biopsy recommendations is low within community and academic settings.[62–64] Other factors that require consideration when using EGD for BE screening include sedation and procedure-related risks, albeit small, as well as direct and indirect costs of the procedure which may be up to $2000.[65]

Unsedated transnasal endoscopy. Transnasal endoscopy (TNE) uses an ultrathin endoscope, which is passed via nasal passages into the esophagus, requiring only topical anesthesia rather than conscious sedation or monitored anesthesia care for the examination. In a randomized crossover investigation of cases and controls comparing TNE to standard endoscopy, both performed by expert endoscopists also trained in TNE, BE was diagnosed by TNE with sensitivity of 98% and specificity of 100% compared to standard endoscopy.[66] Portability of BE screening via a traveling research unit performing TNE demonstrated similar performance to either standard endoscopy and hospital-based TNE with regard to effectiveness, safety, and patient participation.[67] In addition, TNE had decreased procedure and recovery times along with high patient disposition to repeat the procedure if needed.[67] Recently, a second-generation disposable TNE unit was found to have high (>0.9) BE-detection sensitivity and specificity compared to standard endoscopy.[68] Moreover, TNE with the second-generation unit was clearly preferred among participants.[68] One limitation to the second-generation device is the lack of a biopsy channel allowing tissue sampling to provide histologic confirmation. However, the use of the second-generation TNE device for BE screening provides greater opportunity for identifying individuals with endoscopic changes suspicious for BE as the initial step in a 2-step process. Those identified with suspected BE then proceed to standard endoscopy for biopsy and risk stratification. Another potential advantage of TNE for BE screening is reduced direct and indirect costs compared to standard endoscopy especially when a mobile TNE laboratory is used for screening.[69]

Tethered capsule endomicroscopy. Tethered capsule endomicroscopy (TCE) technology is a recently established method of real time microscopy based on optical coherence tomography (OCT) imaging.[70,71] The TCE capsule (approximately 11 by 24 mm) is tethered to a string which is connected to an OCT console, responsible for light generation, collection of data, image processing, and display.[72] After the capsule is swallowed, the device obtains multiple three-dimensional images of the superficial esophageal wall during the descent into the stomach. Images can also be taken on the ascent from distal to proximal esophagus during capsule withdrawal by the tether. A feasibility study tested the TCE device on 38 patients (17 with BE), revealing nearly 90% were able to swallow the capsule.[72] When compared to blinded endoscopic assessment of BE by maximum extent and circumference, robust correlation was reported along with interobserver agreement. Potential advantages of this technology are similar to TNE, reduced direct and indirect costs when compared to standard endoscopic screening, along with possible use for primary care–based BE screening[73]

Nonendoscopic methods
Cell collection systems. Currently there are 3 systems that are FDA cleared for clinical use in the United States: Cytosponge (Medtronic, Minneapolis, MN; https://www.medtronic.com/uk-en/e/cytosponge-healthcare-professionals.html), EsoCheck (Lucid Diagnostics, New York, NY; https://www.luciddx.com/esocheck), and EsophaCap (CapNostics, Concord, NC; https://www.capnostics.com). The Cytosponge is a compressed polyurethane sponge compressed into a gelatinous capsule attached to a thread. Once the capsule is swallowed and reaches the stomach, the capsule dissolves releasing the sponge to expand. After expansion, the sponge is slowly withdrawn by the thread. During extraction, cells are collected from gastric cardia, esophagus, and oropharynx.[74] Collected cells undergo immunohistochemical staining for trefoil factor 3, a biomarker that indicates the presence of intestinal metaplasia.[75] In multiple clinical studies (Barrett's Esophagus Screening Trials [Best] 1, 2, and 3), the Cytosponge was safe, well tolerated, had good BE detection sensitivity/specificity, and diagnosed BE greater than 10 times more frequently than usual care.[76–78] EsoCheck is a surface-textured balloon sampling device which is swallowed in a pill-sized capsule attached to a silicone catheter.[79] Once in the stomach, the balloon is inflated with 5 to 6 cc of air and withdrawn through the lowest 3 to 6 cm of the esophagus to collect epithelial cells. After sampling the distal esophagus as described previously, the balloon is deflated and withdraws back into the capsule protecting the material obtained. The material is tested then for vimentin and cyclin-A1 DNA as both are associated with BE as well as EAC.[79] In a pilot study of EsoCheck, 82% swallowed the capsule successfully with adequate samples obtained in 74%. Sensitivity and specificity of the specimens obtained were 90.3% and 91.7%, respectively, for determining NDBE compared to controls with normal esophageal mucosa, GERD, or erosive esophagitis. EsophaCap is another sampling device comprising a compressed sponge in a gelatin capsule attached to a string. The device is swallowed, and a polyurethane sponge is released in the proximal stomach after dissolution of the capsule. The sponge is then withdrawn via the attached tether with tissue collected for cytology and methylated DNA markers.[80,81] Sensitivities ranged from 68% to 78% with specificity between 91% and 93% in these studies for presence of BE. However, 15% to 30% of patient could not swallow the device.

Blood or breath biomarkers. MicroRNAs (miRNAs) are circulating, small, single-stranded, noncoding ribonucleic acids (RNAs) responsible for physiologic process regulation.[82] Combination of miRNAs have been identified by investigators with potential to differentiate between BE and non-BE patients.[83,84] However, a recent study evaluating variable miRNAs signatures for BE and EAC described a discrepancy among serum and tissue miRNA portfolios.[85] This along with lack of validation in the general population for BE screening limits current applicability. Another potential blood biomarker is doublecortin-like kinase 1 (DCKL1, formally doublecortin and CaM kinase-like 1), a putative tumor stem cell marker identified in multiple gastrointestinal tumors and BE.[86] DCKL1 was found to be elevated in plasma samples of BE and EAC patients compared to normal controls.[87] Furthermore, DCLK1 was found to be elevated in serum samples taken from both BE along with intramucosal or Stage I-II EAC compared to normal controls.[88] In addition, serum DCLK1 decreased after treatment in EAC patients. Validation for use as a potential BE screening tool in the general population has not occurred to date.

Regarding breath sampling analysis for volatile organic compounds (VOC) produced from results of human and gut flora metabolism, 2 current methodologies exist for evaluating BE/EAC. They are gas chromatography-mass spectrometry and an electronic nose apparatus.[89–92] Of note, gas chromatography-mass spectrometry in BE has been evaluated by one study and did not reveal a VOC difference between normal patients and those with BE.[89] Other issues with gas chromatography-mass spectrometry are cost and work intensity required.

The electronic nose apparatus uses a chemical to electrical interface to measure VOC profiles of disease states, combined with machine learning (ML), and is trained in similar fashion as a canine.[93]

The apparatus has been found to have sensitivity of 91% to 96% and specificity of 74% to 80% with patient acceptability of 91% to 95%.[91,92] Other advantages compared to gas chromatography-mass spectrometry are portability and reduced cost. As noted for blood testing, validation for use as a potential BE screening tool in the general population has not occurred to date.

ARTIFICIAL INTELLIGENCE, MACHINE LEARNING, AND COMPUTER-AIDED DIAGNOSIS

Artificial intelligence (AI) application within endoscopy has recently undergone intense study with substantial progress made principally in image and pattern recognition.[94] The aim of AI in endoscopy is to improve patient care during examination, diagnosis, and treatment especially for nonexpert endoscopists. An AI procedure or algorithm initially has to be trained to recognize the item desired in test images so that new image samples are recognized for the desired item. This process, called ML, can occur under supervised, unsupervised, or reinforced conditions. Supervised ML occurs with known patterns, unsupervised/reinforced ML with unknown patterns, and reinforced with trial-and-error processes. Deep learning is based on convolutional neural networks which use nodes (or "neurons") to connect to other nodes in a way that mimics real human neural networking. Several layers of nodes can combine, making a decision to call a grouping of pixels on an image either normal tissue or abnormal.[95] The American Society for Gastrointestinal Endoscopy's Preservation and Incorporation of Valuable Endoscopic Innovations (PIVI) criteria for new technologies recommend that the sensitivity should be at least 0.90, specificity should be at least 0.80, and a negative predictive value of at least 0.98 for detecting HGD or EAC.[96] Most AI and computer-aided diagnosis applications in BE have had a goal of improving detection of dysplastic and early neoplastic lesions in the applicable segment.[97–100] The use of AI has tremendous potential for improving the performance of endoscopists and patient experience while maximizing cost-effectiveness in BE screening/surveillance.

SURVEILLANCE AND TREATMENT

Once BE is discovered and confirmed, the patient moves into a surveillance program. The main goal of BE surveillance is to discover dysplasia and early stage EAC amenable to endoscopic eradication therapy (EET). With the advent of new detection modalities and EET, the current aim of surveillance is to eliminate the predecessors of invasive cancer, HGD, and intramucosal EAC.

Endoscopic Evaluation During Surveillance

The opening assessment of the BE segment by the endoscopist begins with careful determination of anatomic landmarks for orientation purposes. These include the GEJ or top of the gastric folds, squamocolumnar junction, and diaphragmatic hiatus, reported as distance in centimeters from the incisors. As mentioned earlier, the Prague criteria should be used to describe the BE segment along with Paris classification for any visible lesions seen.[21,101] After cautious inspection using HD white light endoscopy, the most recent guideline (ASGE 2019) recommends chromoendoscopy, using an applied dye or electronic.[45] No guideline has recommended the standard employment of other advanced imaging methods including confocal laser endomicroscopy, volumetric laser endomicroscopy, OCT, spectroscopy, or other molecular techniques. Acetic acid and electronic chromoendoscopy (narrow band imaging [NBI]) have met ASGE PIVI criteria for use in surveillance.[102] Acetic acid chromoendoscopy is performed by topical application of acetic acid to the esophageal mucosa and has outstanding operating characteristics for dysplasia detection.[102] Limiting factors in acetic acid chromoendoscopy are the cost of ancillary equipment needed, time necessary for performance, and uneven solution application.[103,104]

There are three electronic chromoendoscopy versions, each associated with its endoscopy platform (NBI; Olympus Americas, Center Valley, PA; Fujinon intelligent color enhancement, Fujinon, Wayne, NJ; i-scan, Pentax Medical, Montvale, NJ). NBI is the most widely studied of the 3 electronic chromoendoscopy versions and has been shown to improve dysplasia detection and decrease biopsy number needed per patient.[105,106] Unfortunately, targeted biopsies via chromoendoscopy have not been recommended by recent guidelines as the preponderance of data favoring electronic chromoendoscopy are from academic centers with BE expertise, limiting generalizability.[1,45]

Assessment of Barrett's Esophagus Segment by Histology

Mucosal abnormalities noted during the endoscopic evaluation should be removed by endoscopic mucosal resection (EMR), if possible, or sampled by biopsy and sent in a separate container for pathologic evaluation.[107] This is due to an association of such abnormalities and malignancy.[108] Mucosal abnormalities do not include erosive esophagitis, which, if found, requires adjustment of acid suppression therapy because of difficulty in distinguishing dysplasia from inflammation at that time. Instead, repeat endoscopy should occur 8 to 12 weeks after therapy optimization. Outside of visible lesion removal, the remaining BE segment should be biopsied using the Seattle protocol: 4 quadrant biopsies every 2 cm for NDBE or every 1 cm for those with known/suspected dysplasia.[22] Despite the time required for completion of the protocol, data indicate diagnostic yield increases with biopsy number obtained and biopsies using a standardized sampling method increases dysplasia/EAC discovery.[109–111] An additional technology for BE tissue assessment during both screening and surveillance is wide-area transepithelial sampling (WATS). This method uses a stiff wire brush to sample the BE segment combined with 3-dimensional computer-assisted analysis to identify concerning tissue for cytopathological review.[112] The ASGE BE guideline in 2019 gave a conditional recommendation for WATS use combined with usual endoscopic biopsy based on a 48% increase in dysplasia detection in 6 studies that included WATS compared to biopsy alone.[42]

Endoscopic Eradication Therapy

EET of BE begins with removal of mucosal lesions by EMR as described previously or endoscopic submucosal dissection at an expert center if not amenable to EMR.[1,17,107,113] If the removed lesion has dysplasia and is confirmed by a gastrointestinal pathologist, ablation of the remaining BE segment should occur with the goal of complete elimination of IM (CE-IM). If EAC confined to the mucosa with a negative deep margin (T1a, curative with low risk of lymph node involvement) is found after successful resection, the remaining BE should be ablated to obtain CE-IM as well. This is due to data indicating that surveillance of the residual BE after resection of visible lesions is associated with high rates of recurrent HGD/EAC.[114–116]

For flat dysplastic BE, multiple ablative modalities have demonstrated high rates of CE-IM including radiofrequency ablation (RFA), photodynamic therapy, cryotherapy, argon plasma coagulation, and hybrid argon plasma coagulation.[117–122] Unfortunately, data comparing modalities to each other in a head-to-head comparison are lacking. Moreover, considerable level 1 evidence exists documenting superiority of RFA to standard surveillance with multiple guidelines indicating that RFA is the therapy of choice for ablation of flat dysplastic BE or residual BE after removal of visible lesions.[1,43,44]

The breakthrough RFA trial indicating that BE with dysplasia could be eradicated was reported by Shaheen and associates in 2009.[117] In this study, BE patients with nonnodular dysplasia were assigned to RFA or sham treatment in a 2:1 ratio with primary outcome variables consisting of complete eradication of dysplasia (CE-D) in LGD/HGD and CE-IM in both groups.

For LGD, CE-D occurred in 90.5% of those undergoing RFA while only 22.7% achieved CE-D in the sham treatment group ($P<.001$). In HGD, CE-D occurred in 81.0% of the RFA subjects, and only 19.0% among sham subjects ($P<.001$). For CE-IM, 77.4% of patients in the ablation group obtained this result, while only 2.3% of those in the control group achieved this endpoint ($P<.001$). Also seen after ablation were decreased progression rates (3.6% vs 16.3%, $P = .03$) and cancer development (1.2% vs 9.3%, $P = .045$) in the RFA group compared to sham.

Phoa and colleagues[118] performed a randomized trial in LGD where 136 patients were assigned to either RFA treatment or endoscopic surveillance. RFA resulted in reduced progression to HGD or EAC compared to standard surveillance (1.5% vs 26.5%, $P<.001$). For CE-D and CE-IM, RFA produced rates of 92.6% and 88.2% compared to surveillance rates of 27% and 0%, respectively, ($P<.001$). The most common adverse event in both studies was stricture formation, successfully resolved after endoscopic dilation.[117,118] Of note, among the cancers found during surveillance after RFA in both studies, all were treatable either endoscopically or via esophagectomy.[117,118] Owing to this, it has been suggested that the decision between EET and surveillance in LGD should be made in a patient-shared decision-making fashion.[123]

For HGD, Shaheen and associates reported a nearly 800% increase in progression to EAC among control patients compared to those receiving RFA.[117] Moreover, a pooled analysis of EMR techniques (focal or complete) combined with RFA in HGD and intramucosal EAC indicated effectiveness of this treatment for CE-D, CE-IM, and EAC.[124] A meta-analysis comparing outcomes of EET to esophagectomy for HGD/intramucosal EAC found no difference in survival up to 5 years or cancer-related deaths between the 2 procedures.[125] Of note, recurrence of dysplasia was higher after EET, but adverse events were lower in the EET group than with esophagectomy. Considering the previous discussion, EET is the preferred treatment for HGD along with intramucosal EAC.

SUMMARY AND FUTURE DIRECTIONS

Diagnosis and management of BE have evolved over time. As technology advances, opportunities arise that could result in better identification of those with BE who do not have GERD symptoms through nonendoscopic methods, using those same methods to maximize benefits of surveillance and EET along with AI to reduce missed lesions at endoscopy. Management of HGD and intramucosal EAC using EET clearly is preferred compared to esophagectomy. Furthermore, determining the best management path for LGD in a patient-centered or outcome-driven fashion will help increase benefit while minimizing harm in those individuals. Once these are possible and available for all, EAC development will be maximally decreased.

CLINICS CARE POINTS

- BE screening/surveillance programs have not provided the anticipated EAC reduction benefit to date.
- Noninvasive sampling devices are increasingly available to screen for BE among those with and without known risk factors.
- Implementation of artificial intelligence platforms to aid the endoscopist during screening and surveillance will soon become routine, minimizing missed lesions during endoscopy.
- BE with low-grade dysplasia can be managed with removal of visible lesions combined with endoscopic eradication therapy or surveillance per recent guidelines.

REFERENCES

1. Shaheen NJ, Falk GW, Iyer PR, et al. ACG clinical guideline: diagnosis and management of Barrett's Esophagus. Am J Gastroenterol 2016;111:30–50.
2. Ronkainen J, Aro P, Storskrubb T, et al. Prevalence of Barrett's esophagus in the general population: an endoscopic study. Gastroenterology 2005;129:1825–31.
3. Zagari RM, Fuccio L, Wallander MA, et al. Gastro-oesophageal reflux symptoms, oesophagitis and Barrett's esophagus in the general population: the Loiano-Mionghidoro study. Gut 2008;57:1354–9.
4. Fan X, Snyder N. Prevalence of Barrett's esophagus in patients with and without GERD symptoms: role of race, age and gender. Dig Dis Sci 2009;54:572–7.
5. Khoury JE, Chisholm S, Jamal MM, et al. African Americans with Barrett's esophagus are less likely to have dysplasia at biopsy. Dig Dis Sci 2012;57:419–23.
6. Lin EC, Holub J, Lieberman D, et al. Low prevalence of suspected Barrett's esophagus in patients with gastroesophageal reflux disease without alarm symptoms. Clin Gastroenterol Hepatol 2019;17:857–63.

7. de Jonge PJ, van Blankenstein M, Looman CW, et al. Risk of malignant progression in patients with Barrett's oesophagus: a Dutch nationwide cohort study. Gut 2010;59:1030-6.

8. Bhat S, Coleman HG, Yousef F, et al. Risk of malignant progression in Barrett's esophagus patients: results from a large population-based study. J Natl Cancer Inst 2011;103:1049-57.

9. Hvid-Jensen F, Pedersen L, Drewes AM, et al. Incidence of adenocarcinoma among patients with Barrett's esophagus. N Engl J Med 2011;365:1375-83.

10. Desai TK, Krishnan K, Samala N, et al. The incidence of oesophageal adenocarcinoma in non- dysplastic Barrett's oesophagus: a meta-analysis. Gut 2012;61: 970-6.

11. Krishnamoorthi R, Ramos GP, Crews N, et al. Persistence of nondysplastic Barrett's esophagus is not protective against progression to adenocarcinoma. Clin Gastroenterol Hepatol 2017;15:950-2.

12. Lim CH, Treanor D, Dixon MF, et al. Low-grade dysplasia in Barrett's esophagus has a high risk of progression. Endoscopy 2007;39:581-7.

13. Curvers WL, ten Kate FJ, Krishnadath KK, et al. Low-grade dysplasia in Barrett's esophagus: overdiagnosed and underestimated. Am J Gastroenterol 2010;105: 1523-30.

14. Duits LC, Phoa KN, Curvers WL, et al. Barrett's oesophagus patients with low-grade dysplasia can be accurately risk-stratified after histological review by an expert pathology panel. Gut 2015;64:700-6.

15. Duits LC, van der Wel MJ, Cotton CC, et al. Patients with Barrett's esophagus and confirmed persistent low-grade dysplasia are at increased risk for progression to neoplasia. Gastroenterology 2017;152:993-1001.e1.

16. Rastogi A, Puli S, El-Serag HB, et al. Incidence of esophageal adenocarcinoma in patients with Barrett's esophagus and high-grade dysplasia: a meta-analysis. Gastrointest Endosc 2008;67:394-8.

17. Sharma P, Shaheen NJ, Katzka D, et al. AGA clinical practice update on endoscopic treatment of Barrett's esophagus with dysplasia and/or early cancer: expert review. Gastroenterology 2020;158:760-9.

18. Wenker TN, Tan MC, Liu Y, et al. Prior diagnosis of Barrett's esophagus is infrequent, but associated with improved esophageal adenocarcinoma survival. Dig Dis Sci 2018;63:3112-9.

19. Sharma P, Morales TG, Sampliner RE. Short Segment Barrett's Esophagus-the need for standardization of the definition and of endoscopic criteria. Am J Gastroenterol 1998;93:1033-6.

20. Jung KW, Talley NJ, Romero Y, et al. Epidemiology and natural history of intestinal metaplasia of the gastroesophageal junction and Barrett's esophagus: a population-based study. Am J Gastroenterol 2011;106:1447-55.

21. Sharma P, Dent J, Armstrong D, et al. The development and validation of an endoscopic grading for Barrett's esophagus: the Prague C & M criteria. Gastroenterology 2006;131:1392-9.

22. Levine DS, Blount PL, Rudolph RE, et al. Safety of a systematic endoscopic biopsy protocol in patients with Barrett's esophagus. Am J Gastroenterol 2000;95: 1152-7.

23. Anaparthy R, Gaddam S, Kanakadandi V, et al. Association between length of Barrett's esophagus and risk of high-grade dysplasia or adenocarcinoma in patients without dysplasia. Clin Gastroenterol Hepatol 2013;11:1430-6.

24. Shaheen N. Is there a "Barrett's iceberg? Gastroenterology 2002;123:636-9.

25. Cameron AJ, Zinsmeister AR, Ballard DJ, et al. Prevalence of columnar-lined (Barrett's) esophagus. comparison of population-based clinical and autopsy findings. Gastroenterology 1990;99:918–22.
26. Hayeck TJ, Kong CY, Spechler SJ, et al. The prevalence of Barrett's esophagus in the US: estimates from a simulation model confirmed by SEER data. Dis Esophagus 2010;23:451–7.
27. Qumseya BJ, Bukannan A, Gendy S, et al. Systematic review and meta-analysis of prevalence and risk factors for Barrett's esophagus. Gastrointest Endosc 2019;90:707–17.e1.
28. Chen YH, Yu HC, Lin KH, et al. Prevalence and risk factors for Barrett's esophagus in Taiwan. World J Gastroenterol 2019;25:3231–41.
29. Prach AT, MacDonald TA, Hopwood DA, et al. Increasing incidence of Barrett's oesophagus: education, enthusiasm, or epidemiology? Lancet 1997;350:933.
30. Conio M, Cameron AJ, Romero Y, et al. Secular trends in the epidemiology and outcome of Barrett's oesophagus in Olmsted County, Minnesota. Gut 2001;48: 304–9.
31. van Soest EM, Dieleman JP, Siersema PD, et al. Increasing incidence of Barrett's oesophagus in the general population. Gut 2005;54:1062–6.
32. Post PN, Siersema PD, Van Dekken H. Rising incidence of clinically evident Barrett's oesophagus in The Netherlands: a nation-wide registry of pathology reports. Scand J Gastroenterol 2007;42:17–22.
33. Sampliner RE. Practice guidelines on the diagnosis, surveillance, and therapy of Barrett's esophagus. The Practice Parameters Committee of the American College of Gastroenterology. Am J Gastroenterol 1998;93:1028–32.
34. Sampliner RE, Practice Parameters Committee of the American College of Gastroenterology. Updated guidelines for the diagnosis, surveillance, and therapy of Barrett's esophagus. Am J Gastroenterol 2002;97:1888–95.
35. Masclee GM, Coloma PM, de Wilde M, et al. The incidence of Barrett's oesophagus and oesophageal adenocarcinoma in the United Kingdom and The Netherlands is levelling off. Aliment Pharmacol Ther 2014;39:1321–30.
36. Petrick JL, Nguyen T, Cook MB. Temporal trends of esophageal disorders by age in the Cerner Health Facts database. Ann Epidemiol 2016;26:151–4.e4.
37. Cook MB, Wild CP, Forman D. A systematic review and meta-analysis of the sex ratio for Barrett's esophagus, erosive reflux disease, and nonerosive reflux disease. Am J Epidemiol 2005;162:1050–61.
38. Corley DA, Kubo A, Levin TR, et al. Race, ethnicity, sex and temporal differences in Barrett's oesophagus diagnosis: a large community-based study, 1994–2006. Gut 2009;58:182–8.
39. Yachimski P, Lee RA, Tramontano A, et al. Secular trends in patients diagnosed with Barrett's esophagus. Dig Dis Sci 2010;55:960–6.
40. Yamasaki T, Sakiani S, Maradey-Romero C, et al. Barrett's esophagus patients are becoming younger: analysis of a large United States dataset. Esophagus 2020;17:190–6.
41. Krishnamoorthi R, Singh S, Ragunathan K, et al. Factors associated with progression of Barrett's esophagus: a systematic review and meta-analysis. Clin Gastroenterol Hepatol 2018;16:1046–55.e8.
42. Qumseya BJ, Bukannan A, Gendy S, et al. Systematic review and meta-analysis of prevalence and risk factors for Barrett's esophagus. Gastrointest Endosc 2019;90:707–17.e1.

43. American Gastroenterological Association, Spechler SJ, Sharma P, Souza RF, et al. American Gastroenterological Association medical position statement on the management of Barrett's esophagus. Gastroenterology 2011;140:1084–91.

44. Fitzgerald RC, Di Pietro M, Ragunath K, et al. British Society of Gastroenterology guidelines on the diagnosis and management of Barrett's oesophagus. Gut 2014;63:7–42.

45. Qumseya B, Sultan S, Bain P, et al. ASGE guideline on screening and surveillance of Barrett's esophagus. Gastrointest Endosc 2019;90:335–59.

46. Saftoiu A, Hassan C, Areia M, et al. Role of gastrointestinal endoscopy in the screening of digestive tract cancers in Europe: European Society of Gastrointestinal Endoscopy (ESGE) Position Statement. Endoscopy 2020;52:293–304.

47. Taylor JB, Rubenstein JH. Meta-analyses of the effect of symptoms of gastroesophageal reflux on the risk of Barrett's esophagus. Am J Gastroenterol 2010;105:1729, 1730–27; [quiz 1738].

48. Singh S, Sharma AN, Murad MH, et al. Central adiposity is associated with increased risk of esophageal inflammation, metaplasia, and adenocarcinoma: a systematic review and meta- analysis. Clin Gastroenterol Hepatol 2013;11:1399–412.

49. Andrici J, Cox MR, Eslick GD. Cigarette smoking and the risk of Barrett's esophagus: a systematic review and meta-analysis. J Gastroenterol Hepatol 2013;28:1258–73.

50. Gerson LB, Edson R, Lavori PW, et al. Use of a simple symptom questionnaire to predict Barrett's esophagus in patients with symptoms of gastroesophageal reflux. Am J Gastroenterol 2001;96:2005–12.

51. Locke GR, Zinsmeister AR, Talley NJ. Can symptoms predict endoscopic findings in GERD? Gastrointest Endosc 2003;58:661–70.

52. Thrift AP, Kendall BJ, Pandeya N, et al. A clinical risk prediction model for Barrett esophagus. Cancer Prev Res (Phila) 2012;5:1115–23.

53. Rubenstein JH, Morgenstern H, Appelman H, et al. Prediction of Barrett's esophagus among men. Am J Gastroenterol 2013;108:353–62.

54. Xie SH, Ness-Jensen E, Medefelt N, et al. Assessing the feasibility of targeted screening for esophageal adenocarcinoma based on individual risk assessment in a population-based cohort study in Norway (The HUNT Study). Am J Gastroenterol 2018;113:829–35.

55. Rubenstein JH, McConnell D, Waljee AK, et al. Validation and comparison of tools for selecting individuals to screen for Barrett's esophagus and early neoplasia. Gastroenterology 2020;158:2082–92.

56. Gerson LB, Shetler K, Triadafilopoulos G. Prevalence of Barrett's esophagus in asymptomatic individuals. Gastroenterology 2002;123:461–7.

57. Rex DK, Cummings OW, Shaw M, et al. Screening for Barrett's esophagus in colonoscopy patients with and without heartburn. Gastroenterology 2003;125:1670–7.

58. Bhat SK, McManus DT, Coleman HG, et al. Oesophageal adenocarcinoma and prior diagnosis of Barrett's oesophagus: a population based study. Gut 2015;64:20–5.

59. Spechler SJ, Katzka DA, Fitzgerald RC. New screening techniques in Barrett's esophagus: great ideas or great practice? Gastroenterology 2018;154:1594–601.

60. Visrodia K, Singh S, Krishnamoorthi R, et al. Magnitude of missed esophageal adenocarcinoma after Barrett's esophagus diagnosis: a systematic review and meta-analysis. Gastroenterology 2016;150:599–607.e7 [quiz e14–5].

61. Visrodia K, Iyer PG, Schleck CD, et al. Yield of repeat endoscopy in Barrett's esophagus with no dysplasia and low-grade dysplasia: a population-based study. Dig Dis Sci 2016;61:158–67.
62. Abrams JA, Kapel RC, Lindberg GM, et al. Adherence to biopsy guidelines for Barrett's esophagus surveillance in the community setting in the United States. Clin Gastroenterol Hepatol 2009;7:736–42 [quiz 710].
63. Westerveld D, Khullar V, Mramba L, et al. Adherence to quality indicators and surveillance guidelines in the management of Barrett's esophagus: a retrospective analysis. Endosc Int Open 2018;6:E300–7.
64. Wani S, Williams JL, Somanduri S, et al. Endoscopists systematically undersample patients with long-segment Barrett's esophagus: an analysis of biopsy sampling practices from a quality improvement registry. Gastrointest Endosc 2019; 90:732–41.
65. Sami SS, Ragunath K, Iyer PG. Screening for Barrett's esophagus and esophageal adenocarcinoma: rationale, recent progress, challenges, and future directions. Clin Gastroenterol Hepatol 2015;13:623–34.
66. Shariff MK, Bird-Lieberman EL, O'Donovan M, et al. Randomized crossover study comparing efficacy of transnasal endoscopy with that of standard endoscopy to detect Barrett's esophagus. Gastrointest Endosc 2012;75:954–61.
67. Sami SS, Dunagan KT, Johnson ML, et al. A randomized comparative effectiveness trial of novel endoscopic techniques and approaches for Barrett's esophagus screening in the community. Am J Gastroenterol 2015;110:148–58.
68. Sami SS, Iyer PG, Pophali P, et al. Acceptability, accuracy, and safety of disposable transnasal capsule endoscopy for Barrett's esophagus screening. Clin Gastroenterol Hepatol 2019;17:638–46.e1.
69. Moriarty JP, Shah ND, Rubenstein JH, et al. Costs associated with Barrett's esophagus screening in the community: an economic analysis of a prospective randomized controlled trial of sedated versus hospital unsedated versus mobile community unsedated endoscopy. Gastrointest Endosc 2018;87:88–94.e2.
70. Gora MJ, Sauk JS, Carruth RW, et al. Tethered capsule endomicroscopy enables less invasive imaging of gastrointestinal tract microstructure. Nat Med 2013;19:238–40.
71. Gora MJ, Sauk JS, Carruth RW, et al. Imaging the upper gastrointestinal tract in unsedated patients using tethered capsule endomicroscopy. Gastroenterology 2013;145:723–5.
72. Gora MJ, Quénéhervé L, Carruth RW, et al. Tethered capsule endomicroscopy for microscopic imaging of the esophagus, stomach, and duodenum without sedation in humans (with video). Gastrointest Endosc 2018;88:830–40.e3.
73. Gora MJ, Simmons LH, Quénéhervé L, et al. Tethered capsule endomicroscopy: from bench to bedside at a primary care practice. J Biomed Opt 2016;21: 104001.
74. Fitzgerald RC. Combining simple patient-oriented tests with state-of-the-art molecular diagnostics for early diagnosis of cancer. United Eur Gastroenterol J 2015;3:226–9.
75. Lao-Sirieix P, Boussioutas A, Kadri SR, et al. Non-endoscopic screening biomarkers for Barrett's oesophagus: from microarray analysis to the clinic. Gut 2009;58:1451–9.
76. Kadri SR, Lao-Sirieix P, O'Donovan M, et al. Acceptability and accuracy of a nonendoscopic screening test for Barrett's oesophagus in primary care: cohort study. BMJ 2010;341:c4372.

77. Ross-Innes CS, Debiram-Beecham I, O'Donovan M, et al. Evaluation of a minimally invasive cell sampling device coupled with assessment of trefoil factor 3 expression for diagnosing Barrett's esophagus: a multi-center case–control study. Plos Med 2015;12:e1001780.

78. Fitzgerald RC, di Pietro M, O'Donovan M, et al. Cytosponge-trefoil factor 3 versus usual care to identify Barrett's oesophagus in a primary care setting: a multicentre, pragmatic, randomized controlled trial. Lancet 2020;396:333–44.

79. Moinova HR, LaFramboise T, Lutterbaugh JD, et al. Identifying DNA methylation biomarkers for non-endoscopic detection of Barrett's esophagus. Sci Transl Med 2018;10:eaao5848.

80. Wang Z, Kambhampati S, Cheng Y, et al. Methylation biomarker panel performance in EsophaCap cytology samples for diagnosing Barrett's esophagus: a prospective validation study. Clin Cancer Res 2019;25:2127–35.

81. Zhou Z, Kalatskaya I, Russell D, et al. Combined EsophaCap cytology and MUC2 immunohistochemistry for screening of intestinal metaplasia, dysplasia and carcinoma. Clin Exp Gastroenterol 2019;12:219–29.

82. Wang H, Peng R, Wang J, et al. Circulating microRNAs as potential cancer biomarkers: the advantage and disadvantage. Clin Epigenet 2018;10:1–10.

83. Mallick R, Patnaik SK, Wani S, et al. A systematic review of esophageal microRNA markers for diagnosis and monitoring of Barrett's esophagus. Dig Dis Sci 2016;61:1039–50.

84. Bus P, Kestens C, Ten Kate FJW, et al. Profiling of circulating microRNAs in patients with Barrett's esophagus and esophageal adenocarcinoma. J Gastroenterol 2016;51:560–70.

85. Craig MP, Rajakaruna S, Paliy O, et al. Differential MicroRNA signatures in the pathogenesis of Barrett's esophagus. Clin Transl Gastroenterol 2020;11:e00125.

86. Vega KJ, May R, Sureban SM, et al. Identification of the putative intestinal stem cell marker doublecortin and CaM kinase-like-1 in Barrett's esophagus and esophageal adenocarcinoma. J Gastroenterol Hepatol 2012;27:773–80.

87. Whorton J, Lightfoot S, Sureban SM, et al. DCLK1 is detectable in plasma of patients with Barrett's esophagus and esophageal adenocarcinoma. Dig Dis Sci 2015;60:509–13.

88. Christman EM, Chandrakesan P, Weygant N, et al. Elevated doublecortin-like kinase 1 serum levels revert to baseline after therapy in early stage esophageal adenocarcinoma. Biomarker Res 2019;7:5.

89. Kumar S, Huang J, Abbassi-Ghadi N, et al. Mass spectrometric analysis of exhaled breath for the identification of volatile organic compound biomarkers in esophageal and gastric adenocarcinoma. Ann Surg 2015;262:981–90.

90. Markar SR, Wiggins T, Antonowicz S, et al. Assessment of a noninvasive exhaled breath test for the diagnosis of oesophagogastric cancer. JAMA Oncol 2018;4: 970–6.

91. Chan DK, Zakko L, Visrodia KH, et al. Breath testing for Barrett's esophagus using exhaled volatile organic compound profiling with an electronic nose device. Gastroenterology 2017;152:24–6.

92. Peters Y, Schrauwen RW, Tan AC, et al. Detection of Barrett's oesophagus through exhaled breath using an electronic nose device. Gut 2020;69:1169–72.

93. Chan DK, Leggett CL, Wang KK. Diagnosing gastrointestinal illnesses using fecal headspace volatile organic compounds. World J Gastroenterol 2016;22: 1639–49.

94. Sinonquel P, Eelbode T, Bossuyt P, et al. Artificial Intelligence and its impact on quality improvement in upper and lower gastrointestinal endoscopy. Dig Endosc 2021;33:242–53.

95. Ebigbo A, Palm C, Probst A, et al. A technical review of artificial intelligence as applied to gastrointestinal endoscopy: clarifying the terminology. Endosc Int Open 2019;7:E1616–23.

96. Sharma P, Savides TJ, Canto MI, et al. The American Society for Gastrointestinal Endoscopy PIVI (Preservation and Incorporation of Valuable Endoscopic Innovations) on imaging in Barrett's Esophagus. Gastrointest Endosc 2012;76: 252–4.

97. Ebigbo A, Mendel R, Probst A, et al. Computer-aided diagnosis using deep learning in the evaluation of early oesophageal adenocarcinoma. Gut 2019; 68:1143–5.

98. Ebigbo A, Mendel R, Probst A, et al. Realtime use of artificial intelligence in the evaluation of cancer in Barrett's oesophagus. Gut 2020;69:615–6.

99. de Groof AJ, Struyvenberg MR, van der Putten J, et al. Deep-learning system detects neoplasia in patients with Barrett's esophagus with higher accuracy than endoscopists in a multistep training and validation study with benchmarking. Gastroenterology 2020;158:915–29.e4.

100. Hashimoto R, Requa J, Dao T, et al. Artificial intelligence using convolutional neural networks for real-time detection of early esophageal neoplasia in Barrett's esophagus (with video). Gastrointest Endosc 2020;91:1264–12671.e1.

101. Endoscopic Classification Review Group. Update on the Paris classification of superficial neoplastic lesions in the digestive tract. Endoscopy 2005;37:570–8.

102. Thosani N, Abu Dayyeh BK, Sharma P, et al. ASGE Technology Committee systematic review and meta-analysis assessing the ASGE preservation and Incorporation of valuable Endoscopic Innovations thresholds for adopting real-time imaging-assisted endoscopic targeted biopsy during endoscopic surveillance of Barrett's esophagus. Gastrointest Endosc 2016;83:684–98.e7.

103. Olliver JR, Wild CP, Sahay P, et al. Chromoendoscopy with methylene blue and associated DNA damage in Barrett's oesophagus. Lancet 2003;362:373–4.

104. Kondo H, Fukuda H, Ono H, et al. Sodium thiosulfate solution spray for relief of irritation caused by Lugol's stain in chromoendoscopy. Gastrointest Endosc 2001;53:199–202.

105. Wolfsen HC, Crook JE, Krishna M, et al. Prospective, controlled tandem endoscopy study of narrow band imaging for dysplasia detection in Barrett's Esophagus. Gastroenterology 2008;135:24–31.

106. Sharma P, Hawes RH, Bansal A, et al. Standard endoscopy with random biopsies versus narrow band imaging targeted biopsies in Barrett's oesophagus: a prospective, international, randomised controlled trial. Gut 2013;62:15–21.

107. Wani S, Qumseya B, Sultan S, et al. Endoscopic eradication therapy for patients with Barrett's esophagus-associated dysplasia and intramucosal cancer. Gastrointest Endosc 2018;87:907–31.e9.

108. Reid BJ, Blount PL, Feng Z, et al. Optimizing endoscopic biopsy detection of early cancers in Barrett's high-grade dysplasia. Am J Gastroenterol 2000;95: 3089–96.

109. Fitzgerald RC, Saeed IT, Khoo D, et al. Rigorous surveillance protocol increases detection of curable cancers associated with Barrett's esophagus. Dig Dis Sci 2001;46:1892–8.

110. Qumseya BJ, Wang H, Badie N, et al. Advanced imaging technologies increase detection of dysplasia and neoplasia in patients with Barrett's esophagus: a

meta-analysis and systematic review. Clin Gastroenterol Hepatol 2013;11: 1562–70, e1–2.

111. Nachiappan A, Ragunath K, Card T, et al. Diagnosing dysplasia in Barrett's oesophagus still requires Seattle protocol biopsy in the era of modern video endoscopy: results from a tertiary centre Barrett's dysplasia database. Scand J Gastroenterol 2020;55:9–13.

112. Kumaravel A, Lopez R, Brainard J, et al. Brush cytology vs. endoscopic biopsy for the surveillance of Barrett's esophagus. Endoscopy 2010;42:800–5.

113. Peters Y, Al-Kaabi A, Shaheen NJ, et al. Barrett oesophagus. Nat Rev Dis Primers 2019;5:35.

114. Manner H, Rabenstein T, Pech O, et al. Ablation of residual Barrett's epithelium after endoscopic resection: a randomized long-term follow-up study of argon plasmacoagulation vs surveillance (APE study). Endoscopy 2014;46:6–12.

115. May A, Gossner L, Pech O, et al. Intraepithelial high-grade neoplasia and early adenocarcinoma in short segment Barrett's esophagus (SSBE): curative treatment using local endoscopic treatment techniques. Endoscopy 2002;34: 604–10.

116. Pech O, Behrens A, May A, et al. Long-term results and risk factor analysis for recurrence after curative endoscopic therapy in 349 patients with high-grade intraepithelial neoplasia and mucosal adenocarcinoma in Barrett's oesophagus. Gut 2008;57:1200–6.

117. Shaheen NJ, Sharma P, Overholt BF, et al. Radiofrequency ablation in Barrett's esophagus with dysplasia. N Engl J Med 2009;360:2277–88.

118. Phoa KN, van Vilsteren FG, Weusten BL, et al. Radiofrequency ablation vs endoscopic surveillance for patients with Barrett esophagus and low-grade dysplasia: a randomized clinical trial. JAMA 2014;311:1209–17.

119. Sie C, Bright T, Schoeman M, et al. Argon plasma coagulation ablation versus endoscopic surveillance of Barrett's esophagus: late outcomes from two randomized trials. Endoscopy 2013;45:859–65.

120. Manner H, May A, Kouti I, et al. Efficacy and safety of hybrid-APC for the ablation of Barrett's esophagus. Surg Endosc 2016;30:1364–70.

121. Shaheen NJ, Greenwald BD, Peery AF, et al. Safety and efficacy of endoscopic spray cryotherapy for Barrett's esophagus with high-grade dysplasia. Gastrointest Endosc 2010;71:680–5.

122. Canto MI, Shaheen NJ, Almario JA, et al. Multifocal nitrous oxide cryoballoon ablation with or without EMR for treatment of neoplastic Barrett's esophagus (with video). Gastrointest Endosc 2018;88:438–46.e2.

123. Krishnamoorthi R. Endoscopic therapy or surveillance for Barrett's esophagus with low-grade dysplasia: time to involve patients in shared decision making. Gastrointest Endosc 2020;92:575–7.

124. Desai M, Saligram S, Gupta N, et al. Efficacy and safety outcomes of multimodal endoscopic eradication therapy in Barrett's esophagus-related neoplasia: a systematic review and pooled analysis. Gastrointest Endosc 2017;85:482–95.e4.

125. Wu J, Pan YM, Wang TT, et al. Endotherapy versus surgery for early neoplasia in Barrett's esophagus: a meta-analysis. Gastrointest Endosc 2014;79:233–41.e2.

Dysphagia
Novel and Emerging Diagnostic Modalities

Amanda J. Krause, MD[a,b], Dustin A. Carlson, MD, MS[a,*]

KEYWORDS

- Esophagus • Motility • Manometry • Achalasia • Impedance

KEY POINTS

- The Chicago Classification version 4.0 represents the state-of-the art diagnostic algorithm for esophageal motility disorders with high-resolution manometry (HRM).
- Provocative HRM maneuvers, including multiple rapid swallows, rapid drink challenge, solid test swallow, solid test meal, pharmacologic provocation, and impedance, can help complement the standard HRM interpretation.
- Timed barium esophagram provides a useful complementary esophageal motility evaluation, especially if initial testing is inconclusive.
- Functional luminal imaging probe panometry evaluates the esophageal response to distension and is a promising modality for the evaluation of esophageal distensibility and motility.

INTRODUCTION

Advances in diagnostic testing for esophageal motility disorders have been substantial over the past 10 to 20 years. The advent of high-resolution manometry (HRM) and esophageal pressure topography (EPT) in the 1990s provided a method to improve depiction of esophageal motor function over conventional line tracing manometry and facilitated organized classification of esophageal motility disorders via the Chicago Classification (CC).[1–3] A novel tool and approach with functional luminal imaging probe (FLIP) panometry, as well as application of barium esophagram, have both helped clinicians to improve diagnostic capabilities. The purpose of this review article is to discuss the current and emerging technologies in the area of esophageal motility and to discuss the authors' approach to diagnosing and managing esophageal motility disorders.

[a] Division of Gastroenterology and Hepatology, Department of Medicine, Northwestern University, Feinberg School of Medicine, 676 St Clair Street, Suite 1400, Chicago, IL 60611-2951, USA; [b] Division of Gastroenterology and Hepatology, Department of Medicine, University of California, San Diego, 9500 Gillman Drive, MC 0956, La Jolla, CA 92093-0956, USA
* Corresponding author.
E-mail address: dustin-carlson@northwestern.edu

Gastroenterol Clin N Am 50 (2021) 769–790
https://doi.org/10.1016/j.gtc.2021.07.003
0889-8553/21/© 2021 Elsevier Inc. All rights reserved.

gastro.theclinics.com

APPROACH TO DYSPHAGIA AND DIAGNOSIS OF ESOPHAGEAL MOTILITY DISORDERS

The clinical evaluation of dysphagia begins with the clinical history with the initial distinction typically related to differentiating between oropharyngeal and esophageal dysphagia. When oropharyngeal dysphagia is suspected, video fluoroscopic swallow examination and evaluation by speech therapy may be considered. With dysphagia that is esophageal in origin, the clinical history for dysphagia may suggest mechanical or motor causes (eg, dysphagia to solids vs liquids), although ultimately that determination will be yielded through objective testing. Thus, the clinical history related to a possible esophageal motility disorder seeks to assess for potential secondary causes of esophageal motor dysfunction, such as previous foregut surgery, as these are essential to incorporate into a subsequent clinical impression. The association of chronic opioid use and esophageal motor dysfunction also garnered recent interest, because of an association with elevated esophagogastric junction (EGJ) outflow pressures on HRM and even spastic achalasia.[4–6]

The initial objective evaluation for esophageal dysphagia is typically endoscopy. A careful endoscopic evaluation is essential to evaluate for mechanical causes of obstruction, including strictures, rings, eosinophilic esophagitis (EoE), advanced erosive esophagitis, hiatal hernias, and, of course (although a vast minority of cases), tumors. In the absence of mechanical obstruction or other alternative cause for dysphagia, an evaluation for esophageal motility disorders should be then pursued.

HIGH-RESOLUTION MANOMETRY AND THE CHICAGO CLASSIFICATION

HRM uses a solid-state catheter assembly with closely spaced pressure sensors (typically 1-cm spacing intervals) that are positioned to traverse the entire length of the esophagus. Software interpolation of this pressure data to EPT allows visualization of esophageal motor function along a space-time-pressure continuum. Furthermore, EPT metrics were developed to quantify components of esophageal motor function, such as deglutitive lower-esophageal sphincter (LES) relaxation via the integrated relaxation pressure (IRP) and peristaltic vigor via the distal contractile integral (DCI).[7,8] These EPT metrics, as well as recognition of pressurization patterns on EPT, facilitated development of a hierarchical classification scheme of esophageal motility disorders: the CC.[2] The CC provides a standard terminology for description of esophageal motility disorders and is used around the world. HRM and the CC provided a method to improve accuracy of interpretation and diagnostic yield for esophageal motility disorders over conventional line tracings.[9,10] The CC was initially published in 2009 and has evolved to reflect advances in the application of HRM through intermittent updates, including the most up-to-date version 4.0 (CCv4.0) published in 2021.[3,11–13] This recent update involved application of RAND methodology to reflect recommendations developed over a 2-year process by the International HRM Working Group, as well as application of the Grading of Recommendations Assessment, Development, and Evaluation process.[3] The working group comprised 52 members selected by 6 international motility societies from 20 different countries.

There were several major updates reflected in the CCv4.0 as compared with the earlier iterations.[3,11,14] One related to standardization of the HRM test protocol, which involved expansion of the protocol and application of complementary provocative maneuvers (**Table 1**). In addition, an important concept sought with CCv4.0 was to identify conclusive and clinically relevant esophageal motility disorders, as compared with

Table 1
High-resolution manometry test maneuvers

Test/Maneuver	Protocol	Diagnostic Utility
Multiple rapid swallows (MRS)	In the upright position, five 2-mL wet swallows using a 10-mL syringe and occurring at 2- to 3-s intervals[3,79]	1. A normal response occurs when no esophageal body contractility is observed (DCI < 100 mm Hg•s•cm) and there is deglutitive inhibition during the repeat swallows, with post-MRS contraction augmentation (DCI post-MRS greater than each single swallow mean DCI)[3,39,79,80] 2. Assessing the inhibitory and excitatory mechanisms within the esophagus and helping to determine peristaltic reserve, especially in association with gastroesophageal reflux[39,79,81] 3. Lack of contractile reserve can be used to support a diagnosis of IEM[3,39] 4. An elevated IRP >12 mm Hg during the MRS and RDC in patients with an elevated IRP in both the supine and upright positions supports a diagnosis of EGJOO[35]
Rapid drink challenge (RDC)	In the upright position, the patient drinks 200 mL of water as quickly as possible through a straw[3,82]	1. A normal response occurs when there is no esophageal body contractility (DCI < 100 mm Hg•s•cm) and complete deglutitive inhibition during this protocol[3,20,82,83] 2. An elevated IRP >12 mm Hg plus panesophageal pressurization during the RDC may be more suggestive of EGJOO[3,20,35,82,83]
Solid test swallow and solid test meal (STM)	Solid test swallow involves 10 swallows of ~1 cm³ of a soft solid and the STM involves consuming 200 g of a soft solid meal and must be completed in 8 min[3]	1. A normal response occurs when the patient is asymptomatic during the study; >20% of pharyngeal swallows are present, and it is followed by a normal esophageal contraction (DCI > 1000 mm Hg•s•cm) and without a significant

(continued on next page)

Table 1 (continued)		
Test/Maneuver	Protocol	Diagnostic Utility
		break of >5 cm in the contractile front[3] 2. Help determine if EGJ obstruction, postprandial rumination, or belching disorder is present[3] 3. An elevated IRP with symptoms of dysphagia is suggestive of EGJOO[3]
Pharmacologic provocation (amyl nitrate & cholecystokinin [CCK])	4–5 sniffs of amyl nitrite in the recumbent position OR administration of 40 ng/kg of CCK intravenously in the recumbent position[3]	1. In achalasia and functional EGJOO, amyl nitrite causes a larger EGJ pressure drop ($\geq$10 mm Hg) when compared with the deglutitive IRP[3] 2. Can help distinguish which patients with EGJOO may have an early form of achalasia and thus may benefit from achalasia treatments[17] 3. With CCK administration, achalasia patients experience an EGJ contraction of >50 mm Hg[3] 4. Can help distinguish between opioid-induced type III achalasia and idiopathic type III achalasia[84]

inconclusive HRM motor patterns. This was based on the recognition that some manometric patterns do not always equate to a clinical disease, that is, are inconclusive. This most notably led to modification to criteria for EGJ outflow obstruction (EGJOO) and ineffective esophageal motility (IEM) and sought to identify HRM findings with increased relevance for these classifications. The HRM pattern of EGJOO, however, was recommended to always be considered an inconclusive *manometric* diagnosis until confirmed by additional complementary testing with barium esophagram or FLIP. Application of clinical (symptom-based) criteria was also applied to the EGJOO classification, as well as to distal esophageal spasm (DES) and hypercontractile esophagus. This was based on recognition that these manometric patterns may not uniformly equate to a clinical disease when they are not associated with noncardiac chest pain and/or dysphagia.

Of note, the diagnosis of primary esophageal motility disorders, and thus the direct application of CCv4.0, is intended for patients with normal foregut anatomy (eg, do not have a large hiatal hernia or paraesophageal hernia) and who have not undergone any previous surgical or invasive foregut interventions.[3] This naturally stipulates that the HRM is interpreted in the context of endoscopic and/or esophagram findings.[3] If manometry is performed in the context of previous foregut surgery or a mechanical obstruction/abnormal anatomy, the CC metrics and interpretation may be used as a standard descriptive method, while recognizing the potential for secondary motor findings.

MANOMETRY TEST PROTOCOL

Previous versions of the CC were based on the cumulative outcome of 10 swallows of 5-mL liquid performed in a single patient position (typically supine).[2,11,14] However, value in performing HRM in 2 patient positions was observed, particularly via the potential to relieve manometric pressure artifact (eg, a false-positive IRP elevation) at the EGJ.[15–17] In addition, provocative HRM maneuvers, such as multiple rapid swallows (MRS), rapid drink challenge (RDC), solid test swallows, solid test meal (STM), pharmacologic challenges, and postprandial monitoring periods, were also reported to complement standard test swallows and potentially increase diagnostic yield of HRM (see **Table 1**).[17–23] Thus, CCv4.0 provided recommendations for a standard HRM protocol, as well as incorporation of complementary maneuvers.

The standard HRM protocol, as discussed in CCv4.0, begins with the patient in a supine position. After a catheter is placed, 60 seconds of time is allotted to ensure a normalization period. A baseline of 30 seconds is captured in order to identify the upper-esophageal sphincter, LES, respiratory inversion point, and basal EGJ pressure.[3] Next, ten 5-mL wet swallows are completed in the primary position (typically supine) and five 5-mL wet swallows are completed in the secondary (typically upright) position. At least 1 MRS and 1 RDC are also recommended (see **Table 1**).[3]

If the above testing is inconclusive, additional maneuvers can be considered (see **Table 1**). Solid test swallows and STM can be used to further evaluate the HRM diagnosis of EGJOO (see **Table 1**).[3,20,21] In patients in whom there is concern for a diagnosis of achalasia (but with an inconclusive HRM) or opioid esophagus, a pharmacologic provocation can be performed.[3,17] Monitoring after a meal (a postprandial study) can also be applied to aid identification of patients suspected to have rumination and/or belching disorder.[23–25] Although if the results of HRM are ambiguous, which in particular includes any case with an HRM classification of EGJOO, a timed barium esophagram (TBE) with a barium tablet swallow and/or FLIP can be used.[3,26,27]

DIAGNOSTIC CRITERIA FOR ESOPHAGEAL MOTILITY DISORDERS

HRM provides a framework for diagnosing disorders of esophageal motility. The CCv4.0, similar to previous iterations of the CC, splits the possible diagnoses into major categories of esophageal dysfunction as disorders of EGJ function (including type I, II, and III achalasia and EGJOO; **Fig. 1**) and disorders of peristalsis (including absent contractility, DES, hypercontractile esophagus, and IEM; **Fig. 2**).

Also of note is that application of the HRM metric values varies related to bolus consistency and volume, patient position, test maneuver, and HRM assembly manufacturer (**Table 2**). Thus, application of these values is imperative for interpretation of the HRM study.

Disorders of EGJ function are categorized by an elevated median IRP, either in the supine or in the upright positions (see **Fig. 1**).

Achalasia

Achalasia represents the prototypical esophageal motility disorder and as such carries effective, targeted treatment options.[28] Achalasia is identified on manometry by elevated LES relaxation pressures and absence of peristalsis. Furthermore, achalasia can be subclassified based on pressurization pattern (type I vs type II) or presence of spastic contraction (type III) (see **Fig. 1**). The achalasia subtypes carry clinical relevance related to prognosis to treatment, such that type II achalasia has the best treatment outcomes.[29–31] More importantly, the achalasia subtypes direct management

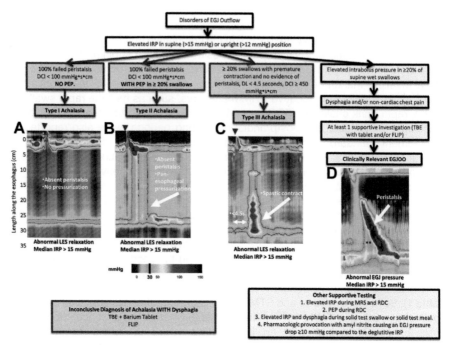

Fig. 1. CCv4.0 disorders of EGJ outflow. The disorders of EGJOO. (*A*) Type I achalasia on HRM. (*B*) Type II achalasia on HRM. (*C*) Type III Achalasia on HRM. (*D*) EGJOO on HRM. [a] DL < 4.5 seconds. [b] Bolus pressurization. DL, distal latency; PEP, panesophageal pressurization. (*Courtesy of* the Esophageal Center of Northwestern, Chicago, IL; with permission.)

decisions in achalasia such that patients with type III achalasia may have better clinical outcomes if preferentially treated with surgical LES myotomy than with pneumatic dilation.[30]

Also worth noting is that patients may have achalasia, but without elevated IRP on HRM. Thus, in these inconclusive cases in which achalasia is clinically suspected, particularly if the IRP values are at the upper limits of normal, complementary evaluation with TBE or FLIP can help confirm an achalasia diagnosis.[3,32]

Esophagogastric Junction Outflow Obstruction

The HRM classification of EGJOO is reached when the IRP is elevated, but peristalsis is present such that criteria for an achalasia subtype are not met. The EGJOO classification was specifically recognized as a limitation in previous versions of the CC related to heterogeneity of clinical diagnosis that could be represented within this HRM pattern. For example, EGJOO on HRM could reflect a variant of achalasia, but could also be related to hiatal hernia, extrinsic esophageal compression, or even artifactual elevation of IRP (in the setting of otherwise normal esophageal motility).[15–17,33,34] Studies suggested that only a minority (<25%) of patients with this HRM pattern represented a primary esophageal motor disorder akin to achalasia and that most patients would instead improve from conservative management alone.[33,34] Thus, the clinical relevance of this HRM pattern was often uncertain.

As a result of this, the classification of EGJOO was modified in CCv4.0 to require that if peristalsis was present such that a conclusive diagnosis of achalasia was not achieved, then a manometric classification of EGJOO required an elevated median

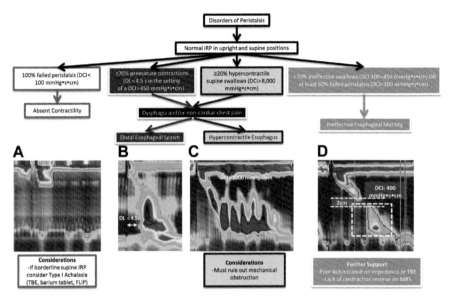

Fig. 2. CCv4.0 disorders of peristalsis. The disorders of peristalsis. (*A*) Absent contractility on HRM. (*B*) DES on HRM. (*C*) Hypercontractile esophagus on HRM. (*D*) IEM on HRM. (*Courtesy of* the Esophageal Center of Northwestern, Chicago, IL; with permission.)

IRP in *both* supine and upright swallows, in addition to the presence of elevated intrabolus pressure with supine wet swallows.[3] An isolated IRP elevation (ie, if IRP normalizes in the second position) likely reflects that the initial IRP elevation was related to pressure artifact, as these isolated IRP elevations were observed to rarely be associated with retention on barium esophagram, that is, rarely clinically significant.[16] The abnormal bolus pressurization provided an additional feature to support the presence of an EGJOO. The HRM classification of EGJOO also required the presence of a relevant symptom (dysphagia or chest pain) to support it as a clinically relevant HRM finding. It was also recommended that the EGJOO classification also be described relative to the pattern of esophageal contractility (eg, spastic or ineffective or normal peristalsis) to further characterize the esophageal motor function. However, the ultimate recommendation from the CCv4.0 was that manometric EGJOO should always be considered an inconclusive clinical diagnosis, and that additional complementary testing with TBE or FLIP be applied to confirm the diagnosis. This is particularly essential before consideration for invasive achalasia-type treatments.

Application of provocative HRM maneuvers may also be useful to complement the overall HRM impression to aid identification of EGJOO (see **Table 1**). Having an elevated IRP greater than 12 mm Hg (Medtronic assembly) during the MRS and RDC in patients with an elevated IRP in both the supine and the upright positions is more likely to be associated with an abnormal esophagram with either retention on the TBE or barium tablet delay, and consequently, a diagnosis of clinically relevant outflow obstruction.[35] In addition, an elevated IRP > 12 mm Hg (Medtronic software) plus panesophageal pressurization during the RDC may be more suggestive of EGJOO.[35]

Disorders of Peristalsis

When EGJ outflow is normal, the CC applies a frequency of swallow types from the primary position of test swallows to seek disorders of peristalsis. The criteria for

Table 2
High-resolution manometry values

Value	Meaning	Interpretation[3]
Integrated relaxation pressure (IRP)	Assess the pressure during relaxation at the level of the esophagogastric junction	• Abnormal if supine median IRP ≥ 15 mm Hg (Medtronic, Inc; Shoreview, MN, USA) • Abnormal if supine median IRP ≥ 22 mm Hg (Laborie/Diverstatek; Portsmouth, NH, USA) • Abnormal if upright median IRP ≥ 12 mm Hg (Medtronic) • Abnormal if upright median IRP ≥ 15 mm Hg (Laborie/Diversatek)
Distal contractile integral (DCI)	Measures the contractile vigor during esophageal peristalsis	• Normal: DCI 450–8000 mm Hg•s•cm • Failed: DCI < 100 mm Hg•s•cm • Hypercontractile: DCI > 8000 mm Hg•s•cm • Ineffective: weak contraction or failed peristalsis. Peristaltic break >5 cm in setting of DCI ≥ 450 mm Hg•s•cm
Distal latency (DL)	Deglutitive inhibition latency	• Premature/spastic: DL < 4.5 s in setting of DCI ≥ 450 mm Hg•s•cm
Isobaric contour	Pressurization	• Panesophageal pressurization: Isobaric contour of ≥30 mm Hg • Intrabolus pressurization: Isobaric contour of ≥20 mm Hg in supine position (Medtronic)

absent contractility have not changed in the current iteration of the CC (see **Fig. 2**).[3] DES and hypercontractile esophagus in CCv4.0 have now been classified as clinically relevant in patients with manometric findings of DES (see **Fig. 2**) as well as symptoms of dysphagia and/or noncardiac chest pain.[3] However, these diagnoses can also be patterns of uncertain clinical significance, such as in association with gastroesophageal reflux disease,[36] secondary manifestation of obstruction,[37] and even potential (albeit) rare overlap with healthy controls.[38] With regards to hypercontractile esophagus, DES and/or achalasia criteria must not be met, and a mechanical obstruction must be ruled out.[3] In addition, achalasia should be considered, particularly if the IRP is near upper limit of normal.[32] Finally, IEM, previously considered a "minor disorder" of peristalsis, now has more rigorous pathologic criteria for diagnosis and includes fragmented peristalsis.[3] This reduced overlap with healthy controls and thus sought to reflect a more clinically relevant phenotype of esophageal hypomotility. Lack of contractile reserve on MRS can be used to further support a diagnosis of IEM (see **Table 1**).[3,39]

IMPEDANCE MANOMETRY

Intraluminal impedance measurements relate to the contents of the esophagus such that impedance decreases with intraluminal liquid and increases with intraluminal air. Thus, impedance-manometry or high-resolution impedance manometry (HRIM) provides methods to objectively assess bolus transit, bolus clearance, intrabolus pressure, and relationships between esophageal pressure and bolus flow.[40–43] However, despite the additional information provided with impedance manometry, the clinical utility remains a topic of debate, and as such, impedance was not included in CCv4.0.

With impedance-manometry, bolus transit and clearance can be evaluated in a dichotomy (complete or incomplete) with previous studies demonstrating abnormal bolus transit among patients with esophageal motility disorders, such as IEM and achalasia.[40,44] An innovative methodology for HRIM interpretation was also developed to objectively measure components of bolus flow timing, bolus retention, pressurization, and luminal distension using a pressure-flow analysis paradigm with demonstrated utility in distinguishing between healthy controls and patient cohorts, including postfundoplication dysphagia and nonobstructive dysphagia.[41,45,46] Additional novel HRIM metrics of the bolus flow time and esophageal impedance integral quantify trans-EGJ bolus flow and esophageal retention, respectively; these metrics correlated with symptom scores and clinical outcomes in patients with achalasia and major motor disorders as well as with symptom scores in patients without major motor disorders.[42,43,47,48] The impedance bolus height, another HRIM metric, quantifies esophageal retention after a 200-mL rapid liquid drink in an upright posture by measuring the height of the residual fluid column after 5 minutes, analogous to a timed-barium esophagram.[49] HRIM can also be applied to a postprandial testing protocol to objectively detect behavioral disorders rumination syndrome and supragastric belching, as both rumination events and supragastric belches have an objective appearance on HRIM.[23–25] Thus, although additional clinical study remains needed to further demonstrate the clinical utility of impedance manometry, this technology also holds potential for diagnostic advances in esophageal disorders.

BARIUM ESOPHAGRAM

Barium esophagram facilitates depiction of esophageal anatomic morphology in addition to evaluating esophageal function. The functional assessment can be objectified by application of standard testing protocols, such as the TBE and use of a standardized solid bolus (eg, 12- to 13-mm barium tablet). The TBE protocol typically involves ingestion of 200 to 236 cc of thin barium with images taken at 1 and 5 minutes after ingestion.[50–53] Esophageal retention can then be quantified as the barium column height superior to the EGJ. TBE carries clinical value for evaluation of treatment outcomes in achalasia,[51,53] although also can be a useful complementary test when assessing patients with dysphagia. TBE can be particularly useful in patients in which an initial evaluation with endoscopy and HRM (and/or FLIP) is inconclusive; the HRM pattern of EGJOO is the prime example.[3,27] TBE thresholds for abnormality were proposed as column height greater than 5 cm at 1 minute (with sensitivity and specificity of 94% and 71%, respectively) and greater than 2 cm at 5 minutes (with sensitivity and specificity of 85% and 86%, respectively) to identify patients with untreated achalasia from nonachalasia.[52] Adding the barium tablet retention increased the accuracy of the test.[52]

FUNCTIONAL LUMINAL IMAGING PROBE

The FLIP uses impedance planimetry technology to measure esophageal luminal dimensions (cross-sectional area ~ diameter) and esophageal distensibility (ie, the dimension/pressure relationship) in response to controlled, volumetric distension. The FLIP study is typically performed during sedated endoscopy. The FLIP is commercially available (Medtronic, Inc, Shoreview, MN, USA) in 2 different sizes: 8 cm or 16 cm. Although the 8-cm FLIP can evaluate EGJ distensibility, the 16-cm FLIP provides simultaneous evaluation of the distal esophageal body and EGJ. Furthermore, by displaying the esophageal diameter changes along a space-time continuum with associated pressure using the FLIP panometry approach, EGJ opening mechanics, esophageal body distensibility, and the contractile response to distension, that is, secondary peristalsis, can all be assessed.[54,55]

Utilization of Functional Luminal Imaging Probe Panometry

As FLIP is used at the time of sedated endoscopy, it can be applied during the initial endoscopy for esophageal symptoms if the endoscopic examination is negative or suggestive of an esophageal motility disorder, thus when an evaluation of esophageal motility is warranted. Alternatively, FLIP with endoscopy may also be considered if an initial evaluation with HRM (or TBE) is inconclusive, and thus additional complementary testing is necessary. Other applications of FLIP may also be considered, such as objective evaluation of luminal diameter and distensibility of the esophageal body and/or strictures, such as in EoE or monitoring at the time of or after therapies, such as in achalasia.[56–60]

Functional Luminal Imaging Probe Study Protocol

Variations in FLIP study protocols have been reported, and thus, efforts are ongoing to standardize the FLIP study protocol (**Table 3**).[61] Although the FLIP study protocol varies slightly whether using the 8- or 16-cm FLIP balloon, both sizes involve maintenance of the adequate positioning of the FLIP relative to the EGJ based on visualization of the EGJ "waist" throughout the duration of the study protocol (**Fig. 3**) and incremental stepwise filling of the FLIP balloon. Real-time interpretation of the FLIP study is possible and is displayed either solely as the instantaneous FLIP "hourglass" with the FLIP 1.0 display or as FLIP panometry with the FLIP 2.0 display (see **Fig. 3**; **Figs. 4** and **5**). In addition, distensibility of the *proximal* esophageal body can also be assessed by, after emptying the FLIP, withdrawing the catheter until the balloon is positioned just below the upper-esophageal sphincter, which may be useful in EoE (see **Fig. 5**).[55]

It can also be worthwhile to archive the FLIP study data for postprocedural review. This can be accomplished through the FLIP system (which creates a TXT file) or via an additional recorder of the real-time FLIP panometry. The customized program that the authors have used for previous research reports uses the TXT files and is available at http://www.wklytics.com/nmgi.[62,63]

Interpretation and Application of Functional Luminal Imaging Probe Panometry

Esophagogastric junction opening

The evaluation of EGJ distensibility on FLIP panometry uses the metric of EGJ-distensibility index (DI), that is calculated as the EGJ-cross-sectional area divided by pressure.[64] The maximum EGJ diameter (ie, the greatest diameter achieved at the EGJ) also provides a useful assessment and can complement the EGJ-DI. The authors observed that with the 16-cm FLIP, the EGJ-DI obtained during the 60-mL fill

Table 3
Functional luminal imaging probe device characteristics and protocol

FLIP Length	16 cm	8 cm
Sensors	• 16 sensors • 1-cm spacing	• 16 sensors • 0.5-cm spacing

Assessment in esophageal syndromes	• EGJ
	• Esophageal body characteristics
	  ○ Contractile response
	  ○ Distensibility
		• EGJ

Balloon length	16 cm	8 cm
Pressure reference	Atmospheric	Atmospheric
Placement	Transoral	Transoral
Baseline positioning	• Balloon should span the EGJ • 2–3 sensors distal to the EGJ	• Balloon should span the EGJ • EGJ waist at midballoon
Baseline fill volume	30 mL	20 mL
Baseline wait time	15 s	15 s
Pressure reference	Atmospheric	Atmospheric
Balloon fill protocol	40 mL, 50 mL, 60 mL, 70 mL	30 mL, 40 mL, 50 mL
Time at each fill level	60 s	30 s
Measurements	• EGJ-DI • EGJ-diameter • Intrabag pressure • Contractile response pattern • Esophageal body distensibility	• EGJ-DI • EGJ-diameter • Intrabag pressure

volume and the maximum EGJ-diameter achieved during the 60- to 70-mL fill volume appeared to provide the most reliable performance for EGJ opening evaluation.[55,63] These fill volumes produced a similar degree of FLIP bag filling (and thus similar distensive stimuli) as the 40- to 50-mL fill volumes with the 8-cm FLIP.

The approach to analyze the EGJ opening using FLIP involves first assessing for whether antegrade contractions are occurring, as this impacts the areas at which EGJ opening measurement is made (see **Fig. 3**). Areas at the EGJ that are affected by *dry catheter artifact*, which is a measurement artifact that impacts diameter measurement when occlusion of the FLIP balloon disrupts the electrical current used for the impedance planimetry technology, need to be recognized (see **Fig. 4**).[62] Because of the artifact, these areas should be excluded from measurement of the EGJ opening. Analysis can instead include other areas of the FLIP study in which the dry catheter artifact does not occur: this may be during a nonoccluding contraction that may occur later during the same fill volume; immediately before or after occlusion occurs related to the antegrade contraction; or at a higher fill volume (eg, 70 mL) during which occluding contractions are less likely to occur. Also of note is that the EGJ-DI value should not be applied if the associated intrabag pressure is less than 15 mm Hg (and be interpreted somewhat cautiously if the pressure is <20–25 mm Hg), as applying low values to the dividend of the calculation can create a misleadingly elevated EGJ-DI value.

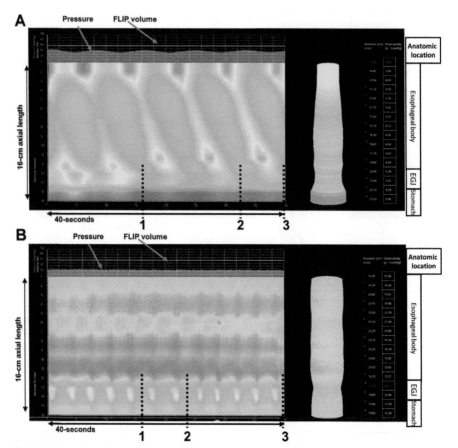

Fig. 3. Evaluation of EGJ opening with FLIP panometry. Real-time FLIP panometry output from 2 patients (*A, B*) as 40 seconds of length (16 cm) × time × color-coded diameter FLIP topography (*bottom left*), with corresponding intraballoon pressure and FLIP fill volume (*top panels*). The hourglass-like image to the right reflects the FLIP at the instant corresponding to the far right of the topography plot; the narrowed region of the balloon ("waist") is at the EGJ. Evaluation of EGJ opening is related to presence (as in panel A) or absence (as in panel B) of antegrade contractions. EGJ opening is assessed at the peak diameter of EGJ opening, reflected by the vertical dashed lines in panels A and B. This occurs related to the pressure ramp or peak associated with contractions in panel A and is measured during expiration (ie, in-between crural contractions) in panel B. The median of 3 values of EGJ-DI is applied to reflect potential dynamic changes in EGJ opening. The patient in panel A had an HRM classified as normal motility; the patient in panel B had systemic sclerosis and an HRM with absent contractility. (*Courtesy of* the Esophageal Center of Northwestern, Chicago, IL; with permission.)

Normal values (ie, those based on testing of asymptomatic volunteers) based on study with the 16-cm FLIP included a median (5–95th) EGJ-DI (60 mL) of 5.8 (3.2–8.4) mm^2/mm Hg and maximum EGJ diameter (60–70 mL) of 20.4 (16.7–21.9) mm.[65] EGJ opening parameters are reduced in esophageal motor disorders of EGJ outflow, such as achalasia; that is, FLIP metrics of EGJ opening are inversely correlated with EGJ pressure measures on HRM.

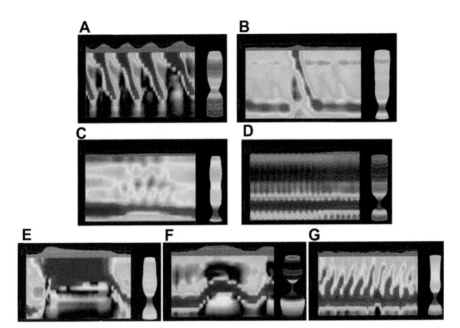

Fig. 4. FLIP panometry contractile response patterns. Real-time FLIP panometry output from 7 different patients (*A–G*). (*A*) Normal contractile response defined by the RAC Rule-of-6s with ≥6 consecutive antegrade contractions of ≥6 cm in axial length occurring at a regular rate of 6 ± 3 antegrade contractions per minute. (*B*) Borderline contractile response defined as presence of a distinct antegrade contraction (≥6 cm in axial length), but not meeting the RAC Rule-of-6s. (*C*) Impaired-disordered contractile response defined as the presence of contractility, but without distinct antegrade contraction and not meeting criteria for a spastic-reactive response (*E–G*). (*D*) Absent contractile response defined by the absence of contractility. A spastic-reactive contractile response was defined by the presence of sustained occluding contraction (SOC) (*E*), a sustained lower-esophageal sphincter contraction (sLESC) (*F*), or repetitive retrograde contractions (RRCs) (*G*). (*E*) SOC, defined as a nonpropagating, occluding contraction of the esophageal body that persisted for greater than 10 seconds, occurred in continuity with the EGJ and was associated with a pressure increase greater than 35 mm Hg. (*F*) sLESC were defined as a transient reduction in diameter attributed to the LES that lasted greater than 5 seconds, was not associated with crural or antegrade contraction, and was associated with an increase in FLIP pressure. (*G*) RRCs were defined by greater than 6 consecutive retrograde contractions at a rate of greater than 9 contractions per minute. Also note the gray-dark blue areas observed concurrently with occluding contractions in panels A, E, and F reflect areas of the FLIP study that are impacted by dry catheter artifact: the esophageal diameters within these affected areas should be omitted from interpretation of the FLIP study. (*Courtesy of* the Esophageal Center of Northwestern, Chicago, IL; with permission.)

Although previous thresholds have been proposed,[61,63] the authors recently proposed and validated an updated approach for assessment of EGJ opening with FLIP based on subsequent evaluation of asymptomatic volunteers and patients with achalasia and normal motility on HRM.[55,62,66] With this approach, 2 parameters, the EGJ-DI at the 60-mL fill volume and the maximum EGJ diameter achieved during the 60- to 70-mL fill volumes (based on 16-cm FLIP) were jointly applied: *reduced EGJ opening* (REO) is defined by EGJ-DI less than 2.0 mm²/mm Hg and a maximum EGJ diameter less than 12 mm. Borderline EGJ opening (BEO) was defined by an EGJ-DI less than 2.0 mm²/mm Hg or a maximum EGJ diameter less than 16 mm (but not

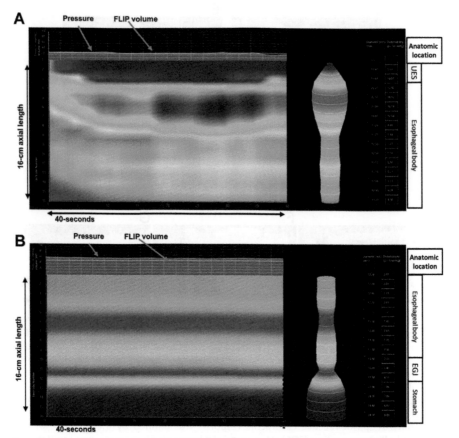

Fig. 5. FLIP panometry in EoE. Real-time FLIP panometry output from a patient (*A*, proximal esophagus; and *B*, distal esophagus) with a narrow caliber esophagus from EoE. The distensibility plateau was 10.2 mm in the distal esophagus (*B*) and 12.2 mm in the proximal esophagus (*A*). UES, upper-esophageal sphincter. (*Courtesy of* the Esophageal Center of Northwestern, Chicago, IL; with permission.)

REO). Normal EGJ opening (NEO) was defined by an EGJ-DI ≥ 2.0 mm^2/mm Hg and ≥ 16 mm. This provided high degrees of certainty for pathology with REO and normality with NEO to improve the application of these findings. This was demonstrated in a validation study of this approach: 94% (218/233 patients) with REO on FLIP panometry had a conclusive disorder of EGJOO based on CCv4.0 (ie, achalasia subtypes I, II, or III; or EGJOO with a confirmatory abnormal TBE), whereas 96% (138/144 patients) with NEO on FLIP panometry had normal EGJ outflow per CCv4.0 (ie, normal supine and upright IRP).[65] Of 466 patients, 89 patients (19%) had a BEO classification and would be recommended to undergo additional complementary evaluation.

Contractile response to distension

The esophageal contractile response to distension, that is, evaluation of secondary peristalsis in response to sustained esophageal distension, is performed during the 50- to 70-mL fill volumes of the 16-cm FLIP study protocol. Unique patterns of this esophageal response occur and are amenable to pattern recognition (see **Fig. 4**).

The normal esophageal response to distension that is observed in 90% of healthy asymptomatic volunteers involves antegrade contractions that occur at a regular repetitive rate: repetitive antegrade contractions (RACs). The normal contractile response pattern is further characterized by the RAC Rule-of-6s.[55,67,68] The classification scheme for the FLIP panometry patterns of the contractile response to distension was recently validated based on demonstration of shared features with primary peristaltic function/dysfunction on HRM.[69]

Evaluation of esophageal motility

Esophageal motility can be assessed and classified with FLIP panometry by application of EGJ opening and the contractile response pattern.[61,63,70]

An important distinction to note is that although similar and shared features are observed in esophageal motor function assessed with FLIP panometry and HRM, these 2 tests evaluate different components of esophageal function. Differences in test outcomes may reflect differences in esophageal function between the esophageal response to swallows (HRM) and the esophageal response to distension (FLIP panometry). This was also previously demonstrated with a difference in primary and secondary peristalsis triggered when evaluated with esophageal manometry.[71,72]

The initial study describing this approach demonstrated that application of a hierarchical classification scheme to evaluate esophageal motility with FLIP panometry (akin to the approach of the CC to HRM) demonstrated that FLIP panometry could accurately evaluate esophageal motility, particularly with detection of achalasia: 70/70 included achalasia patients had an abnormal FLIP panometry study.[63] Subsequent studies have provided additional support to the finding that patients with achalasia will consistently have abnormal EGJ opening and an abnormal contractile response to distension on FLIP panometry.[66,67] In addition, FLIP also was useful to confirm an achalasia diagnosis in patients in which achalasia was strongly suspected based on clinical presentation and abnormal esophagram, but that had normal IRP on HRM.[32] Finally, application of FLIP panometry output to a machine-learning algorithm was able to detect nonspastic (HRM subtype I or II achalasia) from spastic (HRM type III achalasia) with 78% to 90% accuracy.[73]

Another scenario in which FLIP panometry was useful to clarify equivocal esophageal motility evaluations was with the EGJOO classification on HRM.[26,63] A study focused on patients with the EGJOO classification on HRM demonstrated that a normal FLIP panometry study among the HRM-EGJOO cohort was associated with normal esophageal clearance on esophagram and symptom improvement with conservative management.[26] Furthermore, patients with HRM-EGJOO and EGJ-DI less than 2.0 mm^2/mm Hg on FLIP had a higher likelihood of abnormal retention on esophagram and could potentially benefit from LES-targeted treatments.

The implications of a normal FLIP panometry to exclude a major esophageal motor disorder were further described among a cohort of 111 consecutive patients who had also undergone HRM.[68] Of these patients, 70% had normal esophageal motility, and the remainder of the HRM findings were generally considered false positive or equivocal; none had achalasia. This study defined a normal FLIP panometry by an EGJ-DI greater than 3.0 mm^2/mm Hg, lack of repetitive retrograde contractions, and contractile response pattern meeting the RAC Rule-of-6s.[68] In addition, although most patients with normal motility on HRM also had normal findings on FLIP panometry, it should be noted that abnormalities can occur.[62] In a retrospective study of 164 patients with normal esophageal motility on HRM completing FLIP, 27% were found to have abnormal EGJ distensibility, 23% had an abnormal response to distension, and 7% had sustained LES contraction, a pattern during FLIP distension whereby contraction of the LES occurs.[62] However, among the 68 patients who also had undergone an esophagram, abnormal EGJ distensibility was associated with barium retention.[62] Ultimately, a need for future studies to determine the potential for response to targeted therapy was noted.

Overall, FLIP panometry is a valid and useful diagnostic tool for independent and complementary evaluation of esophageal motility at the time of sedated endoscopy. In some scenarios, FLIP panometry could eliminate the need for HRM, for example, a normal FLIP panometry study given the low probability for a major esophageal motor disorder.[68] FLIP panometry can also effectively independently identify achalasia and thus could be sufficient to diagnosis achalasia without HRM, particularly if other clinical information is supportive of the diagnosis (eg, TBE). In other scenarios, FLIP panometry findings may be abnormal, but require clinical correlation with TBE or HRM to clarify (eg, a spastic-reactive contractile response pattern or BEO). Similarly, when HRM findings are inconclusive, application of FLIP panometry can be beneficial to clarify the clinical impression.[3,26,32]

Distensibility of esophageal body

The distensibility plateau, which represents a fixed diameter despite increase in distensive pressure, has been used for evaluation of the esophageal body with FLIP (see **Fig. 5**).[56,74,75] Compliance measures to reflect change in volume relative to pressure have also been applied.[56,76,77] Although these metrics were generated for research purposes via postprocedural analytical data plots, the distensibility plateau of the esophageal body can be estimated on the real-time FLIP panometry by evaluating the esophageal body diameters at the greatest fill volumes. Normal values of distensibility plateau are ≥18 mm at both the distal and the proximal esophageal body.[55]

A previous study evaluating the clinical application of FLIP in EoE demonstrated that reduced distensibility plateau was associated with risk for food impaction (distensibility plateau <17 mm, in particular) and requirement of therapeutic dilation.[57] In addition, improvement in distensibility plateau occurred in response to dietary or medial EoE therapy, and improvement in distensibility plateau was a stronger indicator of symptomatic improvement than mucosal eosinophil counts.[78] Thus, FLIP provides a role to objectively monitor therapy in EoE.

SUMMARY

Ongoing advances in esophageal motility testing are expected as technologies and approaches evolve with ongoing experience to better categorize patients with motility disorders. HRM and EPT combined with the CCv4.0 provide the cornerstone for the diagnosis of esophageal motility disorders. The most recent updates in the CCv4.0 have focused on standardization of the HRM protocol and have refined the diagnosis of clinically relevant esophageal motility disorders. When approaching a patient with esophageal motility disorders, the history is critical, and initial testing typically includes endoscopy to rule out any mechanical causes of obstruction. Apart from the standardized HRM protocol, there are numerous additional testing strategies, such as MRS, RDC, solid test swallow, STM, pharmacologic provocation, impedance, TBE, and FLIP, that can aid clinicians in the diagnosis of esophageal motility disorders. As the field continues to develop and expand, it is hoped that the diagnostic algorithm can be further standardized and simplified and ultimately can direct targeted, effective treatment strategies for patients suffering from esophageal disorders.

CLINICS CARE POINTS

- Initial objective evaluation for esophageal dysphagia is generally endoscopy to rule out mechanical causes of obstruction.

- If endoscopy is unrevealing for an objective diagnosis for a cause of dysphagia, esophageal motility testing with high-resolution manometry (HRM) or functional luminal imaging probe (FLIP) should be considered.

- The Chicago Classification provides the current diagnostic algorithm for esophageal motility disorders and highlights complementary testing strategies for further characterizing these disorders.

- Complementary testing strategies include the MRS, RDC, solid test swallow, STM, pharmacologic provocation, impedance, TBE, and FLIP panometry.

- When HRM findings are inconclusive, the utilization of FLIP panometry can help to clarify the clinical diagnosis.

- FLIP panometry is a useful diagnostic test that can be completed during a sedated endoscopy and could eliminate the need for HRM if normal.

DISCLOSURE

Northwestern University holds shared intellectual property rights and ownership surrounding FLIP Panometry systems, methods, and apparatus with Medtronic Inc. D.A. Carlson: Medtronic (Speaking. Consulting); A.J. Krause: None.

FUNDING

Grant support: This work was supported by P01 DK117824 (P.I. John E. Pandolfino) from the Public Health service and American College of Gastroenterology Junior Faculty Development Award (DAC).

REFERENCES

1. Clouse RE, Parks T, Haroian L, et al. Development and clinical validation of a solid-state high-resolution pressure measurement system for simplified and consistent esophageal manometry: 92. Am Coll Gastroenterol 2003;98:S32–3.
2. Pandolfino JE, Ghosh SK, Rice J, et al. Classifying esophageal motility by pressure topography characteristics: a study of 400 patients and 75 controls. Am J Gastroenterol 2008;103(1):27–37.
3. Yadlapati R, Kahrilas PJ, Fox MR, et al. Esophageal motility disorders on high-resolution manometry: Chicago classification version 4.0((c)). Neurogastroenterol Motil 2021;33(1):e14058.
4. Kraichely RE, Arora AS, Murray JA. Opiate-induced oesophageal dysmotility. Aliment Pharmacol Ther 2010;31(5):601–6.
5. Babaei A, Szabo A, Shad S, et al. Chronic daily opioid exposure is associated with dysphagia, esophageal outflow obstruction, and disordered peristalsis. Neurogastroenterol Motil 2019;31(7):e13601.
6. Ratuapli SK, Crowell MD, DiBaise JK, et al. Opioid-induced esophageal dysfunction (OIED) in patients on chronic opioids. Am J Gastroenterol 2015;110(7): 979–84.

7. Ghosh SK, Pandolfino JE, Zhang Q, et al. Quantifying esophageal peristalsis with high-resolution manometry: a study of 75 asymptomatic volunteers. Am J Physiol Gastrointest Liver Physiol 2006;290(5):G988–97.

8. Ghosh SK, Pandolfino JE, Rice J, et al. Impaired deglutitive EGJ relaxation in clinical esophageal manometry: a quantitative analysis of 400 patients and 75 controls. Am J Physiol Gastrointest Liver Physiol 2007;293(4):G878–85.

9. Roman S, Huot L, Zerbib F, et al. High-resolution manometry improves the diagnosis of esophageal motility disorders in patients with dysphagia: a randomized multicenter study. Am J Gastroenterol 2016;111(3):372–80.

10. Carlson DA, Ravi K, Kahrilas PJ, et al. Diagnosis of esophageal motility disorders: esophageal pressure topography vs. conventional line tracing. Am J Gastroenterol 2015;110(7):967–77 [quiz: 978].

11. Kahrilas PJ, Bredenoord AJ, Fox M, et al. The Chicago classification of esophageal motility disorders, v3.0. Neurogastroenterol Motil 2015;27(2):160–74.

12. Pandolfino JE, Fox MR, Bredenoord AJ, et al. High-resolution manometry in clinical practice: utilizing pressure topography to classify oesophageal motility abnormalities. Neurogastroenterol Motil 2009;21(8):796–806.

13. Bredenoord AJ, Fox M, Kahrilas PJ, et al. Chicago classification criteria of esophageal motility disorders defined in high resolution esophageal pressure topography. Neurogastroenterol Motil 2012;24(Suppl 1):57–65.

14. Bredenoord AJ, Fox M, Kahrilas PJ, et al. Chicago classification criteria of esophageal motility disorders defined in high resolution esophageal pressure topography. Neurogastroenterol Motil 2012;(Suppl 1):57–65.

15. Babaei A, Lin EC, Szabo A, et al. Determinants of pressure drift in Manoscan(TM) esophageal high-resolution manometry system. Neurogastroenterol Motil 2015;27(2):277–84.

16. Triggs JR, Carlson DA, Beveridge C, et al. Upright integrated relaxation pressure facilitates characterization of esophagogastric junction outflow obstruction. Clin Gastroenterol Hepatol 2019;17(11):2218–26.e2.

17. Babaei A, Shad S, Szabo A, et al. Pharmacologic interrogation of patients with esophagogastric junction outflow obstruction using amyl nitrite. Neurogastroenterol Motil 2019;31(9):e13668.

18. Carlson DA, Roman S. Esophageal provocation tests: are they useful to improve diagnostic yield of high resolution manometry? Neurogastroenterol Motil 2018;30(4):e13321.

19. Fornari F, Bravi I, Penagini R, et al. Multiple rapid swallowing: a complementary test during standard oesophageal manometry. Neurogastroenterol Motil 2009;21(7):718–e741.

20. Ang D, Hollenstein M, Misselwitz B, et al. Rapid drink challenge in high-resolution manometry: an adjunctive test for detection of esophageal motility disorders. Neurogastroenterol Motil 2017;29(1). https://doi.org/10.1111/nmo.12902.

21. Ang D, Misselwitz B, Hollenstein M, et al. Diagnostic yield of high-resolution manometry with a solid test meal for clinically relevant, symptomatic oesophageal motility disorders: serial diagnostic study. Lancet Gastroenterol Hepatol 2017;2(9):654–61.

22. Marin I, Cisternas D, Abrao L, et al. Normal values of esophageal pressure responses to a rapid drink challenge test in healthy subjects: results of a multicenter study. Neurogastroenterol Motil 2017;29(6). https://doi.org/10.1111/nmo.13021.

23. Yadlapati R, Tye M, Roman S, et al. Postprandial high-resolution impedance manometry identifies mechanisms of nonresponse to proton pump inhibitors. Clin Gastroenterol Hepatol 2017;16(2):211–8.e1.

24. Kessing BF, Bredenoord AJ, Smout AJ. Mechanisms of gastric and supragastric belching: a study using concurrent high-resolution manometry and impedance monitoring. Neurogastroenterol Motil 2012;24(12):e573–9.

25. Kessing BF, Bredenoord AJ, Smout AJ. Objective manometric criteria for the rumination syndrome. Am J Gastroenterol 2014;109(1):52–9.

26. Triggs JR, Carlson DA, Beveridge C, et al. Functional luminal imaging probe pan-ometry identifies achalasia-type esophagogastric junction outflow obstruction. Clin Gastroenterol Hepatol 2020;18(10):2209–17.

27. Clayton SB, Patel R, Richter JE. Functional and anatomic esophagogastic junc-tion outflow obstruction: manometry, timed barium esophagram findings, and treatment outcomes. Clin Gastroenterol Hepatol 2016;14(6):907–11.

28. Pandolfino JE, Gawron AJ. Achalasia: a systematic review. JAMA 2015;313(18): 1841–52.

29. Pandolfino JE, Kwiatek MA, Nealis T, et al. Achalasia: a new clinically relevant classification by high-resolution manometry. Gastroenterology 2008;135(5): 1526–33.

30. Rohof WO, Salvador R, Annese V, et al. Outcomes of treatment for achalasia depend on manometric subtype. Gastroenterology 2013;144(4):718–25 [quiz: e713–4].

31. Pratap N, Kalapala R, Darisetty S, et al. Achalasia cardia subtyping by high-resolution manometry predicts the therapeutic outcome of pneumatic balloon dilatation. J Neurogastroenterol Motil 2011;17(1):48–53.

32. Ponds FA, Bredenoord AJ, Kessing BF, et al. Esophagogastric junction distensi-bility identifies achalasia subgroup with manometrically normal esophagogastric junction relaxation. Neurogastroenterol Motil 2016;29(1). https://doi.org/10.1111/nmo.12908.

33. van Hoeij FB, Smout AJ, Bredenoord AJ. Characterization of idiopathic esopha-gogastric junction outflow obstruction. Neurogastroenterol Motil 2015;27(9): 1310–6.

34. Schupack D, Katzka DA, Geno DM, et al. The clinical significance of esophago-gastric junction outflow obstruction and hypercontractile esophagus in high res-olution esophageal manometry. Neurogastroenterol Motil 2017;29(10):1–9.

35. Krause AJ, Su H, Triggs JR, et al. Multiple rapid swallows and rapid drink chal-lenge in patients with esophagogastric junction outflow obstruction on high-resolution manometry. Neurogastroenterol Motil 2020;e14000.

36. Crozier RE, Glick ME, Gibb SP, et al. Acid-provoked esophageal spasm as a cause of noncardiac chest pain. Am J Gastroenterol 1991;86(11):1576–80.

37. Burton PR, Brown W, Laurie C, et al. The effect of laparoscopic adjustable gastric bands on esophageal motility and the gastroesophageal junction: analysis using high-resolution video manometry. Obes Surg 2009;19(7):905–14.

38. Rengarajan A, Rogers BD, Wong Z, et al. High-resolution manometry thresholds and motor patterns among asymptomatic individuals. Clin Gastroenterol Hepatol 2020. https://doi.org/10.1016/j.cgh.2020.10.052.

39. Martinucci I, Savarino EV, Pandolfino JE, et al. Vigor of peristalsis during multiple rapid swallows is inversely correlated with acid exposure time in patients with NERD. Neurogastroenterol Motil 2016;28(2):243–50.

40. Tutuian R, Castell DO. Combined multichannel intraluminal impedance and manometry clarifies esophageal function abnormalities: study in 350 patients. Am J Gastroenterol 2004;99(6):1011–9.

41. Nguyen NQ, Holloway RH, Smout AJ, et al. Automated impedance-manometry analysis detects esophageal motor dysfunction in patients who have non-obstructive dysphagia with normal manometry. Neurogastroenterol Motil 2013; 25(3):238–45.e4.

42. Lin Z, Carlson DA, Dykstra K, et al. High-resolution impedance manometry measurement of bolus flow time in achalasia and its correlation with dysphagia. Neurogastroenterol Motil 2015;27(9):1232–8.

43. Carlson DA, Beveridge CA, Lin Z, et al. Improved assessment of bolus clearance in patients with achalasia using high-resolution impedance manometry. Clin Gastroenterol Hepatol 2018;16(5):672–80.e1.

44. Tutuian R, Castell DO. Clarification of the esophageal function defect in patients with manometric ineffective esophageal motility: studies using combined impedance-manometry. Clin Gastroenterol Hepatol 2004;2(3):230–6.

45. Myers JC, Nguyen NQ, Jamieson GG, et al. Susceptibility to dysphagia after fundoplication revealed by novel automated impedance manometry analysis. Neurogastroenterol Motil 2012;24(9):812.e3.

46. Rommel N, Van Oudenhove L, Tack J, et al. Automated impedance manometry analysis as a method to assess esophageal function. Neurogastroenterol Motil 2014;26(5):636–45.

47. Carlson DA, Lin Z, Kahrilas PJ, et al. High-resolution impedance manometry metrics of the esophagogastric junction for the assessment of treatment response in achalasia. Am J Gastroenterol 2016;111(12):1702–10.

48. Carlson DA, Omari T, Lin Z, et al. High-resolution impedance manometry parameters enhance the esophageal motility evaluation in non-obstructive dysphagia patients without a major Chicago Classification motility disorder. Neurogastroenterol Motil 2017;29(3). https://doi.org/10.1111/nmo.12941.

49. Cho YK, Lipowska AM, Nicodeme F, et al. Assessing bolus retention in achalasia using high-resolution manometry with impedance: a comparator study with timed barium esophagram. Am J Gastroenterol 2014;109(6):829–35.

50. de Oliveira JM, Birgisson S, Doinoff C, et al. Timed barium swallow: a simple technique for evaluating esophageal emptying in patients with achalasia. AJR Am J Roentgenol 1997;169(2):473–9.

51. Vaezi MF, Baker ME, Achkar E, et al. Timed barium oesophagram: better predictor of long term success after pneumatic dilation in achalasia than symptom assessment. Gut 2002;50(6):765–70.

52. Blonski W, Kumar A, Feldman J, et al. Timed barium swallow: diagnostic role and predictive value in untreated achalasia, esophagogastric junction outflow obstruction, and non-achalasia dysphagia. Am J Gastroenterol 2018;113(2):196–203.

53. Rohof WO, Lei A, Boeckxstaens GE. Esophageal stasis on a timed barium esophagogram predicts recurrent symptoms in patients with long-standing achalasia. Am J Gastroenterol 2013;108(1):49–55.

54. Carlson DA, Lin Z, Rogers MC, et al. Utilizing functional lumen imaging probe topography to evaluate esophageal contractility during volumetric distention: a pilot study. Neurogastroenterol Motil 2015;27(7):981–9.

55. Carlson DA, Kou W, Lin Z, et al. Normal values of esophageal distensibility and distension-induced contractility measured by functional luminal imaging probe panometry. Clin Gastroenterol Hepatol 2019;17(4):674–81.e1.

56. Kwiatek MA, Hirano I, Kahrilas PJ, et al. Mechanical properties of the esophagus in eosinophilic esophagitis. Gastroenterology 2011;140(1):82–90.

57. Nicodeme F, Hirano I, Chen J, et al. Esophageal distensibility as a measure of disease severity in patients with eosinophilic esophagitis. Clin Gastroenterol Hepatol 2013;11(9):1101–7.e1.

58. Wu PI, Szczesniak MM, Craig PI, et al. Novel intra-procedural distensibility measurement accurately predicts immediate outcome of pneumatic dilatation for idiopathic achalasia. Am J Gastroenterol 2018;113(2):205–12.

59. Jain AS, Carlson DA, Triggs J, et al. Esophagogastric junction distensibility on functional lumen imaging probe topography predicts treatment response in achalasia-anatomy matters! Am J Gastroenterol 2019;114(9):1455–63.

60. Holmstrom AL, Campagna RAJ, Cirera A, et al. Intraoperative use of FLIP is associated with clinical success following POEM for achalasia. Surg Endosc 2020; 35(6):3090–6.

61. Savarino E, di Pietro M, Bredenoord AJ, et al. Use of the functional lumen imaging probe in clinical esophagology. Am J Gastroenterol 2020;115(11):1786–96.

62. Carlson DA, Baumann AJ, Donnan E, et al. Evaluating esophageal motility beyond primary peristalsis: assessing esophagogastric junction opening mechanics and secondary peristalsis in patients with normal manometry. Neurogastroenterol Motil 2021. https://doi.org/10.1111/nmo.14116.

63. Carlson DA, Kahrilas PJ, Lin Z, et al. Evaluation of esophageal motility utilizing the functional lumen imaging probe. Am J Gastroenterol 2016;111(12):1726–35.

64. Pandolfino JE, Shi G, Curry J, et al. Esophagogastric junction distensibility: a factor contributing to sphincter incompetence. Am J Physiol Gastrointest Liver Physiol 2002;282(6):G1052–8.

65. Carlson D, Prescott J, Baumann A, et al. Validation of clinically relevant thresholds of esophagogastric junction obstruction using FLIP panometry. Clin Gastroenterol Hepatol 2021. https://doi.org/10.1016/j.cgh.2021.06.040.

66. Rooney KP, Baumann AJ, Donnan E, et al. Esophagogastric junction opening parameters are consistently abnormal in untreated achalasia. Clin Gastroenterol Hepatol 2020;19(5):1058–60.e1.

67. Carlson DA, Kou W, Pandolfino JE. The rhythm and rate of distension-induced esophageal contractility: a physiomarker of esophageal function. Neurogastroenterol Motil 2020;32:e13794.

68. Baumann AJ, Donnan EN, Triggs JR, et al. Normal functional luminal imaging probe panometry findings associate with lack of major esophageal motility disorder on high-resolution manometry. Clin Gastroenterol Hepatol 2021;19(2): 259–268 e251.

69. Carlson D, Baumann AJ, Prescott J, et al. Validation of secondary peristalsis classification using FLIP panometry in 741 subjects undergoing manometry. Neurogastroenterol Motil 2021. https://doi.org/10.1111/nmo.14192.

70. Carlson DA, Gyawali CP, Kahrilas PJ, et al. Esophageal motility classification can be established at the time of endoscopy: a study evaluating real-time functional luminal imaging probe panometry. Gastrointest Endosc 2019;90(6):915–23.e1.

71. Schoeman MN, Holloway RH. Secondary oesophageal peristalsis in patients with non-obstructive dysphagia. Gut 1994;35(11):1523–8.

72. Schoeman MN, Holloway RH. Integrity and characteristics of secondary oesophageal peristalsis in patients with gastro-oesophageal reflux disease. Gut 1995;36(4):499–504.

73. Carlson DA, Kou W, Rooney KP, et al. Achalasia subtypes can be identified with functional luminal imaging probe (FLIP) panometry using a supervised machine learning process. Neurogastroenterol Motil 2020;33:e13932.

74. Carlson DA, Lin Z, Hirano I, et al. Evaluation of esophageal distensibility in eosinophilic esophagitis: an update and comparison of functional lumen imaging probe analytic methods. Neurogastroenterol Motil 2016;28(12):1844–53.

75. Menard-Katcher C, Benitez AJ, Pan Z, et al. Influence of age and eosinophilic esophagitis on esophageal distensibility in a pediatric cohort. Am J Gastroenterol 2017;112(9):1466–73.

76. Hassan M, Aceves S, Dohil R, et al. Esophageal compliance quantifies epithelial remodeling in pediatric patients with eosinophilic esophagitis. J Pediatr Gastroenterol Nutr 2019;68(4):559–65.

77. Carlson DA, Kou W, Masihi M, et al. Repetitive antegrade contractions: a novel response to sustained esophageal distension is modulated by cholinergic influence. Am J Physiol Gastrointest Liver Physiol 2020. https://doi.org/10.1152/ajpgi.00305.2020.

78. Carlson DA, Hirano I, Zalewski A, et al. Improvement in esophageal distensibility in response to medical and diet therapy in eosinophilic esophagitis. Clin Transl Gastroenterol 2017;8(10):e119.

79. Shaker A, Stoikes N, Drapekin J, et al. Multiple rapid swallow responses during esophageal high-resolution manometry reflect esophageal body peristaltic reserve. Am J Gastroenterol 2013;108(11):1706–12.

80. Elvevi A, Mauro A, Pugliese D, et al. Usefulness of low- and high-volume multiple rapid swallowing during high-resolution manometry. Dig Liver Dis 2015;47(2):103–7.

81. Daum C, Sweis R, Kaufman E, et al. Failure to respond to physiologic challenge characterizes esophageal motility in erosive gastro-esophageal reflux disease. Neurogastroenterol Motil 2011;23(6):517.e200.

82. Woodland P, Gabieta-Sonmez S, Arguero J, et al. 200 mL rapid drink challenge during high-resolution manometry best predicts objective esophagogastric junction obstruction and correlates with symptom severity. J Neurogastroenterol Motil 2018;24(3):410–4.

83. Marin I, Serra J. Patterns of esophageal pressure responses to a rapid drink challenge test in patients with esophageal motility disorders. Neurogastroenterol Motil 2016;28(4):543–53.

84. Babaei A, Shad S, Massey BT. Motility patterns following esophageal pharmacologic provocation with amyl nitrite or cholecystokinin during high-resolution manometry distinguish idiopathic vs opioid-induced type 3 achalasia. Clin Gastroenterol Hepatol 2020;18(4):813–21.e1.

Early Esophageal Cancer
What the Gastroenterologist Needs to Know

Mike T. Wei, MD[a,b,*,1], Shai Friedland, MD[a,b,1]

KEYWORDS

- Esophageal cancer • Endoscopic mucosal resection
- Endoscopic submucosal dissection • Early esophageal cancer
- Squamous cell carcinoma • Adenocarcinoma • Radiofrequency ablation

KEY POINTS

- Although symptoms such as dysphagia and weight loss may occur with esophageal cancer, this is generally associated with late-stage disease.
- Most patients with early esophageal cancer are asymptomatic. As such, it is important to maintain an observant eye and a methodical examination during any upper endoscopy.
- Early esophageal cancer, defined as cancer limited to the mucosa (T1a) or submucosa (T1b), has decreased risk of metastasis compared with deeper disease. As such, early esophageal cancer in the right context may allow for endoscopic removal with subsequent surveillance.

INTRODUCTION

Worldwide, GLOBOCAN estimated 572,034 new cases of esophageal cancer in 2018, with 508,585 deaths from esophageal cancer.[1] In the United States, the Surveillance Epidemiology and End Results (SEER) Program estimated that 18,440 new esophageal cases and 16,170 deaths from esophageal cancer occurred in 2020.[2] Men are at higher risk for esophageal cancer compared with women. Within the United States, the incidence of esophageal cancer was 7.2 for men compared with 1.6 new cases per 100,000 persons for women in 2017.[2,3] In addition, non-Hispanic White patients have the highest incidence (4.8 new cases per 100,000 persons), followed by Native Americans or Alaska Natives (3.6), Black (3.5), Hispanic (2.6), and Asian (2.3).[2,3]

Treatment differs significantly depending on the stage at diagnosis. In this review, we will focus on the detection and management of early esophageal cancer, defined as cancer limited to the mucosa and submucosa.[4] We will discuss the staging of esophageal cancer, treatment guidelines, techniques for removal, and prevention of complications.

[a] Stanford University, Stanford, CA, USA; [b] Veterans Affairs Palo Alto Health Care System, Palo Alto, CA, USA
[1] Present address: 420 Broadway D, Redwood City, CA 94063.
* Corresponding author.
E-mail address: mtwei@stanford.edu

Gastroenterol Clin N Am 50 (2021) 791–808
https://doi.org/10.1016/j.gtc.2021.07.004
0889-8553/21/Published by Elsevier Inc.

SYMPTOMS

Although symptoms such as dysphagia, weight loss, chest discomfort, and worsening heartburn can occur with esophageal cancer, they are generally associated with advanced disease.[5] Most patients with early esophageal cancer are asymptomatic, and as such frequently identified incidentally on endoscopy performed for other indications or on routine surveillance endoscopies in patients with Barrett's esophagus. Endoscopic findings in early squamous esophageal cancer (**Figs. 1** and **2**) and early cancer within Barrett's esophagus (**Fig. 3**) are often subtle and require careful inspection and meticulous endoscopic examination.[6]

THE ENDOSCOPIC EVALUATION

During any upper endoscopy, an endoscopist must evaluate for features concerning esophageal cancer. The esophagus must first be cleared of debris, bubbles, and mucous. We recommend a slow methodical examination upon withdrawal from the stomach, with additional attention to any concerning areas. High-definition endoscopy systems are strongly preferred over standard-definition systems.[7] During the

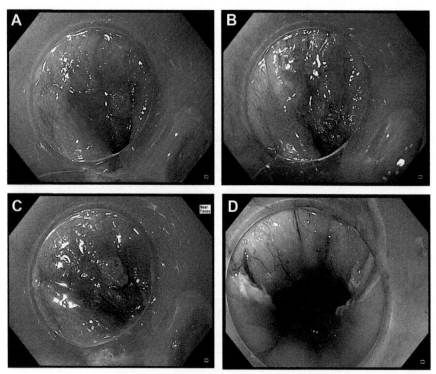

Fig. 1. Intramucosal esophageal squamous cell cancer. (*A*) White light view of the proximal portion of the tumor. Squamous dysplasia is typically more erythematous than the surrounding normal mucosa. A diminutive slightly raised nodular area is noted within the erythematous lesion. (*B*) Narrow-band imaging accentuates the abnormalities. (*C*) Near focus provides a more detailed view of the surface of the tumor, including the slightly raised nodular portion. (*D*) View of the half circumferential resection site after ESD. The pathology was Intramucosal Cancer with clear margins (R0).

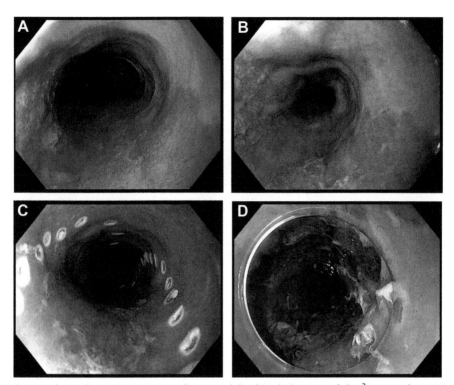

Fig. 2. T1b esophageal squamous cell cancer. (*A*) White light view of the ³/₄ circumferential tumor. There is a small area of normal pale esophageal mucosa on the top right side of the screen. Most of the tumor is flat and more erythematous than the normal mucosa, but the lower left side is nodular. (*B*) Narrow-band imaging highlights the tumor, which is darker than the normal mucosa on the top right side of the screen. The nodularities—variation in the thickness of the mucosa—are also more easily seen on the left and lower left portions of the screen. Significant nodularity is associated with submucosal invasion. (*C*) Cautery marking dots have been placed around the lesion in preparation for ESD. (*D*) The lesion has been resected *en bloc* by ESD, leaving a thin strip of unresected mucosa along the length of the esophagus (bottom right side of the screen). Leaving a strip of unresected normal mucosa can reduce the severity of postresection stricture formation compared with circumferential resection. However, this patient did develop a significant stricture despite prophylactic treatment with steroids. The pathology was T1b with clear margins but significant submucosal invasion and lymphovascular invasion.

examination, we recommend critically evaluating the mucosa for surface pattern (smooth, irregular, round, villous, ridged, ulcerated) and mucosal vascular pattern (normal vs abnormal).[8]

Whenever possible, visible lesions should be described using the Paris classification.[9,10] Barrett's mucosa should be characterized using Prague criteria.[11] Chromoendoscopy can be used to further delineate lesions. Lugol's solution is primarily used in the evaluation for squamous cell carcinoma (SCC)[12]; some endoscopists advocate using acetic acid to improve visualization of neoplastic lesions in patients with Barrett's esophagus.[8] Virtual chromoendoscopy can also be deployed, such as with narrow-band imaging (NBI)[13–15] or digital processing techniques such as i-Scan (Pentax) or Fujinon Intelligent Chromoendoscopy (Fujinon).[11,16] NBI uses narrowed bandwidths of blue

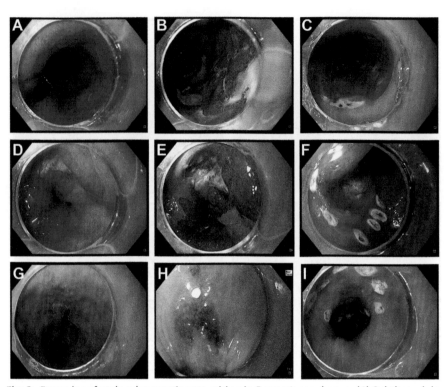

Fig. 3. Examples of early adenocarcinoma arising in Barrett's esophagus. (A) Subtle nodular T1a cancer involving ¹/₄ of circumference located on the lower right corner of the screen. The pale-colored squamous mucosa proximal to the Barrett's is visible on the far right side of the screen. A few pale squamous islands (sites of prior biopsies) are visible just distal to the lesion. (B) The same lesion is viewed with narrow-band imaging. The nodularity of the tumor is more pronounced. The squamous islands lateral and distal to the nodular tumor are nearly white and stand out against the darkly colored Barrett's. (C) Cautery dots have been placed around the tumor (bottom of the screen) in preparation for ESD. The resection will include a margin of a few millimeters outside of the cautery dots. (D) The T1a cancer is visible on white light near the top of the screen. It is partially covered by a white exudate and there is a subtle nodular area distal to the exudate. (E) The same tumor is visualized with narrow-band imaging. The nodular portion of the tumor distal to the white exudate is more pronounced. (F) Cautery dots have been placed around the proximal portion of the tumor in preparation for ESD (note that the endoscope has been rotated to facilitate placement of the dots so the tumor is now on the bottom left side of the screen). (G) T1a cancer at the proximal end of a tongue of Barrett's, near the top of the screen. The tumor is partially covered by squamous mucosa. (H) Magnified narrow-band imaging view of the proximal portion of the tumor where it is surrounded and partially covered by squamous mucosa. (I) Cautery dots have been placed around the tumor in preparation for ESD.

(440–460 nm) and green (540–560 nm) visible light to optimize visualization of capillaries, veins, and other tissues.[14] In one randomized controlled trial (RCT) comparing NBI with Lugol chromoendoscopy in evaluating for esophageal SCC, both had similar sensitivity but NBI had higher specificity. We recommend evaluating first under white light with a high-definition endoscope, followed by an examination with NBI or another imaging enhancing modality. If needed, and especially if there is a history of prior SCC, we recommend examining the esophagus with Lugol's solution.

In 2015, the Barrett's International NBI Group (BING) created a set of characteristics to evaluate Barrett's epithelium under NBI to help determine the presence of dysplasia. In this system, regular mucosa was characterized as circular, tubular, ridged, or villous pattern. In contrast, irregular mucosa was categorized by irregular or absent surface patterns. Furthermore, regular mucosa is characterized by blood vessels following mucosal ridges and having long branching patterns. In contrast, irregular vascular mucosa does not follow ridges and has an irregular pattern. Using this system, in the initial study, patients were identified with dysplasia with 85% accuracy.[17]

When dysplasia is suspected, we recommend performing 1or 2 targeted biopsies of the abnormal area and review with a pathologist specialized in evaluating gastrointestinal diseases. Biopsy guidance is recommended before endoscopic resection.[11] More than 2 biopsies of the target lesion may unnecessarily increase submucosal fibrosis, making future endoscopic resection more challenging.[11] In selected cases, separate biopsies of other areas of the esophagus may be helpful in planning treatment, such as planning the longitudinal and circumferential extent of the endoscopic resection.

STAGING OF EARLY ESOPHAGEAL CANCER

The 8th edition of the American Joint Committee on Cancer (AJCC) was released in 2017, providing updated guidelines regarding TNM staging for esophageal cancer (**Tables 1** and **2**). The staging provided differs slightly from the Japan Esophageal Society, whose classification we have included as well.[19,20]

Options for staging include endoscopic evaluation (upper endoscopy, endoscopic resection, and endoscopic ultrasound (EUS)–fine needle aspiration) as well as cross-sectional imaging (PET/CT).[18] Cross-sectional imaging and EUS can be useful for evaluating advanced esophageal cancer by assessing for muscularis propria invasion or lymph node metastasis. However, they cannot reliably distinguish T1a from T1b tumors; endoscopic resection is, therefore, the primary diagnostic and therapeutic modality for early esophageal cancer.[21–23] Endoscopic evaluation as the initial step provides the opportunity to provide curative treatment if an early enough esophageal cancer is identified and treated.[18,24]

Many studies have further characterized mucosal or submucosal disease using m1-m3 for mucosal tumors and sm1-sm3 for submucosally invasive cancer, respectively (**Fig. 4**). For the purposes of our discussion, early esophageal cancer is defined as cancer limited to the mucosa (T1a) or submucosa (T1b).[4]

RISK OF DISEASE SPREAD

Depth and type of esophageal cancer are important as they correlate to the risk of disease spread.[25] Overall, SCC has a higher risk of lymph node spread compared with adenocarcinoma. In several studies evaluating surgical specimens for SCC, lymph node metastasis was identified in 3% to 15% of esophageal cancer confined to the mucosa and 37% to 41% of cases involving the submucosa.[26–28] Lymph node metastasis was 0% for lesions confined to the lamina propria but increased to 40% to 61% in sm3 lesions.[25–28] For esophageal adenocarcinoma, in one systematic review, lymph node metastasis occurred in 1.93% of intramucosal carcinomas. In contrast, lymph node metastasis was 9% to 20% for sm1 and 24% to 50% for sm3 lesions.[29]

Table 1
Cancer staging in the esophagus and esophagogastric junction

	AJCC[18]	Japan Esophageal Society[19,20]
TX	Unable to assess	Unable to assess
T0	No evidence of neoplasia	No evidence of neoplasia
Tis	High-grade dysplasia	Carcinoma in situ
Tumor depth		
T1	Lamina propria, muscularis mucosae, or submucosa	
T1a	Lamina propria or muscularis mucosae	Mucosa: T1a-LPM: lamina propria mucosae; T1a-MM: muscularis mucosae
T1b	Submucosa	Submucosa: T1b-SM1: upper third of submucosa; T1b-SM2: middle third; T1b-SM3 bottom third
T2	Muscularis propria	Muscularis propria
T3	Adventitia	Adventitia
T4	Tumor invades adjacent structures	Tumor invades adjacent structures
T4a	Invades azygos vein, diaphragm, peritoneum, pericardium, or pleura	Invades azygos vein, diaphragm, peritoneum, pericardium, or pleura
T4b	Invades aorta, trachea, or vertebral body	Invades aorta, trachea, or vertebral body
N category		
NX	Regional lymph nodes cannot be assessed	Regional lymph nodes cannot be assessed
N0	No regional lymph node metastasis	No regional lymph node metastasis
N1	1–2 regional lymph nodes	Group 1 lymph nodes only
N2	3–6 regional lymph nodes	Group 2 lymph nodes
N3	7 or more regional lymph nodes	Group 3 lymph nodes
N4	Not applicable	Group 4 lymph nodes
M category		
MX	Not applicable	Distant metastases cannot be assessed
M0	No metastasis	No metastasis
M1	Yes metastasis	Yes metastasis

Table 2
AJCC clinical staging of esophageal and esophagogastric cancers, by squamous cell carcinoma or adenocarcinoma

Stage Group	Squamous Cell Carcinoma	Adenocarcinoma
0	TisN0M0	TisN0M0
I	T1N0-1M0	T1N0M0
II	T2N0-1M0 T3N0M0	IIA: T1N1M0 IIB: T2N0M0
III	T3N1M0 T1-3N2M0	T2N1M0 T3-4aN0-1M0
IVA	T4N0-2M0 T1-4N3M0	T1-4aN2M0 T4bN0-2M0 T1-4N3M0
IVB	T1-4N0-3M1	T1-4N0-3M1

TREATMENT GUIDELINES

Overall, we recommend consideration for endoscopic management of early esophageal cancer at high-volume centers if possible.[30] Given the steep curve inherent in managing esophageal cancer and need of surgical capability, we believe that the performance of endoscopic resection at high-volume centers may reduce complications and optimize patient outcomes. Consistent with American Gastroenterological Association (AGA) guidelines, we feel that patients with esophageal cancer should be presented at a multidisciplinary tumor board consisting of an oncologist, gastroenterologist, GI pathologist, and thoracic surgeon.[31]

Adenocarcinoma

Intramucosal esophageal adenocarcinoma (T1a) has minimal risk of metastasis or lymph node involvement (<2%). For T1a lesions, the AGA recommends endoscopic therapy over esophagectomy (**Fig. 5**).[31] In one meta-analysis, endotherapy for high-grade dysplasia or intramucosal adenocarcinoma had a higher recurrence rate (Relative risk [RR], 9.50; 95% confidence interval [CI], 3.26–27.75), fewer major adverse events (RR, 0.38; 95% CI, 0.20–0.73), and had similar overall survival compared to esophagectomy.[32] For submucosal esophageal adenocarcinoma (T1b), esophagectomy or

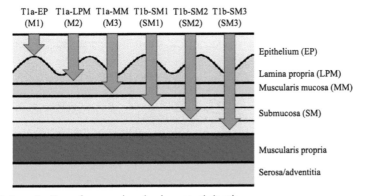

Fig. 4. Categorization of mucosal and submucosal depth.

endoscopic therapy can be considered. In particular, endoscopic management can be considered if the lesion has low-risk features (sm1, good to moderate differentiation, no lymphatic invasion).[31] The National Comprehensive Cancer Network (NCCN) recommends that endoscopic therapies can be considered for up to T1b adenocarcinoma for patients not considered to be surgical candidates.[33] To date, there are no RCTs directly comparing esophagectomy to endoscopic therapy for intramucosal adenocarcinoma.[34]

According to the European Society for Gastrointestinal Endoscopy (ESGE), the management of Barrett's esophagus neoplasia is dependent on the presence of visible lesions. Patients with high-grade dysplasia or intramucosal cancer without visible lesions can be managed by ablative techniques, including radiofrequency ablation (RFA).[11] These techniques are particularly attractive for the commonly encountered scenario of circumferential Barrett's esophagus, where endoscopic resection carries a very high risk of severe stricture formation. However, it should be noted that dysplastic lesions may be subtle and one study from the Netherlands demonstrated that 76% of patients referred to an expert center after random biopsies of Barrett's detected high-grade dysplasia or adenocarcinoma were found to have a visible dysplastic lesion that was missed on the index endoscopy and therefore required endoscopic resection rather than ablation.[35]

When lesions are visible, endoscopic resection is preferred for 2 reasons. The first is that lesions may be upstaged to T1b cancer, which may require definitive surgery. The second is that ablation is often too superficial to reliably eliminate visible lesions that may be thicker than flat Barrett's mucosa. Endoscopic resection can be achieved by endoscopic mucosal resection (EMR) or endoscopic submucosal dissection (ESD) (see below). After resection of the cancer and healing of the resection site, any residual Barrett's is treated by ablation, most commonly by RFA, to reduce the considerable risk of development of new cancers in untreated residual Barrett's.[11]

Squamous Cell Carcinoma

The NCCN suggests endoscopic therapies or esophagectomy as preferred options for patients with Tis or T1a SCC. However, endoscopic therapy can be considered for up to T1b for patients who are not surgical candidates.[33] The AGA currently does not have guidelines related to the management of esophageal SCC.

The Japan Esophageal Society recommends that endoscopy can potentially be considered in cancer localized to the mucosa. Their recommendations are based primarily on experience with managing SCC, given relative scarcity of adenocarcinoma cases in Japan. According to the Japanese guidelines, endoscopic resection should be considered where there is uncertainty regarding depth of tumor invasion, and for patients who are not good surgical candidates. Circumferential extent of the lesion should be considered in the management, given the increased risk of stenosis

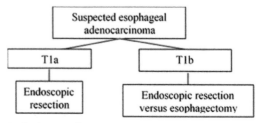

Fig. 5. Management of adenocarcinoma.

formation with circumferential and near-circumferential resections. For patients with T1b disease, radiotherapy or chemoradiation is recommended (**Fig. 6**).[36]

For m1 and m2 SCC, the ESGE recommends ESD as the first choice for management, though EMR can be considered for lesions less than 10 mm. For patients with comorbidities or who are unwilling to receive esophagectomy, ESD can be considered for m3 or sm1 disease with less aggressive features, such as well-differentiated cancers without lymphovascular invasion.[11]

ENDOSCOPIC TECHNIQUE FOR EARLY ESOPHAGEAL CANCER REMOVAL

Endoscopic management of early esophageal cancer primarily involves EMR or ESD. EMR is generally performed via cap-EMR or band-EMR (also referred to as multiband mucosectomy [MBM]).[37] An earlier technique, the strip-biopsy method, involved submucosal injection to lift the lesion followed by hot snare resection.[38] This technique is generally no longer used because of its decreased efficacy and technical challenges, given the flatness of the lesions. Other proposed techniques include use of RFA, photodynamic therapy (PDT), argon plasma coagulation (APC), and cryoablation. However, because these ablative techniques preclude the opportunity to precisely stage early cancers, they should be reserved for Barrett's esophagus without visible lesions or other clinical scenarios such as circumferential squamous high-grade dysplasia, where the benefits from endoscopic resection outweigh the risk of severe stricture formation.[37]

CAP-ASSISTED EMR

During cap-assisted EMR, a specially designed clear plastic cap with a distal ridge is attached to the tip of the endoscope. The ridge allows an opened electrosurgical snare to be seated near the distal end of the cap in preparation for resection. After submucosal injection of fluid to lift the lesion, the cap is placed over the lesion, which is then suctioned into the cap. The snare is then closed around the lesion and cautery is applied to remove it.[39,40] The size of the resected specimen is limited by the size of the cap and is typically less than 15 mm.

In a study in 2007, Esaki and colleagues reviewed EMR (strip-biopsy or cap-EMR) of 106 patients with esophageal cancer limited to mucosa and submucosa. Local recurrence was identified in 21.9% cases, with recurrence at 13% for lesions limited to the lamina propria and 31% for lesions involving muscularis mucosa and upper

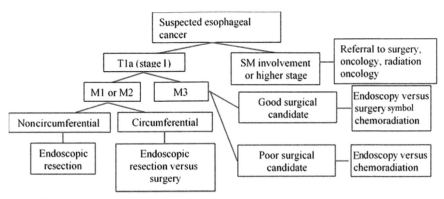

Fig. 6. Management of SCC.

one-third of submucosa.[41] In another study by Shimzu and colleagues[42] in 2002, there was a similar 5-year overall survival rate between patients with ESCC invading the muscularis mucosa or upper submucosa receiving EMR (77.4%) or surgery (84.5%).

BAND-EMR (MULTIBAND MUCOSECTOMY)

MBM uses modified variceal band ligator with a channel that allows passage of a specially designed electrosurgical snare (**Fig. 7**).[43] Cautery dots are sometimes placed around the lesion because visualization may be difficult. Similar to variceal banding, the lesion is suctioned into the cap followed by release of the band onto the lesion.[43,44] The hexagonal snare is placed below the band and the lesion is removed using cautery. Specimens resected by band mucosectomy are typically approximately 10 mm in size. Unlike cap-assisted EMR, submucosal injection is commonly not performed, which simplifies the procedure and saves time.

In one study, patients with Barrett's esophagus with high-grade intraepithelial neoplasia (HGIN) or esophageal cancer underwent cap-assisted EMR or MBM.[43] MBM had a higher rate of negative vertical margin compared with cap-assisted EMR, although this was not statistically significant ($P = .11$). There were 4 T1m3-T1sm cancers that were resected by MBM, all of which had negative vertical margins.[43] Although there are other studies reporting success with removal of intramucosal adenocarcinoma,[45] the relatively small specimen size has made the performance of RCTs challenging. In one controlled trial evaluating cap-assisted

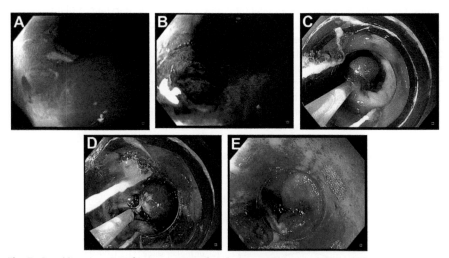

Fig. 7. Band ligation EMR for treatment of early Barrett's cancer. (*A*) A subtle lesion is visible on the bottom left side of the lumen under white light. It is partially covered by white exudate. (*B*) The same lesion is slightly more pronounced on narrow-band imaging. (*C*) Part of the lesion has been captured by a black-colored rubber band and a snare has been positioned on the bottom of the band in preparation for cutting with electrocautery. (*D*) The remainder of the lesion (the distal portion) has been captured by a second band and the snare is nearly in position around the bottom of the band. (*E*) The resection site is visible on the bottom left side of the screen. There is a small dark circle of cautery effect visible within the resection site where a coagulation forceps was used to treat a bleeding vessel immediately after resection of the second piece.

EMR and band-EMR in piecemeal EMR of Barrett's neoplasia, there was no significant difference in complication rate but band-EMR was significantly faster (34 vs 50 minutes, $P = .02$).[40]

Endoscopic Submucosal Dissection

ESD, initially developed in the 1990s, can overcome some of the technical limitations of EMR. However, ESD is a more time-consuming procedure and has a significantly steeper learning curve compared to EMR. Although esophageal EMR is limited to en bloc resection of less than 10 to 15 mm, lesions larger than 2 cm can be removed en bloc with ESD.[30]

Endoscopic submucosal dissection generally involves the following steps

1. Mark the boundary of the lesion with cautery dots[39]
2. Lift the lesion with a submucosal injection solution, often stained blue to facilitate recognition of the submucosal layer
3. Use an electrosurgical knife to cut the mucosa circumferentially around the lesion (or semicircumferentially around the lesion if a pocket or tunneling technique is used)
4. Use an electrosurgical knife to dissect through the submucosa beneath the lesion, thereby separating it from the muscle layer

ENDOSCOPIC SUBMUCOSAL DISSECTION VERSUS EMR

Compared with ESD, EMR achieves higher rates of en bloc removal, leading to improved histologic evaluation of the resection margins, lower recurrence, and higher rate of cure.[46,47] In 2014, Guo and colleagues[48] in a meta-analysis found that ESD had higher en bloc resection rate (97.1% vs 49.3%, odds ratio 52.8 [95% CI, 25.6–108.8]) and curative resection rate (92.3% vs 52.7%, odds ratio 13.9 [95% CI, 4.84–39.95]). In one study performing pathologic review of EMR compared to ESD specimen of Barrett's-related neoplasia, EMR was noted to have significantly more equivocal horizontal as well as lateral margin margins, leading to greater inability to reach definitive diagnosis.[49]

In 2017, Terheggen and colleagues performed an RCT evaluating patients with HGIN or early adenocarcinoma ≤ 3 cm to EMR or ESD. The relatively small cohort of 40 patients were randomized 1:1 to EMR and ESD. Although overall mean procedural duration was longer for ESD (54 vs 22 min, $P = .0002$), ESD had higher en bloc resection (100% vs 15%, $P<.0001$), complete resection (58.8% vs 11.8%, $P = .01$), and curative resection (52.9% vs 11.8%, $P = .03$). Although there were 2 cases of perforation (10%) for ESD compared to none for EMR, this was not statistically significant. This to date remains the only randomized clinical trial available comparing EMR to ESD in the management of early esophageal cancer. Further studies are needed to better compare ESD to EMR, particularly as the tools and techniques of ESD evolve.

EMR is technically simpler and less time-consuming but is typically limited to en bloc resection of less than 10 to 15 mm. ESD is particularly suitable for en bloc resection of tumors larger than 15 mm. ESD is also effective for tumors that are difficult or impossible to remove by EMR, such as those with significant submucosal fibrosis which impairs capture of the lesion by the snares and band ligation devices used in EMR. In addition, the depth of resection can be controlled precisely during ESD so the resection specimen includes sufficient submucosa to achieve a clear deep margin.[11]

OTHER TECHNIQUES

Beyond EMR or ESD, other techniques explored include RFA, PDT, APC, and cryoablation. The AIM dysplasia trial and its follow-up have demonstrated the effectiveness as well as durability of RFA in patients with low-grade dysplasia or high-grade dysplasia Barrett's.[50,51] RFA is commonly used to ablate residual Barrett's esophagus after endoscopic resection of early cancer to prevent the development of metachronous cancers in the residual Barrett's. RFA has been demonstrated to be a possible treatment strategy for squamous cell neoplasia (moderate/HGIN, SCC) in work by Bergman and colleagues,[52] though the one patient with SCC included in this clinical trial was unable to achieve a complete histologic response.

PDT involves activation of a photosensitizer administered intravenously with certain wavelengths targeted at the cancerous tissue. To reduce the risk of phototoxicity, patients are advised to avoid sun exposure for a minimum of 6 weeks.[53] The use of PDT for ablation of Barrett's esophagus has largely been supplanted by newer techniques such as RFA. Similarly, although several early studies have demonstrated its utility in managing early SCC, this has become less popular with the availability of ESD and EMR.[54,55] APC has also been explored in small studies of SCC but with overall disappointing results.[56] There has been some suggestion that APC can be used for superficial SCC in the residual esophagus following esophagectomy.[57]

Cryoablation has been found to help in managing dysplastic Barrett's esophagus.[58,59] Cryoablation may allow sufficient depth of treatment to treat nodular areas in Barrett's esophagus, but endoscopic resection in these cases is generally preferable so that accurate staging can be performed to identify patients who may require additional treatment for potential lymph node metastasis.

Although further studies are needed, we recommend ESD in the primary management of SCC. For adenocarcinoma, we recommend EMR and ESD as primary management, with RFA or cryoablation serving as adjunctive therapy for the treatment of residual Barrett's esophagus after endoscopic resection.

ENDOSCOPIC THERAPY VERSUS SURGERY

In an early analysis of the SEER database, Das and colleagues[60] evaluated 742 cases of stage 0 and I esophageal cancer diagnosed between 1998 and 2003, with 13.3% that underwent endoscopic therapy (EMR alone, EMR with PDT, EMR with thermal ablation, thermal ablation only) and 86.7% surgery. Median cancer-free survival was not significantly different between endoscopic therapy compared to surgery. However, endoscopic therapy was associated with decreased costs,[61] fewer adverse events,[62] decreased hospital readmissions, shortened length of stay, and decreased 30 and 90-day mortality.[63]

PREVENTION OF STENOSIS

Although ESD has significant advantages in the management of early esophageal cancer, stricture development is the most common complication after ESD,[64] and has been reported in 5% to 17% of cases.[65] Strictures are significantly more likely to form with ESD of esophageal cancers with circumferential extent greater than 3/4, and depth of invasion greater than m2.[66] Stricture rates have been described at 100% for circumferential resection and 56% to 76% for noncircumferential resection.[67] In a meta-analysis conducted by the Japan Esophageal Society, comparing lesions involving greater than 3/4 circumference compared to less than 3/4 circumference, there was a risk ratio of 30.9 (95% CI, 18.85–50.76) of developing stenosis (P<.001).[52] Overall, there was no significant difference in the development of esophageal stricture between ESD and EMR (odds ratio, 1.14; 95% CI, 0.71–1.84; P = .59).[48] As such, given the significant difference in outcome for postprocedural stenosis, the Japan Esophageal Society emphasizes the importance of assessing the circumferential extent of esophageal cancer lesions before resection.[52]

Many efforts have been made to limit the development of stenosis including steroids, balloon dilation, and stent placement.[68] Several studies have evaluated the use of oral or local injection of steroids, balloon dilation, or stenting.[49,67,69–71] Other strategies explored include use of modified steroid treatment (instilling saline solution of triamcinolone in the esophagus), polyglycolic acid sheets, tranilast, 5-fluorouracil, botulinum toxin type A, tissue engineering, and transplantation of esophageal mucosa.[67] In 2019, the Japan Gastroenterological Endoscopy Society recommended steroid injections for lesions greater than 1/2 to 3/4 and oral steroids for lesions greater than 1/2 circumferential extent, with consideration of combination oral and injection route of steroid for lesions involving the entire circumference.[71] Esophageal balloon dilation without steroid injection is felt to be inferior to steroid therapy; however, strictures commonly develop despite steroid treatment and multiple dilation procedures may be required after near-circumferential or circumferential resections.[71,72] At present, stricture development is a major impediment to the treatment of Barrett's esophagus with early cancer by circumferential ESD. By limiting the extent of the resection to cancer (with an adequate margin) and subsequently ablating the residual Barrett's esophagus after healing of the resection site, it is usually possible to avoid the development of severe or refractory strictures.

SURVEILLANCE

After curative resection of SCC, the ESGE recommends a follow-up endoscopy at 3 to 6 months, and then annually thereafter. For Barrett-associated adenocarcinoma, the ESGE does not have specific guidelines for the intervals required for surveillance. For Tis or T1a disease, The NCCN recommends EGD every 3 months for 1 year, then every 6 months for the second year, and then annually thereafter. This recommendation applies to both SCC and adenocarcinoma. However, this type of aggressive surveillance schedule may be more suitable after piecemeal resections, which have a relatively high recurrence rate and potential for histologic staging inaccuracies rather than R0 resections with ESD.

SUMMARY

Endoscopic findings in early esophageal cancer are often subtle and require careful inspection and meticulous endoscopic examination. When early esophageal cancer is suspected, we recommend consideration for endoscopic management at high-volume centers if possible. We recommend endoscopic resection (ESD or EMR) of visible lesions to provide the possibility of curative treatment as well as pathologic staging. In the case of adenocarcinoma, after resection of any visible cancer and healing of the resection site, residual Barrett's can be treated by ablation, most commonly by RFA, to reduce the risk of developing new cancers in untreated residual Barrett's. Overall, further studies are needed to evaluate the management of circumferential and near-circumferential lesions as well as tools and techniques to facilitate the performance of ESD and EMR.

CLINICS CARE POINTS

- During any upper endoscopy, an endoscopist must evaluate for features concerning esophageal cancer.
- When dysplasia is suspected, we recommend performing 1 or 2 targeted biopsies of the abnormal area and review with a pathologist specialized in evaluating gastrointestinal diseases.
- Overall, we recommend consideration for endoscopic management of early esophageal cancer at high-volume centers if possible.

DISCLOSURE

M.T. Wei has nothing to disclose. S. Friedland is a consultant for Capsovision.

REFERENCES

1. Bray F, Ferlay J, Soerjomataram I, et al. Global cancer statistics 2018: GLOBO-CAN estimates of incidence and mortality worldwide for 36 cancers in 185 countries. CA Cancer J Clin 2018;68(6):394–424.
2. Howlader N, Noone A, Krapcho M, et al. SEER Cancer Statistics Review (CSR) 1975-2016. Bethesda, Md: National Cancer Institute; 2019.
3. Uhlenhopp DJ, Then EO, Sunkara T, et al. Epidemiology of esophageal cancer: update in global trends, etiology and risk factors. Clin J Gastroenterol 2020; 13(6):1010–21.
4. Wani S, Drahos J, Cook MB, et al. Comparison of endoscopic therapies and surgical resection in patients with early esophageal cancer: a population-based study. Gastrointest Endosc 2014;79(2):224–32.e1.
5. Bhatt A, Kamath S, Murthy SC, et al. Multidisciplinary evaluation and management of early stage esophageal cancer. Surg Oncol Clin North Am 2020;29(4): 613–30.
6. Ahmed O, Ajani JA, Lee JH. Endoscopic management of esophageal cancer. World J Gastrointest Oncol 2019;11(10):830–41.
7. Mannath J, Ragunath K. Role of endoscopy in early oesophageal cancer. Nat Rev Gastroenterol Hepatol 2016;13(12):720–30.
8. Longcroft-Wheaton G, Duku M, Mead R, et al. Acetic acid spray is an effective tool for the endoscopic detection of neoplasia in patients with Barrett's esophagus. Clin Gastroenterol Hepatol 2010;8(10):843–7.
9. Group ECR. Update on the paris classification of superficial neoplastic lesions in the digestive tract. Endoscopy 2005;37(6):570–8.
10. The Paris endoscopic classification of superficial neoplastic lesions: esophagus, stomach, and colon: November 30 to December 1, 2002. Gastrointest Endosc 2003;58(6 Suppl):S3–43.
11. Pimentel-Nunes P, Dinis-Ribeiro M, Ponchon T, et al. Endoscopic submucosal dissection: European Society of Gastrointestinal Endoscopy (ESGE) guideline. Endoscopy 2015;47(9):829–54.
12. Gruner M, Denis A, Masliah C, et al. Narrow-band imaging versus Lugol chromoendoscopy for esophageal squamous cell cancer screening in normal endoscopic practice: randomized controlled trial. Endoscopy 2020. https://doi.org/10.1055/a-1224-6822.

13. Takenaka R, Kawahara Y, Okada H, et al. Narrow-band imaging provides reliable screening for esophageal malignancy in patients with head and neck cancers. Am J Gastroenterol 2009;104(12):2942–8.

14. Mannath J, Subramanian V, Hawkey CJ, et al. Narrow band imaging for characterization of high grade dysplasia and specialized intestinal metaplasia in Barrett's esophagus: a meta-analysis. Endoscopy 2010;42(5):351–9.

15. Iwagami H, Kanesaka T, Ishihara R, et al. Features of Esophageal Adenocarcinoma in Magnifying Narrow-Band Imaging. Dig Dis 2021;39(2):89–95.

16. Lipman G, Bisschops R, Sehgal V, et al. Systematic assessment with I-SCAN magnification endoscopy and acetic acid improves dysplasia detection in patients with Barrett's esophagus. Endoscopy 2017;49(12):1219–28.

17. Sharma P, Bergman JJ, Goda K, et al. Development and validation of a classification system to identify high-grade dysplasia and esophageal adenocarcinoma in barrett's esophagus using narrow-band imaging. Gastroenterology 2016; 150(3):591–8.

18. Rice TW, Patil DT, Blackstone EH. 8th edition AJCC/UICC staging of cancers of the esophagus and esophagogastric junction: application to clinical practice. Ann Cardiothorac Surg 2017;6(2):119–30.

19. Society JE. Japanese Classification of esophageal cancer, 11th edition: part I. Esophagus 2017;14(1):1–36.

20. Society JE. Japanese classification of esophageal cancer, 11th edition: part II and III. Esophagus 2017;14(1):37–65.

21. Zuccaro G, Rice TW, Vargo JJ, et al. Endoscopic ultrasound errors in esophageal cancer. Am J Gastroenterol 2005;100(3):601–6.

22. Thota PN, Sada A, Sanaka MR, et al. Correlation between endoscopic forceps biopsies and endoscopic mucosal resection with endoscopic ultrasound in patients with Barrett's esophagus with high-grade dysplasia and early cancer. Surg Endosc 2017;31(3):1336–41.

23. Pouw RE, Heldoorn N, Alvarez Herrero L, et al. Do we still need EUS in the workup of patients with early esophageal neoplasia? A retrospective analysis of 131 cases. Gastrointest Endosc 2011;73(4):662–8.

24. Berry MF. Esophageal cancer: staging system and guidelines for staging and treatment. J Thorac Dis 2014;6(Suppl 3):S289–97.

25. Naveed M, Kubiliun N. Endoscopic treatment of early-stage esophageal cancer. Curr Oncol Rep 2018;20(9):71.

26. Endo M, Yoshino K, Kawano T, et al. Clinicopathologic analysis of lymph node metastasis in surgically resected superficial cancer of the thoracic esophagus. Dis Esophagus 2000;13(2):125–9.

27. Shimada H, Nabeya Y, Matsubara H, et al. Prediction of lymph node status in patients with superficial esophageal carcinoma: analysis of 160 surgically resected cancers. Am J Surg 2006;191(2):250–4.

28. Akutsu Y, Uesato M, Shuto K, et al. The overall prevalence of metastasis in T1 esophageal squamous cell carcinoma: a retrospective analysis of 295 patients. Ann Surg 2013;257(6):1032–8.

29. Dunbar KB, Spechler SJ. The risk of lymph-node metastases in patients with high-grade dysplasia or intramucosal carcinoma in Barrett's esophagus: a systematic review. Am J Gastroenterol 2012;107(6):850–62 [quiz 863].

30. Draganov PV, Wang AY, Othman MO, et al. AGA institute clinical practice update: endoscopic submucosal dissection in the United States. Clin Gastroenterol Hepatol 2019;17(1):16–25.e1.

31. Sharma P, Shaheen NJ, Katzka D, et al. AGA clinical practice update on endoscopic treatment of barrett's esophagus with dysplasia and/or early cancer: expert review. Gastroenterology 2020;158(3):760–9.

32. Wu J, Pan YM, Wang TT, et al. Endotherapy versus surgery for early neoplasia in Barrett's esophagus: a meta-analysis. Gastrointest Endosc 2014;79(2): 233–41.e2.

33. Ajani JA, D'Amico TA, Bentrem DJ. Esophageal and esophagogastric junction cancers, version 4.2021, NCCN clinical practice guidelines in oncology. J. Natl. Compr. Cancer Netw 2021.

34. Rouphael C, Anil Kumar M, Sanaka MR, et al. Indications, contraindications and limitations of endoscopic therapy for Barrett's esophagus and early esophageal adenocarcinoma. Therap Adv Gastroenterol 2020;13. 1756284820924209.

35. Schölvinck DW, van der Meulen K, Bergman JJGH, et al. Detection of lesions in dysplastic Barrett's esophagus by community and expert endoscopists. Endoscopy 2017;49(2):113–20.

36. Kitagawa Y, Uno T, Oyama T, et al. Esophageal cancer practice guidelines 2017 edited by the Japan Esophageal Society: part 1. Esophagus 2019;16(1):1–24.

37. Alsop BR, Sharma P. Esophageal cancer. Gastroenterol Clin North Am 2016; 45(3):399–412.

38. Karita M, Tada M, Okita K, et al. Endoscopic therapy for early colon cancer: the strip biopsy resection technique. Gastrointest Endosc 1991;37(2):128–32.

39. Ahmed Y, Othman M. EMR/ESD: techniques, complications, and evidence. Curr Gastroenterol Rep 2020;22(8):39.

40. Pouw RE, van Vilsteren FG, Peters FP, et al. Randomized trial on endoscopic resection-cap versus multiband mucosectomy for piecemeal endoscopic resection of early Barrett's neoplasia. Gastrointest Endosc 2011;74(1):35–43.

41. Esaki M, Matsumoto T, Hirakawa K, et al. Risk factors for local recurrence of superficial esophageal cancer after treatment by endoscopic mucosal resection. Endoscopy 2007;39(1):41–5.

42. Shimizu Y, Tsukagoshi H, Fujita M, et al. Long-term outcome after endoscopic mucosal resection in patients with esophageal squamous cell carcinoma invading the muscularis mucosae or deeper. Gastrointest Endosc 2002;56(3): 387–90.

43. Peters FP, Kara MA, Curvers WL, et al. Multiband mucosectomy for endoscopic resection of Barrett's esophagus: feasibility study with matched historical controls. Eur J Gastroenterol Hepatol 2007;19(4):311–5.

44. Chen ZY, Yang YC, Liu LM, et al. Comparison of the clinical value of multi-band mucosectomy versus endoscopic mucosal resection for the treatment of patients with early-stage esophageal cancer. Oncol Lett 2015;9(6):2716–20.

45. Bhat YM, Furth EE, Brensinger CM, et al. Endoscopic resection with ligation using a multi-band mucosectomy system in barrett's esophagus with high-grade dysplasia and intramucosal carcinoma. Therap Adv Gastroenterol 2009;2(6): 323–30.

46. Sgourakis G, Gockel I, Lang H. Endoscopic and surgical resection of T1a/T1b esophageal neoplasms: a systematic review. World J Gastroenterol 2013;19(9): 1424–37.

47. Harlow C, Sivananthan A, Ayaru L, et al. Endoscopic submucosal dissection: an update on tools and accessories. Ther Adv Gastrointest Endosc 2020;13. 2631774520957220.

48. Guo HM, Zhang XQ, Chen M, et al. Endoscopic submucosal dissection vs endoscopic mucosal resection for superficial esophageal cancer. World J Gastroenterol 2014;20(18):5540–7.
49. Podboy A, Kolahi KS, Friedland S, et al. Endoscopic submucosal dissection is associated with less pathologic uncertainty than endoscopic mucosal resection in diagnosing and staging Barrett's-related neoplasia. Dig Endosc 2020;32(3): 346–54.
50. Shaheen NJ, Sharma P, Overholt BF, et al. Radiofrequency ablation in Barrett's esophagus with dysplasia. N Engl J Med 2009;360(22):2277–88.
51. Shaheen NJ, Overholt BF, Sampliner RE, et al. Durability of radiofrequency ablation in Barrett's esophagus with dysplasia. Gastroenterology 2011;141(2):460–8.
52. Bergman JJ, Zhang YM, He S, et al. Outcomes from a prospective trial of endoscopic radiofrequency ablation of early squamous cell neoplasia of the esophagus. Gastrointest Endosc 2011;74(6):1181–90.
53. Wu H, Minamide T, Yano T. Role of photodynamic therapy in the treatment of esophageal cancer. Dig Endosc 2019;31(5):508–16.
54. Okunaka T, Kato H, Conaka C, et al. Photodynamic therapy of esophageal carcinoma. Surg Endosc 1990;4(3):150–3.
55. Yoshida K, Suzuki S, Mimura S, et al. [Photodynamic therapy for superficial esophageal cancer: a phase III study using PHE and excimer dye laser]. Gan To Kagaku Ryoho 1993;20(13):2063–6.
56. Wang GQ, Hao CQ, Wei WQ, et al. [Long-term outcomes of endoscopic argon plasma coagulation (APC) therapy for early esophageal cancer and precancerous lesions]. Zhonghua Zhong Liu Za Zhi 2013;35(6):456–8.
57. Saisho K, Tanaka T, Matono S, et al. Argon plasma coagulation for superficial squamous cell carcinoma in the residual esophagus after esophagectomy. Esophagus 2020;17(4):448–55.
58. Dumot JA, Vargo JJ, Falk GW, et al. An open-label, prospective trial of cryospray ablation for Barrett's esophagus high-grade dysplasia and early esophageal cancer in high-risk patients. Gastrointest Endosc 2009;70(4):635–44.
59. Canto MI, Trindade AJ, Abrams J, et al. Multifocal cryoballoon ablation for eradication of barrett's esophagus-related neoplasia: a prospective multicenter clinical trial. Am J Gastroenterol 2020;115(11):1879–90.
60. Das A, Singh V, Fleischer DE, et al. A comparison of endoscopic treatment and surgery in early esophageal cancer: an analysis of surveillance epidemiology and end results data. Am J Gastroenterol 2008;103(6):1340–5.
61. Wirsching A, Boshier PR, Krishnamoorthi R, et al. Endoscopic therapy and surveillance versus esophagectomy for early esophageal adenocarcinoma: a review of early outcomes and cost analysis. Am J Surg 2019;218(1):164–9.
62. Zhang Y, Ding H, Chen T, et al. Outcomes of endoscopic submucosal dissection vs esophagectomy for T1 esophageal squamous cell carcinoma in a real-world cohort. Clin Gastroenterol Hepatol 2019;17(1):73–81.e3.
63. Marino KA, Sullivan JL, Weksler B. Esophagectomy versus endoscopic resection for patients with early-stage esophageal adenocarcinoma: a National Cancer Database propensity-matched study. J Thorac Cardiovasc Surg 2018;155(5): 2211–8.e1.
64. Jain D, Singhal S. Esophageal stricture prevention after endoscopic submucosal dissection. Clin Endosc 2016;49(3):241–56.
65. Kim GH, Jee SR, Jang JY, et al. Stricture occurring after endoscopic submucosal dissection for esophageal and gastric tumors. Clin Endosc 2014;47(6):516–22.

66. Shi Q, Ju H, Yao LQ, et al. Risk factors for postoperative stricture after endoscopic submucosal dissection for superficial esophageal carcinoma. Endoscopy 2014;46(8):640–4.
67. Ishihara R. Prevention of esophageal stricture after endoscopic resection. Dig Endosc 2019;31(2):134–45.
68. Hikichi T, Nakamura J, Takasumi M, et al. Prevention of stricture after endoscopic submucosal dissection for superficial esophageal cancer: a review of the literature. J Clin Med 2020;10(1):20.
69. Yang J, Wang X, Li Y, et al. Efficacy and safety of steroid in the prevention of esophageal stricture after endoscopic submucosal dissection: a network meta-analysis. J Gastroenterol Hepatol 2019;34(6):985–95.
70. Kadota T, Yoda Y, Hori K, et al. Prophylactic steroid administration against strictures is not enough for mucosal defects involving the entire circumference of the esophageal lumen after esophageal endoscopic submucosal dissection (ESD). Esophagus 2020;17(4):440–7.
71. Yamamoto Y, Kikuchi D, Nagami Y, et al. Management of adverse events related to endoscopic resection of upper gastrointestinal neoplasms: review of the literature and recommendations from experts. Dig Endosc 2019;31(Suppl 1):4–20.
72. Yamaguchi N, Isomoto H, Nakayama T, et al. Usefulness of oral prednisolone in the treatment of esophageal stricture after endoscopic submucosal dissection for superficial esophageal squamous cell carcinoma. Gastrointest Endosc 2011;73(6):1115–21.

Endoscopic and Surgical Management of Gastroesophageal Reflux Disease

Christopher J. Zimmermann, MD, Anne Lidor, MD, MPH*

KEYWORDS

- GERD • Nissen • Fundoplication • LINX • Stretta • ARMS • TIF

KEY POINTS

- GERD is common worldwide and leads to decreased quality of life and reflux-associated complications.
- Diagnosis of GERD is complex and involves barium swallow, esophageal pH measurement, EGD, and manometry.
- Surgical fundoplication is the gold standard operative intervention for GERD. Despite high patient satisfaction rates, many patients return to PPI therapy postoperatively.
- Newer technologies and techniques do not supplant fundoplication but offer safe alternatives with similar outcomes.

INTRODUCTION

Gastroesophageal reflux disease (GERD) is the result of refluxing stomach contents reaching the esophagus, causing symptoms and complications over time.[1] The estimated prevalence of weekly GERD symptoms ranges from 10% to 14.9% in the United States and from 2.5% to 52% globally, leading to decreased health-related quality of life, particularly among patients with disruptive symptoms.[2–4] Complications of GERD include erosive esophagitis, esophageal stricture, Barrett's esophagus, and esophageal adenocarcinoma, as well as the development or worsening of extraesophageal problems such as hoarseness, cough, and asthma.[1] In addition to quality of life implications, GERD and GERD treatments leave a significant economic footprint through direct costs such as the cost of proton pump inhibitor (PPI) therapy and hospital admissions/readmissions, as well as indirect costs through work absenteeism.[5–7] Acid reducing measures are the mainstay of nonsurgical GERD treatment and can be accompanied by lifestyle modification such as the avoidance of certain foods (low level of evidence) and weight loss.[8] However, surgical management of GERD is an

Department of Surgery, University of Wisconsin- Madison, Clinical Science Center, 600 Highland Avenue, Madison, WI 53792-7375, USA
* Corresponding author. Department of Surgery, University of Wisconsin- Madison, Clinical Science Center, 600 Highland Avenue, K4/744, Madison, WI 53792-7375.
E-mail address: lidor@surgery.wisc.edu

Gastroenterol Clin N Am 50 (2021) 809–823
https://doi.org/10.1016/j.gtc.2021.07.005
0889-8553/21/© 2021 Elsevier Inc. All rights reserved.

gastro.theclinics.com

effective long-term treatment for patients whose symptoms are recalcitrant to medical therapy, particularly in patients with typical acid reflux symptoms and those whose symptoms initially/partially respond well to PPI therapy.[9–11]

The indications for antireflux procedures are listed in **Box 1**.[12] The most common indication is GERD symptoms that are refractory to medical treatment. However, recent evidence for the negative effects of chronic PPI use (chronic kidney disease, community-acquired pneumonia, *Clostridium difficile* colitis, lower bone density) may lead patients and surgeons to increasingly consider antireflux procedures.[13]

PREOPERATIVE WORKUP

Several studies are used preoperatively in working up the patient with GERD. The four studies used most frequently are listed in **Box 2**. Although society guidelines do not make strong recommendations,[12] a US Esophageal Diagnostic Advisory Panel was convened in 2012 and developed consensus guidelines around the use of four studies based on available evidence and expert opinion.[14] The panel recommended the use of all four studies in evaluating patients before antireflux surgery. Similar recommendations were made by an international consensus group in 2019.[15] Although these recommendations represent the ideal, surgeons often do not obtain all four studies preoperatively—they are invasive, costly, and can delay surgical treatment for patients who are suffering. Surgeons more commonly use a selective, graded approach: for example, ordering manometry only when dysmotility is suggested on an interview or on a barium swallow.

Direct visualization of the esophagus via esophagogastroduodenoscopy (EGD) is paramount as it provides objective evidence of reflux (mucosal breaks, Los Angeles [LA] grading of esophagitis, peptic strictures, Barrett's esophagus), delineates anatomy (can suggest the presence/absence of hiatal hernia), and assesses for malignancy which would preclude an antireflux operation. A barium swallow study can further delineate anatomy (differentiate between type I and III paraesophageal hernias, identify diverticula and esophageal strictures, measure esophageal length) and can relay esophageal functional information (bolus transport, peristalsis, presence of reflux, reducibility of paraesophageal hernias) and can suggest achalasia and other underlying esophageal dysmotility issues. Esophageal manometry is used to rule out achalasia and identify esophageal dysmotility. Surgeons can use manometric data to tailor the type of procedure offered (partial vs complete fundoplication, determine candidacy for magnetic sphincter augmentation [MSA]). In addition, manometry facilitates placement of the pH probe or impedance catheter for pH testing by precisely identifying the gastroesophageal junction (GEJ). Lastly, pH testing with or without impedance, either via transnasal 24-h ambulatory study or through the

---

Box 1
Indications for antireflux procedures

Failed medical management (inadequate symptom control or severe symptoms despite acid-suppressing medications, medication side effects)

Patient desires operative management despite successful medical management (due to quality-of-life considerations, the lifelong need for medication intake, or the expense of medications)

GERD with complications (Barrett's esophagus, peptic stricture)

Extraesophageal manifestations secondary to GERD (new or worsening asthma, hoarseness, cough, chest pain, aspiration)

Box 2
Preoperative evaluations for antireflux procedures

Study	Description	Data
Esophagogastroduodenoscopy	Flexible endoscopic examination of the esophageal, gastric, and proximal duodenal lumens	Provides objective evidence of pathologic reflux, delineates anatomy, detects GERD complications, and rules out malignancy
Barium swallow	Radiographic and fluoroscopic imaging of the esophagus and stomach with oral contrast	Delineates anatomy and may detect esophageal motility disorders
Esophageal manometry	Intraluminal catheter-detected esophageal pressure recordings	Measures esophageal motility and can detect motility disorders
pH monitoring with or without impedance testing	Intraluminal esophageal pH monitoring via transnasal catheter or clip probe placed during endoscopy	Provides objective evidence of acid reflux and can correlate reflux episodes with symptoms when combined with impedance

wireless pH system (BRAVO capsule by Medtronic, Inc, Minneapolis, MN[16]), is considered the gold standard test to diagnose pathologic GERD and can be used to identify patients who will have a good response to antireflux surgery by way of associating symptoms with reflux events. Patients with long-segment Barrett's esophagus ($\geq$three cm) or LA grade C and D esophagitis on EGD do not require pH testing as the chance of a positive test is $\sim$ 100%.[17]

PATIENT SELECTION

The selection of patients for antireflux surgery is challenging because of the number of studies used in the preoperative workup outlined earlier and the paucity of high-quality data available linking the results of these preoperative studies to postoperative outcomes. The most consistent predictor of a good response to antireflux surgery is the presence of pathologic GERD with reflux-symptom concordance and a good response to PPI therapy.[12,14,15] However, there are subgroups of individuals with low reflux-symptom concordance, those with functional gastrointestinal disorders, and those with extraesophageal symptoms who may benefit from antireflux surgery, albeit with worse outcomes. It is our practice to offer antireflux surgery to patients who feel that their quality of life is so negatively impacted by their symptoms that they are willing to accept the (relatively low) risks and side effects of the operation in exchange for a chance at symptom improvement or resolution. This is a difficult decision to make, particularly for patients presenting with primarily atypical symptoms and poor response to PPIs. We are transparent with all patients that the procedure may not improve their symptoms, and that they may return to medical therapy in time. Ultimately, the decision to offer surgery must occur on an individual basis by clarifying patient goals and using shared decision-making to clearly set postoperative expectations.[15]

PROCEDURES FOR GASTROESOPHAGEAL REFLUX DISEASE

Compared to medical therapy, which merely alkalinizes the esophageal refluxate, antireflux procedures aim to create or reinforce a physical barrier to acidic stomach contents refluxing from the stomach into the lower esophagus. Each procedure outlined in the following achieves this through a different mechanism.

Fundoplication

Multiple randomized controlled trials have compared fundoplication to medical therapy.[10,18] The initial of these occurred in the late 1980s as part of a multicenter Veteran's Administration (VA) study which compared fundoplication to then-standard ranitidine-based medical therapy.[19] Medical therapy was found to be significantly less effective, popularizing fundoplication for GERD. Subsequent long-term follow-up demonstrated that 62% of patients who received surgery ultimately returned to PPI therapy for symptom control.[20] These results cast doubt on the efficacy of fundoplication for definitive management of GERD with a concomitant reduction in the performance of fundoplications.[21] More recent Randomized Controlled Trials (RCTs) have demonstrated similar results regarding return to PPI use after surgery, though select populations may benefit from surgery without long-term reliance on antacid medications. For example, one VA-funded study demonstrated that surgery was significantly superior to both active medical treatment and control medical treatment arms in a highly-selected subgroup of veterans with PPI-refractory-related and reflux-related heartburn.[11] This is also consistent with the findings of a Cochrane systematic review, which, despite overall low-level of evidence from the four included studies, concluded that patients undergoing fundoplication experienced less heartburn and reflux symptoms at short-term and medium-term intervals compared to medical management.[18] This follows given the mechanism of fundoplication and the reconstitution of the lower esophageal sphincter (LES). The LOTUS trial, a multi-institution exploratory randomized open parallel-group trial in Europe found that acid regurgitation symptoms were less frequent in the surgery group, whereas dysphagia and bloating were more frequent compared with the medicine group at five years. Ultimately, the authors found that the difference in GERD remission rates between the two groups was comparable.[10]

The fundoplication has been and remains the gold standard for surgical treatment of GERD. Fundoplication addresses reflux by reinforcing the LES by wrapping the gastric fundus around the esophagus and suturing it to itself and the esophagus (**Fig. 1**). Today, this operation is performed via a laparoscopic approach with studies showing similar or better control of GERD symptoms in long-term follow-up over the open approach, as well as shorter hospital stay and lower ventral hernia rates.[22,23] There has been much debate in the literature regarding full (Nissen, **Fig. 2**) or partial (Toupet, **Fig. 3**) fundic wraps. The outcomes of multiple randomized controlled trials demonstrate similar or better control of GERD symptoms in patients who received a total wrap at the expense of higher rates of postoperative dysphagia compared to patients with a partial wrap.[24–27] However, dysphagia rates and reflux symptom scores are

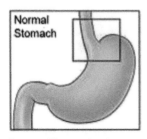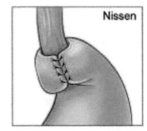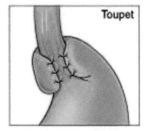

Fig. 1. Different fundic wraps.

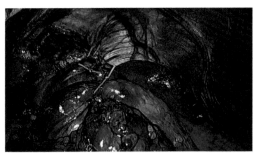

Fig. 2. Intraoperative photo of a Nissen fundoplication. Note the sutures in the foreground approximating the fundus of the stomach (*dagger*) about the esophagus (*asterisk*) as it projects through the diaphragmatic hiatus. ‡, left diaphragm; S, spleen; L, left segment of the liver.

similar on long-term follow-up[28,29] and any differences seen in randomized controlled trials between full or partial fundic wraps are not corroborated in systematic reviews and meta-analyses.[30,31] As a result, many surgeons exclusively perform full or partial wraps, whereas others tailor the choice of wrap to the patient, favoring partial fundoplication for those with concern for dysmotility on preoperative workup.[32] Interestingly, this approach has been called into question as it has not been borne out in the literature.[33] Our preferred approach is to tailor the wrap to the patient as earlier.

Acute complications such as 30-day mortality, infection, bleeding, and esophageal perforation are rare following fundoplication, while dysphagia affects approximately half of all patients.[34] However, long-term complications such as structural issues due to wrap failure or migration with subsequent return of GERD symptoms are much more common. In a survey of patients 20 years status postfundoplication by an expert in the field, 17% required revisional surgery. Notably, the average time between index and redo fundoplication was 11 years and 77.8% had complete resolution of symptoms after revision. Despite this revision rate, 90% of patients in this study were satisfied with surgical treatment of their GERD.[29]

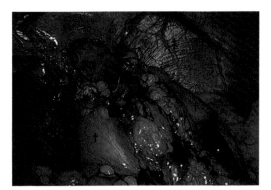

Fig. 3. Intraoperative photo of a Toupet fundoplication. Note the sutures affixing the gastric fundus (*dagger*) to the esophagus (*asterisk*), creating a partial wrap ("hot dog in a bun"). The arrowhead indicates sutures used to reapproximate the diaphragmatic crura following reduction of a concurrent hiatal hernia in this patient. ‡, diaphragm.

Magnetic Sphincter Augmentation

MSA is a new technology developed in 2002 by Torax Medical, Inc (Shoreview, MN, USA) with their proprietary LINX Reflux Management System.[35] The device consists of a string of spherical magnets placed laparoscopically about the GEJ (**Figs. 4** and **5**). At rest, the magnetic beads maintain the LES in a closed position and avoid the reflux of gastric contents into the esophagus. The beads rest against each other to reduce esophageal compression. When esophageal or gastric pressure is high enough, the attractive force between the magnets is overcome and the LES opens—allowing passage of a swallowed bolus, or other functions such as belching and vomiting. In this way, MSA is a dynamic augmentation of the LES compared to traditional fundoplication. Placement of the device occurs under general anesthesia, is achieved in under one hour with minimal hiatal dissection, and patients are started on a general diet immediately after the operation (compared to fundoplication, after which most patients are typically kept on a liquid diet for several weeks before slow advancement). FDA approval for LINX was granted in 2012 after trials suggested good safety and efficacy profiles. The exclusion criteria were strict, however, and patients with a hiatal hernia larger than three cm were excluded. This is reflected in the relative contraindications to MSA, which include hiatal hernias >three cm, presence of Barrett's esophagus or LA grade C or D esophagitis, major motility disorders, and other specific conditions such as BMI greater than 35 kg/m^2, scleroderma, and esophageal stricture.[35] However, more recent studies are pushing out these contraindications, with regression of Barrett's esophagus and decrease in hiatal hernia recurrence for patients with hernias >three cm in size seen in two studies published by a high-volume group.[36,37] Since gaining FDA approval, multiple prospective observational trials have been conducted, which also suggest that the device is safe with no reported deaths and a very low rate of intraoperative and postoperative complications (0.1%).[35,38] Prospective and retrospective studies show generally good effect of the device in controlling GERD symptoms, with ~85% reporting no PPI use at five years, reduced reflux symptoms, and improved GERD-HRQL.[39,40] The most common complications are dysphagia, with ~70% experiencing symptoms perioperatively. However, this is transient in most patients, with 11% having persistent dysphagia at one year and 4% at three years in the pivotal study of the device.[41] A

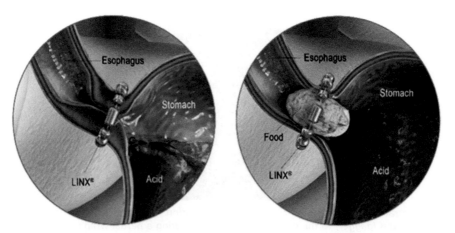

Fig. 4. Graphical representation of the LINX device. (*Courtesy of* J&J Medical Devices, Irvine, CA; with permission.)

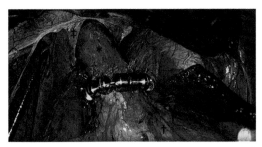

Fig. 5. Intraoperative photo of the LINX device in place about the esophagus. *, Esophagus; ‡, right crus; S, spleen; †, stomach.

more recent retrospective review over a five-year period describes a persistent dysphagia rate of 15.5% at three or more months after surgery, with ~30% of the 380 patients studied requiring dilation for dysphagia, chest pain, or both.[40] Erosions are rare, as is persistent dysphagia requiring removal of the device.[35,40] Although there are multiple comparative studies pitting MSA against fundoplication, no prospective randomized controlled trial data exist to date. The impact of MSA on quality of life, reduction in GERD symptoms, and postoperative dysphagia are at least similar to fundoplication based on these studies, with a reduction in gas bloat and an increase in the ability to belch.[35,42] One Torax-funded randomized controlled trial evaluating the effectiveness of MSA versus double-dose PPI therapy in moderate to severe regurgitation has been conducted using a small group of 152 patients.[43] At six months, 89% of the MSA group reported regurgitation relief compared to 10% of the BID PPI group ($P<.001$), 81% of the MSA group reported $\geq$50% improvement in GERD-HRQL scores compared to 8% in the BID PPI group, and 91% of the MSA group remained off of PPI therapy. Twenty-eight percent of the MSA group reported transient dysphagia and 4% reported ongoing dysphagia. Overall, MSA is another safe and effective tool within the GERD treatment armamentarium and is a reasonable option for appropriately selected patients.

Transoral Incisionless Fundoplication

Transoral incisionless fundoplication (TIF) is an endoluminal approach to GERD using the EsophyX device developed by Endogastric Solutions (Redwood City, WA) that was approved by the FDA in 2007.[44] The EsophyX device augments the LES by placing a series of H-shaped fasteners at the posterior and anterior sides of the lesser curvature, creating a full-thickness fundic plication at the GEJ (**Fig. 6**). This technique requires no abdominal or thoracic incision and is performed under general anesthesia by a surgeon and/or an endoscopist, typically in under one hour. Endogastric Solutions lists several contraindications to TIF on their Web site, including a BMI greater than 35 kg/m^2, LA grade C or D esophagitis, Barrett's esophagus, portal hypertension and/or varices, hiatal hernias greater than two cm in size, esophageal strictures, and previous esophageal or gastric surgery.[45] Multiple observational and randomized controlled trials have been conducted evaluating the efficacy of TIF compared to PPI controls.[44] A systematic review[46] including 18 of these studies between 2007 and 2015 reported a relative risk of response rate to TIF versus PPIs or sham treatment of 2.44 (95% confidence interval, 1.25–4.79; $P = .0009$). TIF was found to reduce the total number of reflux events, though the acid exposure time and the number of acid reflux episodes after TIF were not significantly improved. Furthermore, PPI usage increased with time after the procedure, albeit at lower doses on long-term follow-up. Adverse events were rare. To date, no trial has

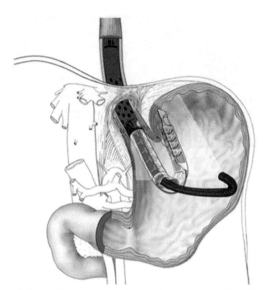

Fig. 6. Cross-sectional view of the stomach during deployment of the Esophyx device during transoral incisionless fundoplication. The endoscope is placed through the device and retro-flexed to provide visualization during the procedure. (*Courtesy of* EndoGastric Solutions, Redmond, WA; with permission.)

directly compared TIF to surgical fundoplication. A systematic review and network meta-analysis by Richter and colleagues[47] in 2018 identified seven trials with a total of 1128 patients to compare the outcomes between TIF, laparoscopic Nissen fundoplication, sham procedure, and PPIs. This study found that TIF had the highest chance of increasing GERD-health-related quality of life (GERD-HRQL) (0.96) followed by fundoplication (0.66), sham procedure (0.35), and PPIs (0.042). However, TIF also had the highest chance for persistent esophagitis next to sham procedure and was less likely to reduce esophageal acid exposure time compared to fundoplication and PPIs. The authors did not recommend TIF as a long-term alternative to PPIs or laparoscopic Nissen fundoplication for the treatment of GERD. The impact of failed TIF on subsequent surgical fundoplication is a potential concern that is understudied, though the scarce observational studies in the literature describe challenging but safe operations with positive outcomes.[44,48] Interestingly, TIF is being used in combination with laparoscopic hiatal hernia repair to expand the accessibility of TIF to patients with GERD and hiatal hernias greater than two cm in size. Although this clearly is no longer an "incisionless" approach, proponents argue this hybrid surgical and endoscopic procedure may provide an alternative antireflux option for patients with large hiatal hernias who wish to avoid gas bloating symptoms more commonly experienced after traditional fundoplication.[49]

Radiofrequency Ablation

Radiofrequency ablation (RFA) therapy by way of the Stretta system (Mederi Therapeutics, Greenwich, CT, USA) cyclically heats the tissues at the LES with the goal of remodeling the sphincter musculature to treat GERD symptoms. The device was approved by the FDA in 2000. The exact mechanism of action is unclear, though it is postulated that heat-induced neurolysis or tissue necrosis leads to local inflammation and muscular thickening of the LES, decreasing transient relaxation.[50] The Stretta system is composed of a transoral catheter with a balloon wielding radially placed needles that is positioned at the LES under conscious sedation (**Fig. 7**). Radiofrequency energy is then applied through the needles to the muscularis propria for approximately 60 seconds to a target temperature of 65° to 85° Fahrenheit circumferentially.[44,50] The procedure takes under one hour to complete. Multiple observational and randomized controlled trials have evaluated the efficacy of RFA, leading to multiple systematic reviews and meta-analyses. The quality and rigor of the science in these studies varies, leading to discordant results from the systematic reviews, and ultimately controversial recommendations from different societies, namely the

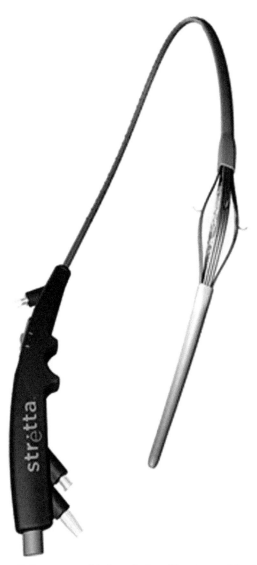

Fig. 7. The Stretta radiofrequency ablation device. (*Courtesy of* Stretta Centre, United Kingdom; with permission.)

American College of Gastroenterology (recommending against its use due to low level of evidence) and the Society of American Gastrointestinal and Endoscopic Surgeons (recommending its use based on a long safety record, improvement in GERD-HRQL scores, and decreased PPI use despite diminished effectiveness over time).[8,44,51–54]

Roux-en-Y Gastric Bypass

Roux-en-Y gastric bypass (RYGB) is perhaps the most aggressive surgical treatment for recalcitrant GERD and can serve as a last-resort salvage operation after multiple failed attempts at symptom control using other methods as long as the stomach remains robust and viable after undergoing multiple previous operations. In the patient with symptomatic GERD and concurrent obesity, RYGB may be the most appropriate first-line treatment and is considered gold-standard. RYGB for GERD is a large topic deserving of its own chapter and will not be discussed in detail here.

Antireflux Mucosectomy

Antireflux mucosectomy (ARMS) is an emerging new endoscopic antireflux technique developed by Inoue and colleagues in Japan. Their group discovered an improvement in reflux symptoms after a patient underwent endomucosal resection for Barrett's esophagus.[55] The fully endoscopic technique involves the injection of indigo carmine dye into the submucosa of the gastric cardia, elevating the mucosa and lifting it off the remaining layers of the gastric wall beneath. The lifted mucosa is then snared and cauterized off. This process is repeated multiple times to create mucosal defects in a "butterfly" shape, sparing the mucosa along the axis of the lesser and greater curvatures of the stomach (**Fig. 8**). The procedure takes place under general anesthesia, lasts between 30 minutes to one and a half hours, and virtually all patients are discharged home the same day. Healing of the affected area induces scarring, which is thought to reinforce and tighten the incompetent LES, leading to reduced reflux and GERD symptoms. Early retrospective studies show that the technique is well tolerated, safe, and has promising outcomes comparable to Nissen fundoplication with improved postoperative recovery and less gas bloat.[56,57] The technique does

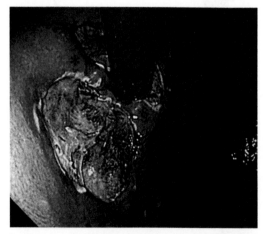

Fig. 8. An endoscopic photograph with the endoscope in retroflexion showing a completed antireflux mucosectomy. Note the "butterfly" shape created about the gastroesophageal junction on the gastric side. * Marks the lesser curvature of the stomach; § marks the greater curvature.

not appear to preclude subsequent antireflux procedures if symptoms return.[56] Prospective studies are needed, but this technique may provide yet another effective therapy for selected patients.

SUMMARY

GERD is a prevalent and challenging disease—in its diagnosis, workup, and treatment. The preponderance of evolving, well-intentioned evidence at times illuminates a clear path for the clinician as often as it clouds. There are multiple surgical and endoscopic interventions for GERD that offer an alternative to medical therapy, with the gold standard laparoscopic fundoplication as the most effective and most studied of all. Complications and risks accompany surgical fundoplication's success rates, and many patients return to PPI use long-term. Evolving and new technologies such as MSA, TIF, RFA, and ARMS do not entirely supplant surgical fundoplication. Rather, they provide alternatives with similar outcomes for the interventionalist's growing toolbox with which to serve the suffering GERD patient.

CLINICS CARE POINTS

- Obtain objective evidence of pathologic GERD before recommending an antireflux procedure.
- Esophagoduodenoscopy, esophageal manometry, pH monitoring with/without impedance, and barium swallow are all recommended by consensus in the workup of GERD.
- Patients with pathologic GERD, strong reflux-symptom concordance, and who exhibit a good response to PPI therapy are most likely to have a good response to antireflux procedures.
- Antireflux procedures are safe and improve GERD symptoms over PPI therapy in the majority of patients and patient satisfaction rates are high.
- Dysphagia, gas bloat, and return to PPI use after antireflux procedures is common.
- Surgical fundoplication has the strongest, most long-standing supporting evidence. Magnetic sphincter augmentation, transoral incisionless fundoplication, radiofrequency ablation, and antireflux mucosectomy are novel and emerging procedures with outcomes similar to fundoplication.

DISCLOSURE

The authors have nothing to disclose.

REFERENCES

1. Vakil N, van Zanten SV, Kahrilas P, et al. The Montreal definition and classification of gastroesophageal reflux disease: a global evidence-based consensus. Am J Gastroenterol 2006;101(8):1900–20 [quiz 1943].
2. Eusebi LH, Ratnakumaran R, Yuan Y, et al. Global prevalence of, and risk factors for, gastro-oesophageal reflux symptoms: a meta-analysis. Gut 2018;67(3): 430–40.
3. Tack J, Becher A, Mulligan C, et al. Systematic review: the burden of disruptive gastro-oesophageal reflux disease on health-related quality of life. Aliment Pharmacol Ther 2012;35(11):1257–66.
4. King A, MacDonald C, Orn C. Understanding gastro-oesophageal reflux disease: a patient-cluster analysis. Int J Clin Pract 2008;62(12):1838–43.

5. Peery AF, Crockett SD, Murphy CC, et al. Burden and cost of gastrointestinal, liver, and pancreatic diseases in the United States: Update 2018. Gastroenterology 2019;156(1):254–272 e211.

6. Fedorak RN, Veldhuyzen van Zanten S, Bridges R. Canadian digestive health foundation public impact series: gastroesophageal reflux disease in Canada: incidence, prevalence, and direct and indirect economic impact. Can J Gastroenterol 2010;24(7):431–4.

7. Funk LM, Zhang JY, Drosdeck JM, et al. Long-term cost-effectiveness of medical, endoscopic and surgical management of gastroesophageal reflux disease. Surgery 2015;157(1):126–36.

8. Katz PO, Gerson LB, Vela MF. Guidelines for the diagnosis and management of gastroesophageal reflux disease. Am J Gastroenterol 2013;108(3):308–28 [quiz 329].

9. Oelschlager BK, Quiroga E, Parra JD, et al. Long-term outcomes after laparoscopic antireflux surgery. Am J Gastroenterol 2008;103(2):280–7 [quiz 288].

10. Galmiche JP, Hatlebakk J, Attwood S, et al. Laparoscopic antireflux surgery vs esomeprazole treatment for chronic GERD: the LOTUS randomized clinical trial. JAMA 2011;305(19):1969–77.

11. Spechler SJ, Hunter JG, Jones KM, et al. Randomized trial of medical versus surgical treatment for refractory heartburn. N Engl J Med 2019;381(16):1513–23.

12. SAGES. Guidelines for surgical treatment of gastroesophageal reflux disease (GERD) 2010. https://www.sages.org/publications/guidelines/guidelines-for-surgical-treatment-of-gastroesophageal-reflux-disease-gerd/. Accessed February 27, 2021.

13. Maret-Ouda J, Markar SR, Lagergren J. Gastroesophageal reflux disease: a review. JAMA 2020;324(24):2536–47.

14. Jobe BA, Richter JE, Hoppo T, et al. Preoperative diagnostic workup before antireflux surgery: an evidence and experience-based consensus of the Esophageal Diagnostic Advisory Panel. J Am Coll Surg 2013;217(4):586–97.

15. Pauwels A, Boecxstaens V, Andrews CN, et al. How to select patients for antireflux surgery? The ICARUS guidelines (international consensus regarding preoperative examinations and clinical characteristics assessment to select adult patients for antireflux surgery). Gut 2019;68(11):1928–41.

16. Medtronic. BRAVO calibration-free reflux testing system. Available at: https://www.medtronic.com/covidien/en-us/products/reflux-testing/bravo-reflux-testing-system.html. Accessed March 18, 2019.

17. Schwameis K, Lin B, Roman J, et al. Is pH testing necessary before antireflux surgery in patients with endoscopic erosive esophagitis? J Gastrointest Surg 2018; 22(1):8–12.

18. Garg SK, Gurusamy KS. Laparoscopic fundoplication surgery versus medical management for gastro-oesophageal reflux disease (GORD) in adults. Cochrane database Syst Rev 2015;(11):CD003243.

19. Spechler SJ. Comparison of medical and surgical therapy for complicated gastroesophageal reflux disease in veterans. The Department of Veterans Affairs Gastroesophageal Reflux Disease Study Group. N Engl J Med 1992;326(12): 786–92.

20. Spechler SJ, Lee E, Ahnen D, et al. Long-term outcome of medical and surgical therapies for gastroesophageal reflux disease: follow-up of a randomized controlled trial. JAMA 2001;285(18):2331–8.

21. Spechler SJ. The durability of antireflux surgery. JAMA 2017;318(10):913–5.

22. Salminen PT, Hiekkanen HI, Rantala AP, et al. Comparison of long-term outcome of laparoscopic and conventional nissen fundoplication: a prospective random-ized study with an 11-year follow-up. Ann Surg 2007;246(2):201–6.

23. Chrysos E, Tsiaoussis J, Athanasakis E, et al. Laparoscopic vs open approach for Nissen fundoplication. A comparative study. Surg Endosc 2002;16(12):1679–84.

24. Varin O, Velstra B, De Sutter S, et al. Total vs partial fundoplication in the treat-ment of gastroesophageal reflux disease: a meta-analysis. Arch Surg 2009; 144(3):273–8.

25. Nijjar RS, Watson DI, Jamieson GG, et al. Five-year follow-up of a multicenter, double-blind randomized clinical trial of laparoscopic Nissen vs anterior 90 de-grees partial fundoplication. Arch Surg 2010;145(6):552–7.

26. Kurian AA, Bhayani N, Sharata A, et al. Partial anterior vs partial posterior fundo-plication following transabdominal esophagocardiomyotomy for achalasia of the esophagus: meta-regression of objective postoperative gastroesophageal reflux and dysphagia. JAMA Surg 2013;148(1):85–90.

27. Hakanson BS, Lundell L, Bylund A, et al. Comparison of laparoscopic 270 de-grees posterior partial fundoplication vs total fundoplication for the treatment of gastroesophageal reflux disease: a randomized clinical trial. JAMA Surg 2019; 154(6):479–86.

28. Gunter RL, Shada AL, Funk LM, et al. Long-term quality of life outcomes following nissen versus toupet fundoplication in patients with gastroesophageal reflux dis-ease. J Laparoendosc Adv Surg Tech A 2017;27(9):931–6.

29. Robinson B, Dunst CM, Cassera MA, et al. 20 years later: laparoscopic fundopli-cation durability. Surg Endosc 2015;29(9):2520–4.

30. Du X, Hu Z, Yan C, et al. A meta-analysis of long follow-up outcomes of laparo-scopic Nissen (total) versus Toupet (270 degrees) fundoplication for gastro-esophageal reflux disease based on randomized controlled trials in adults. BMC Gastroenterol 2016;16(1):88.

31. Broeders JA, Mauritz FA, Ahmed Ali U, et al. Systematic review and meta-analysis of laparoscopic Nissen (posterior total) versus Toupet (posterior partial) fundopli-cation for gastro-oesophageal reflux disease. Br J Surg 2010;97(9):1318–30.

32. Kauer WK, Peters JH, DeMeester TR, et al. A tailored approach to antireflux sur-gery. J Thorac Cardiovasc Surg 1995;110(1):141–6 [discussion 146–7].

33. Booth MI, Stratford J, Jones L, et al. Randomized clinical trial of laparoscopic total (Nissen) versus posterior partial (Toupet) fundoplication for gastro-oesophageal reflux disease based on preoperative oesophageal manometry. Br J Surg 2008;95(1):57–63.

34. Yadlapati R, Hungness ES, Pandolfino JE. Complications of Antireflux Surgery. Am J Gastroenterol 2018;113(8):1137–47.

35. Telem DW, Shah A, Hutter P. LINX reflux management system: SAGES Tehcnol-ogy and Value Assessment Committee (TAVAC) safety and effectiveness analysis 2017. Available at: https://www.sages.org/publications/tavac/tavac-safety-and-effectiveness-analysis-linx-reflux-management-system/. Accessed March 20, 2021.

36. Dunn CP, Henning JC, Sterris JA, et al. Regression of Barrett's esophagus after magnetic sphincter augmentation: intermediate-term results. Surg Endosc 2020.

37. Dunn CP, Zhao J, Wang JC, et al. Magnetic sphincter augmentation with hiatal hernia repair: long term outcomes. Surg Endosc 2020.

38. Lipham JC, Taiganides PA, Louie BE, et al. Safety analysis of first 1000 patients treated with magnetic sphincter augmentation for gastroesophageal reflux dis-ease. Dis esophagus 2015;28(4):305–11.

39. Ganz RA, Edmundowicz SA, Taiganides PA, et al. Long-term outcomes of patients receiving a magnetic sphincter augmentation device for gastroesophageal reflux. Clin Gastroenterol Hepatol 2016;14(5):671–7.

40. Ayazi S, Zheng P, Zaidi AH, et al. Magnetic sphincter augmentation and postoperative dysphagia: characterization, clinical risk factors, and management. J Gastrointest Surg 2020;24(1):39–49.

41. Ganz RA, Peters JH, Horgan S. Esophageal sphincter device for gastroesophageal reflux disease. N Engl J Med 2013;368(21):2039–40.

42. Guidozzi N, Wiggins T, Ahmed AR, et al. Laparoscopic magnetic sphincter augmentation versus fundoplication for gastroesophageal reflux disease: systematic review and pooled analysis. Dis Esophagus 2019;32(9):doz031.

43. Bell R, Lipham J, Louie B, et al. Laparoscopic magnetic sphincter augmentation versus double-dose proton pump inhibitors for management of moderate-to-severe regurgitation in GERD: a randomized controlled trial. Gastrointest Endosc 2019;89(1):14–22 e11.

44. Stefanidis DR, Dunkin B. Endoluminal Treatments for Gastroesophageal Reflux Disease (GERD). Clinical Spotlight Review; 2017. Available at: https://www.sages.org/publications/guidelines/endoluminal-treatments-for-gastroesophageal-reflux-disease-gerd/.

45. Solutions E. Policy/Criteria: transoral Incisionless Fundoplication (TIF) procedure with EsophyX device. Available at: https://www.endogastricsolutions.com/wp-content/uploads/2017/12/Policy-Criteria-for-EsophyX-TIF-Procedure.pdf. Accessed 3/20/21, 2021.

46. Huang X, Chen S, Zhao H, et al. Efficacy of transoral incisionless fundoplication (TIF) for the treatment of GERD: a systematic review with meta-analysis. Surg Endosc 2017;31(3):1032–44.

47. Richter JE, Kumar A, Lipka S, et al. Efficacy of laparoscopic nissen fundoplication vs transoral incisionless fundoplication or proton pump inhibitors in patients with gastroesophageal reflux disease: a systematic review and network meta-analysis. Gastroenterology 2018;154(5):1298–308, e1297.

48. Puri R, Smith CD, Bowers SP. The spectrum of surgical remediation of transoral incisionless fundoplication-related failures. J Laparoendosc Adv Surg Tech A 2018;28(9):1089–93.

49. Choi AY, Roccato MK, Samarasena JB, et al. Novel interdisciplinary approach to GERD: concomitant laparoscopic hiatal hernia repair with transoral incisionless fundoplication. J Am Coll Surg 2021;232(3):309–18.

50. Hopkins J, Switzer NJ, Karmali S. Update on novel endoscopic therapies to treat gastroesophageal reflux disease: a review. World J Gastrointest Endosc 2015;7(11):1039–44.

51. Fass R, Cahn F, Scotti DJ, et al. Systematic review and meta-analysis of controlled and prospective cohort efficacy studies of endoscopic radiofrequency for treatment of gastroesophageal reflux disease. Surg Endosc 2017;31(12):4865–82.

52. Lipka S, Kumar A, Richter JE. No evidence for efficacy of radiofrequency ablation for treatment of gastroesophageal reflux disease: a systematic review and meta-analysis. Clin Gastroenterol Hepatol 2015;13(6):1058–67.e1.

53. Richardson WS, Stefanidis D, Fanelli RD. Society of American gastrointestinal and endoscopic surgeons response to "no evidence for efficacy of radiofrequency ablation for treatment of gastroesophageal reflux disease: a systematic review and meta-analysis. Clin Gastroenterol Hepatol 2015;13(9):1700–1.

54. Kumar A, Lipka S, Richter JE. Reply: to PMID 25459556. Clin Gastroenterol Hepatol 2015;13(9):1701.

55. Satodate H, Inoue H, Yoshida T, et al. Circumferential EMR of carcinoma arising in Barrett's esophagus: case report. Gastrointest Endosc 2003;58(2):288–92.

56. Wong HJ, Su B, Attaar M, et al. Anti-reflux mucosectomy (ARMS) results in improved recovery and similar reflux quality of life outcomes compared to laparoscopic Nissen fundoplication. Surg Endosc 2020.

57. Sumi K, Inoue H, Kobayashi Y, et al. Endoscopic treatment of proton pump inhibitor-refractory gastroesophageal reflux disease with anti-reflux mucosectomy: experience of 109 cases. Dig Endosc 2021;33(3):347–54.

Eosinophilic Esophagitis

Incidence, Diagnosis, Management, and Future Directions

Nielsen Q. Fernandez-Becker, MD, PhD

KEYWORDS

- Eosinophilic esophagitis • Proton pump inhibitors • Swallowed topical steroids
- Elimination diets

KEY POINTS

- Eosinophilic esophagitis is a clinicopathologic disease.
- Allergic inflammation underlies pathogenesis.
- Natural history of Eosinophilic esophagitis: inflammation causes tissue remodeling and fibrosis.
- Prevalence of Eosinophilic esophagitis has increased.
- Treatment: Drugs, diet, and dilation.

INTRODUCTION

Eosinophilic esophagitis (EoE) is a clinicopathologic disease, whereby tissue eosinophilia causes symptoms of esophageal dysfunction. In adults, this esophageal dysfunction most commonly manifests as dysphagia, and EoE is the leading cause of food impaction requiring emergent endoscopic intervention.[1–3] The diagnosis requires the following: (i) the presence of esophageal eosinophilia, (ii) characteristic symptoms, and (iii) the exclusion of other causes.[1–4] The incidence and prevalence of EoE has grown in the last quarter century, and EoE is associated with significant burden on our health care system, costing approximately $1.4 billion per year in the United States.[5]

EoE is a complex multifactorial disease that involves an interaction between host factors, genetics, environment, and immunity. Atopy, a genetic predisposition to allergy, is an important factor as many patients with EoE have other allergic conditions.[6] Several genetic EoE risk variants have been identified including genes whose products affect eosinophilic migration (CCL26/eotaxin-3 and IL-13), activate Th2 cells [thymic stromal lymphopoietin (TSLP)], affect barrier function [Desmoglein −1 and filaggrin], and promote esophageal remodeling [periostin].[7–9]

Department of Medicine, Stanford University, Redwood City, CA, USA
E-mail address: Nfernan1@stanford.edu

Gastroenterol Clin N Am 50 (2021) 825–841
https://doi.org/10.1016/j.gtc.2021.08.001
0889-8553/21/© 2021 Elsevier Inc. All rights reserved.

gastro.theclinics.com

In EoE, eosinophils infiltrate the esophageal mucosa in response to allergen exposure. Ingested substances including food components, microbial factors, and airborne allergens promote production of cytokines that activate T cells and affect eosinophil production and trafficking via an inflammatory pathway that involves the cytokines/chemokines TSLP, IL-4, IL5, IL-13, and eotaxin-3.[7-10] The resulting inflammation causes gross inflammatory changes to the esophageal lining and ultimately leads to fibrostenotic complications such as esophageal strictures and narrow caliber esophagus.[3,11-13] Natural history studies indicate that EoE is a chronic disease that if untreated results in continued inflammation, subepithelial fibrosis, and esophageal remodeling.[12,14-16] Consistent with this, patients with delayed diagnosis are more likely to present with fibrostenotic disease.[15,16] Treatment involves pharmacologic or dietary control of inflammation and endoscopic therapy of fibrostenotic disease. The purpose of this review article is to provide the practicing gastroenterologist with critical information and updates on epidemiology, diagnosis, and management of EoE.

DIAGNOSIS

As discussed previously, the diagnosis of EoE requires both the presence of esophageal dysfunction and esophageal eosinophilia. A major focus of the first diagnostic guidelines in 2007 was to distinguish EoE from gastroesophageal reflux (GERD), which can also cause esophageal eosinophilia.[17] In 2011, the term proton pump inhibitor (PPI) responsive esophageal eosinophilia (PPI-REE) was introduced to describe patients with esophageal eosinophilia who met criteria for EoE but demonstrated a symptomatic and histologic response to PPI therapy.[18] At the time, the definition of EoE required a lack of response to PPI. This criterion was later abandoned when PPI-REE and EoE were found to be indistinguishable with respect to clinical manifestations, histology, and molecular analysis.[3,19-21] Now PPI-REE is recognized as a subset of EoE. The current international consensus guidelines define EoE as follows (**Box 1**)[3,4,20]:

(1) symptoms of esophageal dysfunction such as dysphagia and (2) the presence of greater than $\geq$15 eosinophils per high power field (hpf) on esophageal biopsy. Eosinophilia should be limited to the esophagus and other potential causes of eosinophilia must be excluded (**Box 2**).

INCIDENCE

In the last two decades, EoE moved from rare case reports to recent prevalence estimates of 34.4 cases/100,000 inhabitants.[22] Although there has been increased recognition of EoE, it does not solely account for the increased incidence. Multiple single center studies in the United States and Europe reported incidence as high as 10 cases/100,000 cases.[23-26] Systemic analyses of studies in the United States, Europe, and Australia have reported a significant increase in the incidence of EoE in studies performed after 2008 compared with those that were carried out before.[22,27] The

---

Box 1
EoE diagnostic criteria

1. Symptoms of esophageal dysfunction
2. Evidence of eosinophilic inflammation 15 $\geq$ Eos/HPF
3. Exclusion of other causes of Eosinophilia

Box 2
Causes of esophageal eosinophilia other than EoE

Causes of Esophageal Eosinophilia
  GERD
  Achalasia
  Eosinophilic gastrointestinal disease
  Crohn's disease
  Celiac disease
  Graft versus host disease
  Drug reaction
  Connective tissue disorder
  Vasculitis

---

incidence of EoE continues to rise without foreseeable signs of deceleration. A population-based study in Denmark analyzed incidence of EoE during 1997 to 2012 found a 19.5-fold increase in the incidence of EoE, ranging from 0.13 cases/ 100,000 to 2.6/100,000 cases over the 15-year period.[23] Most recently, a Dutch study also demonstrated a dramatic rise in EoE incidence from 1995 to 2019. The incidence rate increased modestly from 0.1 to 0.08 new cases per 100,000 persons from 1995 to 2004 and in comparison, accelerated in the interval between 2005 and 2019 as it rose from 0.14 to 3.16 new cases per 100,000 inhabitants.[28] The factors driving this rise are likely multifactorial and remain elusive.

CLINICAL PRESENTATION

EoE has been described in all age groups with a predilection for men in the third to fourth decade of life.[29,30] Epidemiologic studies have demonstrated that other atopic diseases including allergic rhinitis (57%–70%), asthma (27%–60%), atopic dermatitis (6%–46%), and IgE-mediated food allergy (24%–68%) are highly prevalent in patients with EoE.[6,31] Therefore, presence of dysphagia and other atopic conditions should raise clinical suspicion for EoE, but it is important to recognize that the clinical presentation may vary. For instance, the presenting symptoms in children often differ compared with adults. Children typically present with reflux-like symptoms, abdominal pain, nausea, vomiting, failure to thrive, and food intolerance, whereas adolescents and adults usually experience dysphagia and food impaction (**Table 1**).[12,30,32] The reason for this difference may be that the symptoms in children are the result of the inflammatory phase of the disease and adults suffer from fibrostenotic consequences, presumably directly proportional to disease duration. However, this does not apply to all cases and different clinical phenotypes of EoE may exist. Recent studies have shown that chest pain and heartburn can be prominent symptoms in adults with EoE, and that young children may also present with dysphagia.[17,29,33,34] It is likely that EoE, like other atopic diseases, is heterogenous. Sallis and colleagues, compared mRNA expression profile of esophageal biopsies from children with EoE who developed food impactions and those that did not.[35] Although the two groups could not be distinguished by clinical characteristics including histology or age, they differed in their expression profile.[35] This supports the concept that different molecular EoE phenotypes exist but their relevance to the disease process remains to be established. A deeper understanding of mechanisms underlying different disease phenotypes can open a window into a more personalized approach to treatment and disease monitoring.

Table 1
Clinical characteristics and presentation of EoE

EoE Clinical Characteristics	Symptoms
Male > Female	Children:
White race	Failure to thrive
History of atopy (allergic rhinitis, asthma, atopic dermatitis, food allergy)	Nausea and Vomiting
	Picky eating
Family history of atopy	Heartburn
Family history of dysphagia	Abdominal pain
Family history of EoE	Adults:
	Dysphagia
	Heartburn
	Chest pain
	Food avoidance
	Slow eating

Patients with EoE may engage in compensatory behaviors that may contribute to delayed diagnosis. These patients may underreport symptoms but on direct questioning will admit to certain behaviors such as food modification, avoidance, slow eating, crushing pills, drinking water excessively to "wash food down" and in extreme cases fear of eating and avoiding restaurants due to fear of food impaction. In a small prospective study, 10 EoE and 10 control patients were asked to rate eating difficulty and quality of life and were directly observed eating a standardized meal. On direct observation patients with active EoE took longer to eat, consumed more water, took more single bites, and chewed more per bite compared with controls and patients with inactive EoE.[36] Therefore, it is important to ask specific questions about adaptive eating behaviors to elicit an accurate assessment of severity.

DIAGNOSTIC MODALITIES
Endoscopy

In patients with symptoms of esophageal dysfunction, an endoscopy is recommended for direct visualization of the mucosa, as well as collection of biopsies for histologic analysis. The practice of taking at least six biopsies from proximal, mid, and distal esophagus, paying attention to target abnormal mucosa is 99% sensitive at detecting EoE.[37]

Endoscopically EoE may have normal appearance; however there are often mucosal changes which should increase suspicion for EoE. These have been described by an Endoscopic Reference Score (EREFS). EREFS uses endoscopic findings including exudates, rings, edema, furrows, and strictures to generate a score that has been clinically validated and used to assess efficacy of therapy[11,13] (**Fig. 1**). The presence of EREFS is not pathognomonic for EoE and a substantial number of patients will have normal or near normal appearance, thus it is important to biopsy if clinical suspicion exists.[38–40] Other features include mucosal fragility and narrow caliber esophagus.

Histology

Esophageal eosinophilia is the hallmark of EoE but not the only histologic feature. Eosinophil density is the most widely used histologic criterion expressed either as eosinophil load or peak eosinophil count (PEC). A PEC of 15 eos/HPF has 100% sensitivity in detecting EoE and specificity of 96%.[41] There is concern, however, that

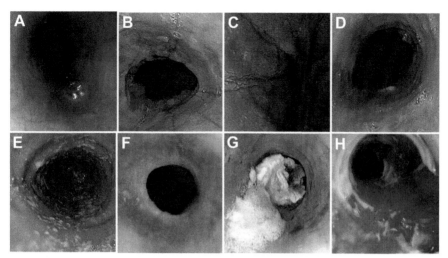

Fig. 1. Endoscopic findings in EoE. (*A*) Normal esophagus, mucosa is thin and smooth allowing visualization of blood vessels. (*B, C*) Edema and longitudinal furrows. (*D*) Rings and edema. (*E*) Narrow caliber esophagus and white exudates, (*F*) Stricture, (*G*) Food impaction. (*H*) Mucosal disruption following dilation.

reliance solely on esophageal density may miss other important indicators of disease severity such as barrier dysfunction and esophageal remodeling.[7–9] The EoE Histologic Scoring System (EoEHSS) was developed as a quantitative tool to measure efficacy in clinical practice and pharmacologic trials. It takes into account 8 different features of EoE including eosinophilic inflammation, basal zone hyperplasia, eosinophil abscesses, eosinophil surface layering, dilated intracellular spaces, surface epithelial alteration, dyskeratotic epithelial cells, and lamina propria fibrosis[42] (**Fig. 2**). A composite score is generated by rating the severity (grade) and extent of mucosal involvement (stage).[42] EoEHSS was found to have excellent intra- and inter-rater reliability and was shown to be highly sensitive to treatment in several recent clinical trials.[43–46] Before the EoEHSS can be incorporated into clinical practice, more research is needed to determine how EoEHSS correlates with EoE disease activity and clinical outcomes such as food impaction, fibrosis, and stricture formation.

Esophagram

Stricture formation and narrow caliber esophagus are fibrostenotic consequence of inflammation and the cause of dysphagia and food impaction. Many patients remain symptomatic despite resolution of esophageal inflammation. Remarkably, strictures are often missed with endoscopy and esophagram can serve as a complementary test that can assist in tailoring therapy.[33]

Functional Lumen Imaging Probe

Similar to esophagram, the functional lumen imaging probe (FLIP) can be a useful adjunct diagnostic test to endoscopy. FLIP uses high-resolution impedance planimetry to determine the three-dimensional geometry of the luminal esophagus, as well as distensibility of the esophageal wall as a function of progressive volume distension. FLIP can accurately measure esophageal diameter and wall stiffness and can be useful to detect fibrostenotic manifestations of EoE such as subtle strictures and narrow caliber esophagus. While upper endoscopy and esophagram and FLIP can assess

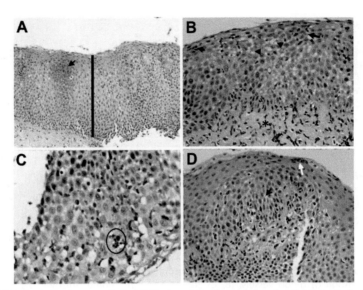

Fig. 2. Histologic Features or EoE. (*A*) Eosinophilia (*arrow*) basal cell hyperplasia (*bar*). (*B*) Eosinophilia (*arrow*), dilated intracellular spaces (*arrowhead*) and LP fibrosis (*asterisk*). (*C*) Eosinophilic abscesses (*circle*). (*D*) Eosinophilia dilated intracellular spaces (*black arrow*), eosinophilic surface layering and surface alteration (*white arrow*). Histology slides courtesy of Dr. Neeraja Kambham.

EoE-related fibrostenotic disease, only FLIP has been shown to accurately predict likelihood of food impaction.[47] In a prospective study of 70 patients with EoE, it was demonstrated that reduced distensibility was proportionally associated with need for dilation and increased risk of food impaction.[47] It has been suggested that FLIP can be used to monitor EoE disease activity and may correlate better with symptoms than histology.[48] FLIP, with ability to measure esophageal diameter and predict risk for food impactions, can allow for real-time decisions regarding need for dilation. FLIP is not widely available, thus limiting its use in the community setting. Establishing standard procedural techniques and stronger normative values will improve use of FLIP in routine management of EoE.

Mucosal Impedance

Mucosal impedance (MI), also referred to as mucosal integrity, measures epithelial cell barrier integrity and has been proposed as a test that can distinguish between GERD and EoE, which can be challenging.[49,50] MI is measured using a specialized balloon catheter in direct contact with the esophageal mucosa and is inversely proportional to barrier dysfunction. Therefore, MI is high in normal individuals, where esophageal mucosal barrier is intact compared with patients with GERD and EoE.[49,50] However, the distribution of barrier dysfunction differs such that patients with EoE exhibit low MI uniformly throughout the entire length of the esophagus (or with a patchy distribution of irregularity) compared with those with GERD, where MI is low in the distal esophagus and normalizes proximally.[51] This is a promising technology, but it is not yet widely available.

Minimally Invasive Esophageal Sampling Alternatives

The diagnosis of EoE requires interrogation of esophageal mucosa and histologic analysis. Endoscopy is invasive, associated with procedural and sedation/anesthesia risks, costly and inconvenient as patients have to take time off work. Furthermore, management of EoE may require multiple endoscopies. For these reasons, use of less invasive tests has been examined including, transnasal endoscopy, esophageal string test, and Cytosponge.[33] These tools are largely experimental and currently not widely used in clinical practice but may become options in the near future.

MANAGEMENT
Treatment Goals

After the diagnosis is established, the goals of therapy are as follows: (1) symptom resolution, (2) treatment of eosinophil-rich inflammation, and (3) prevention of fibrostenotic complications. Resolution of symptoms can be achieved by treatment of inflammation and fibrostenotic disease with the end points of esophageal eosinophilia $\leq$ 15 eos/hpf and esophageal luminal diameter greater than 15 mm.[3,4,52] The treatment of EoE can be summarized by "3 D's" as drugs, diet, and dilation.[53] As per current guidelines, PPI, topical steroids, and exclusion diets are all considered therapeutic options for first-line therapy. Choice depends on a variety of factors, including age, symptom severity, and lifestyle. Lack of response to one therapy leads to consideration of one of the remaining alternatives[3,4,20,54] **(Fig. 3)**. If patients progress to fibrosis, then dilation may be necessary to treat strictures and narrow caliber esophagus, which may not respond to pharmacologic intervention.[3,4,20]

Proton Pump Inhibitors

Distinguishing eosinophilia due to GERD versus EoE was at the heart of using response to PPIs as a diagnostic criterion for EoE.[17,18] However, it was recognized that the relationship between GERD and EoE is complex, and both entities can coexist in the same patient.[3,20] The efficacy of PPI in EoE has been reported in multiple

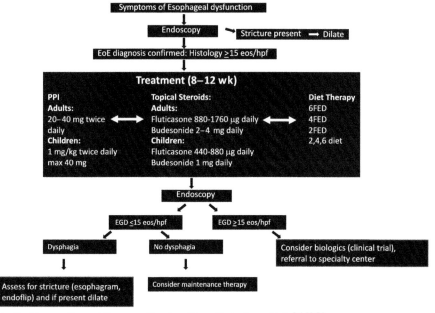

Fig. 3. Diagnostic and therapeutic algorithm. *Data from Refs* [3,4,20,54].

studies to be in the range of 33% to 50% depending on criteria used to define histo-logic remission (<5–7 eosinophils/HPF or < 15 eosinophils/HPF).[55,56] Both *in vivo* and *in vitro* studies suggest that the underlying mechanism for the efficacy of PPIs in EoE is anti-inflammatory and independent of their acid suppression qualities.[57] Analogous to topical steroids, PPIs downregulate expression of eotaxin-3 and other Th2-dependent cytokines in the esophageal mucosa.[57] Furthermore, PPIs were also shown to partially restore mucosal barrier dysfunction in *in vitro* studies using esophageal biopsies from patients with EoE.[58,59] A meta-analysis of 619 patients which included both children and adults found an overall histologic remission and clinical response of 50.5% and 60.8%, respectively.[60] Twice daily dosing was more effective than daily dosing.[60] Both European guidelines and the AGREE international consensus proposed PPIs as first-line therapy, recommending a dose of 20 to 40 mg twice daily for 8 weeks to induce remission.[3,20] Rank and colleagues in a technical review from the AGA Insti-tute and Joint Task Force on Allergy-Immunology Practice Parameters reported a response rate of 42% after evaluation of twenty-three observational studies; however, precise benefit was difficult to discern because studies were highly variable with re-gard to study design, patient selection criteria, PPI dosing, and trial duration.[61] Based on this, the latest AGA guidelines for active EoE downgraded PPI therapy to a condi-tional recommendation. Nonetheless, PPI can be suitable primary therapy for select patients. The safety profile and ease of administration is attractive to many patients compared with topical corticosteroids and dietary therapy.

Swallowed Topical Steroids

Multiple studies including placebo-controlled randomized clinical trials have demon-strated efficacy of swallowed topical steroids (STEs) in various forms in inducing his-tologic and symptomatic remission.[34,62,63] Early concerns for long-term safety limited their use; however, available evidence suggests that chronic use of these agents is safe and well tolerated.[3,4,64–67] Adrenal suppression was of concern in children where is it is reported to be a rare complication.[68] A recent systematic review found that the risk of adrenal insufficiency was low and reported mostly in small uncontrolled obser-vational studies but not in high quality ones.[69] Candidal esophagitis is the most com-mon adverse effect of STEs; however, it is usually mild, and patients are frequently asymptomatic.[66]

Currently in the United States, there is no FDA-approved pharmacologic therapy for EoE and ingested STE formulations designed to be inhaled for the treatment of asthma are often used in clinical practice. Fluticasone meter dose inhaler at a dose of 220 mcg 2 puffs twice a day is a common treatment.[33,70] However, patients often have difficulty swallowing the medication directly from the inhaler and thus distribution to the esoph-agus can be affected. Dellon and colleagues showed that a viscous slurry of budeso-nide performed better than a nebulized form for the treatment of EoE in a prospective study.[71] This was attributed to the distribution and duration of exposure of the esoph-ageal mucosa to the drug. Scintigraphy demonstrated that the nebulized form had lower contact time with esophageal mucosa and was present more in the lungs compared with viscous form. In a subsequent study, it appears that this could be over-come by increasing the drug dose and providing patients with instructions to maxi-mize esophageal contact and decrease lung exposure.[72] Budesonide slurry at a dose of 1 mg twice daily is indeed an effective therapy, but the formulation that is currently available is for nebulization which is required for treating asthma.[33,70] To in-crease the viscosity and improve esophageal contact time, patients are asked to mix the budesonide liquid with sucralose or honey. This is cumbersome, inconvenient, and unpalatable to many patients leading to medication nonadherence. To improve delivery of the drug to the esophagus and ease of use, multiple STE formulations designed to be swallowed have been under investigation including an oral dispersible fluticasone tablet and budesonide in the form of effervescent tablet and premixed solution. All have been found to be safe and highly effective in clinical trials.[70,73] Some of these have already been approved in Europe and will hopefully be available in the United States soon.

Rank and colleagues, evaluated eight double-blind placebo-controlled studies involving 437 patients that tested efficacy of topical budesonide and fluticasone formulations.[61] These trials included both investigational STE designed for esophageal delivery (tablet or fluid) and ingested STEs that were intended for treatment of asthma as discussed previously. Histologic remission was achieved in two-thirds of patients compared with less than 15% in patients treated with placebo (RR: 0.39; 95% CI: 0.26–0.58).[61] The 2020 AGA guidelines designated STE as a strong recommendation for treatment of EoE based on moderate quality evidence.[4]

Dietary Therapy

Dietary exclusion therapy is an effective treatment alternative to PPI and STE for the treatment of EoE. Three dietary approaches including elemental diet, empiric elimination diet, and allergy testing–directed elimination diet have been used. Elemental diet, which eliminates all food except for an amino acid formula, is the most efficacious (94%); however, it is limited by poor adherence and high cost.[74] Empiric elimination diets, involving systematic elimination of the most common food allergens, are attractive to patients who are concerned with medication side effects and who are interested in an intervention aimed at the "root cause" of the disease. The six-food elimination diet (6FED) is most standard dietary EoE therapy. In this approach, patients simultaneously exclude the 6 most common allergens associated with EoE (dairy, wheat, eggs, soy, nuts, and sea food) for 6 to 8 weeks.[75–77] If histologic remission is achieved, this is followed by systematic reintroduction of food items and repeat endoscopy to identify a patient's specific food trigger(s). In general food items statistically most likely to induce a reaction (gluten and dairy) are reintroduced last.[75] The sequence of food introduction may also be influenced by patient's historic response to the various food items. Although less effective than the elemental diet, the aggregate efficacy rate was reported to be 72.1% in a meta-analysis published in 2014.[78] The disadvantages of this approach include cost, inconvenience, and risk of multiple endoscopies.

Given the restrictive nature of 6FED diets, diets requiring exclusion of fewer food items have been explored. Cow's milk, wheat, egg, and soy were identified as allergens most likely to trigger inflammation.[75] Kagalwalla and colleagues assessed the efficacy of a diet eliminating these four food items [four food elimination diet (4FED)] in 78 children with persistent eosinophilia following an 8-week PPI trial.[79] The response rate was 68%. Reintroduction of food items identified milk as the most potent trigger, eliciting eosinophilia in 85% of patients.[79] Other studies have explored the efficacy of eliminating just a single item of milk [one food elimination diet (1FED)].[80,81] In one study involving 17 children, eliminating dairy resulted in a remission rate of 65% in children.[80] Another study that directly compared 1FED with a 4FED found similar histologic remission rates 44% with 1FED versus 41.2% in 4FED and comparable improvement of symptom scores.[81] These studies were limited by low sample size and although results are promising, studies involving more patients and validation in adults are required to understand the true efficacy of 1FED.

In 2018, Molina-Infante et al investigated the use of a structured and sequential dietary exclusion approach referred to as "2-4-6 diet".[82] One hundred thirty patients with EoE were first subjected to 2FED diet (dairy and gluten). The diet was broadened to 4FED in nonresponders (additional elimination of eggs and legumes) and then full 6FED in those who continued to exhibit active inflammation. The overall remission rate was 79%, with 43% achieving remission with exclusion of dairy and wheat alone.[82] Shared decision-making with your patient is recommended when deciding the appropriate dietary therapy approach (**Fig. 4**).

The rationale behind allergy testing–directed diet is that elimination of allergens identified by conventional allergy tests would effectively treat EoE. However, allergy testing has been unreliable and either no better or less efficacious than empiric diets.[78]

Maintenance Therapy

EoE is a progressive chronic disease, where spontaneous resolution is very rare and natural history studies indicate that continued inflammation results in fibrostenosis. An argument has been made for maintenance therapy because stopping treatment results in relapse in most patients.[66] Straumann and colleagues treated 28 patients with EoE who were in clinical remission with 0.25 mg twice daily or placebo for a period of 50 weeks and found that while higher than the placebo-treated patients, only 50% of those in the treatment arm maintained a complete or partial remission.[67] The most compelling evidence in support of maintenance therapy comes from a 48-week, placebo-controlled, randomized study of 204 patients using varying doses of budesonide oral-dispersible tablet (BOT).[83] The efficacy of 1 mg BID (full treatment dose) and 0.5 mg BID dosing in maintaining remission was similar (75% vs 73.5%, respectively) compared with placebo (4.4%).[83] The fact that a quarter of subjects treated with full treatment dose failed to maintain a remission suggests loss of response to steroids. The study lacks generalizability, given that the formulation used is only available in

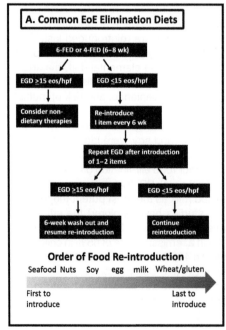
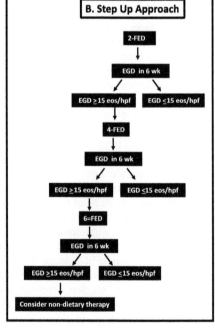

Fig. 4. Dietary therapeutic approaches.

Europe and dosing may not apply to currently available formulations in the United States. Shared decision-making between physician and patient is recommended and should include discussion about the pros and cons of long-term topical steroids (**Table 2**).

PPIs and elimination diet can also be considered for maintenance therapy; however, they have not been well studied for this use. For dietary therapy, there are reports that after food elimination, patients can experience de novo IgE-mediated reactions in the reintroduction phase; however, this seems to be very rare.[4] In PPI, responders using the lowest effective dose for maintenance have been reported.[20]

Dilation

In many patients with EoE, the risk of discrete strictures and narrow caliber esophagus rises with disease duration.[12] Pharmacologic therapy and diet address inflammation but do not reverse fibrosis which may explain persistence of symptoms despite effective treatment of inflammation. Dilation is an effective treatment for fibrostenotic disease in EoE. The goal of dilation is lumen diameter of 15 to 18 mm, which allows patients to tolerate a regular diet free of dysphagia in most cases.[52,84] Early studies indicated that dilation posed significant risk of perforation and was recommended against in the initial guidelines. However, more recent studies have shown that by adopting a more conservative approach, esophageal dilation is safe and effective with risk of serious complications estimated to be less than 1%.[52,84–86] Both balloon and bougie dilations have proven to be effective, although savary dilations are preferred by many to treat long strictures. The duration of symptoms relief is variable, but a recent metanalysis reported that three-quarters of patients with EoE who underwent dilation had durable resolution of dysphagia.[87] Severe chest pain following dilation is common and thus patients should be warned about it, and pain should be managed with pain medications if necessary.[52]

FUTURE DIRECTIONS

A deeper understanding of the molecular basis of EoE has led to the discovery of several potential therapeutic targets. IL-5 is one such target, given its role in eosinophil development and maturation. Unfortunately, results from three randomized clinical trials using agents designed to block IL-5 (mepolizumab and reslizumab) were disappointing with less than 10% of subjects achieving histologic remission and none

Table 2
Pros/cons of maintenance therapy with topical steroids

Pro	Cons
Highly effective inducing histologic remission	Costly
Highly effective at treating symptoms	Lack of long-term safety data
May decrease need for dilation	Risk of Candida esophagitis
Reduces risk of relapse	No FDA approved formulation
	Inconvenient
	Potential for steroid resistance
	Unclear benefit in patients with mild disease phenotype
	Ideal maintenance dose is unknown

experiencing improvement of symptoms[4,73,88] Anti-IgE has also been studied as a potential therapy but was not found to be efficacious either histologically or symptomatically.[4,73,88] IL-4 and IL-13 are also attractive targets, given the central role of these cytokines in eosinophil production and trafficking to the esophageal mucosa. Three different agents have been investigated, QAX570 and RPC4046, both monoclonal antibodies that block IL-13, and dupilumab, a monoclonal antibody the blocks the receptor to IL-4α. Although QAX576 was not found to be effective in clinical trials, a phase II trial on RPC4046 found the agent to significantly improve histologic and endoscopic disease activity.[4,73,88] A phase II trial on dupilumab also had positive results demonstrating improvement in dysphagia symptoms and histology compared with placebo.[4,73,88] Phase III trials on both of these agents are either currently underway (dupilumab) or about to start (RPC4046), suggesting that biologic therapies may be available for patients with EoE in the near future.

SUMMARY

The field of EoE has rapidly evolved in the last two decades, and now there is a better understanding of the pathophysiology, natural history, relationship to GERD, and efficacy of various treatments. However, significant knowledge gaps remain that are the focus of ongoing investigation. PPIs, STE, and exclusion diets are all appropriate first-line therapies, and the decision of which therapy to use is largely driven by patient preference. The implementation of less invasive modalities to monitor disease activity such as transnasal endoscopy, Cytosponge, and string test should allow easier optimization of therapy, especially with regard to tailoring dietary therapy. Ideally, prospective natural history studies, aided by biomarkers, will help predict disease course and identify patients who will benefit from a particular therapy. The hope is that better characterization of EoE disease phenotypes will lead to a more personalized and targeted therapeutic approach.

CLINICS CARE POINTS

- EoE is a chronic disease that is left untreated leads to fibrosis and development of strictures, resulting in dysphagia and food impaction.
- Definition of EoE no longer requires PPI response as a diagnostic criterion.
- PPI, swallowed topical steroids, and dietary elimination therapy are all appropriate first line.
- Shared decision-making between physician and patient is important when choosing therapy.
- 4-Food and 6-food elimination and step-up 2,4,6 diet are different but effective strategies for dietary treatment.
- Novel pharmacologic therapies are under development.

DISCLOSURE

The author has nothing to disclose.

REFERENCES

1. Dellon ES, Gonsalves N, Hirano I, et al. ACG clinical guideline: evidenced based approach to the diagnosis and management of esophageal eosinophilia and eosinophilic esophagitis (EoE). Am J Gastroenterol 2013;108(5):679–92, quiz 693.

2. Dellon ES, Liacouras CA. Advances in clinical management of eosinophilic esophagitis. Gastroenterology 2014;147(6):1238–54.
3. Dellon ES, Liacouras CA, Molina-Infante J, et al. Updated international consensus diagnostic criteria for eosinophilic esophagitis: proceedings of the AGREE conference. Gastroenterology 2018;155(4):1022–1033 e1010.
4. Hirano I, Chan ES, Rank MA, et al. AGA institute and the joint task force on allergy-immunology practice parameters clinical guidelines for the management of eosinophilic esophagitis. Gastroenterology 2020;158(6):1776–86.
5. Jensen ET, Kappelman MD, Martin CF, et al. Health-care utilization, costs, and the burden of disease related to eosinophilic esophagitis in the United States. Am J Gastroenterol 2015;110(5):626–32.
6. Capucilli P, Hill DA. Allergic comorbidity in eosinophilic esophagitis: mechanistic relevance and clinical implications. Clin Rev Allergy Immunol 2019;57(1):111–27.
7. Davis BP. Pathophysiology of eosinophilic esophagitis. Clin Rev Allergy Immunol 2018;55(1):19–42.
8. O'Shea KM, Aceves SS, Dellon ES, et al. Pathophysiology of eosinophilic esophagitis. Gastroenterology 2018;154(2):333–45.
9. Sherrill JD, Rothenberg ME. Genetic and epigenetic underpinnings of eosinophilic esophagitis. Gastroenterol Clin North Am 2014;43(2):269–80.
10. Ryu S, Lee KH, Tizaoui K, et al. Pathogenesis of eosinophilic esophagitis: a comprehensive review of the genetic and molecular aspects. Int J Mol Sci 2020;21(19).
11. Dellon ES, Cotton CC, Gebhart JH, et al. Accuracy of the eosinophilic esophagitis endoscopic reference score in diagnosis and determining response to treatment. Clin Gastroenterol Hepatol 2016;14(1):31–9.
12. Dellon ES, Hirano I. Epidemiology and natural history of eosinophilic esophagitis. Gastroenterology 2018;154(2):319–32.e313.
13. Hirano I. Role of advanced diagnostics for eosinophilic esophagitis. Dig Dis 2014;32(1–2):78–83.
14. Dellon ES, Kim HP, Sperry SL, et al. A phenotypic analysis shows that eosinophilic esophagitis is a progressive fibrostenotic disease. Gastrointest Endosc 2014; 79(4):577–85.e574.
15. Schoepfer AM, Safroneeva E, Bussmann C, et al. Delay in diagnosis of eosinophilic esophagitis increases risk for stricture formation in a time-dependent manner. Gastroenterology 2013;145(6):1230–6, e1231-1232.
16. Warners MJ, Oude Nijhuis RAB, de Wijkerslooth LRH, et al. The natural course of eosinophilic esophagitis and long-term consequences of undiagnosed disease in a large cohort. Am J Gastroenterol 2018;113(6):836–44.
17. Furuta GT, Liacouras CA, Collins MH, et al. Eosinophilic esophagitis in children and adults: a systematic review and consensus recommendations for diagnosis and treatment. Gastroenterology 2007;133(4):1342–63.
18. Liacouras CA, Furuta GT, Hirano I, et al. Eosinophilic esophagitis: updated consensus recommendations for children and adults. J Allergy Clin Immunol 2011;128(1):3–20.e26, quiz 21-22.
19. Dellon ES, Speck O, Woodward K, et al. Clinical and endoscopic characteristics do not reliably differentiate PPI-responsive esophageal eosinophilia and eosinophilic esophagitis in patients undergoing upper endoscopy: a prospective cohort study. Am J Gastroenterol 2013;108(12):1854–60.
20. Lucendo AJ, Molina-Infante J, Arias Á, et al. Guidelines on eosinophilic esophagitis: evidence-based statements and recommendations for diagnosis and management in children and adults. United European Gastroenterol J 2017;5:335–58.

21. Moawad FJ, Schoepfer AM, Safroneeva E, et al. Eosinophilic oesophagitis and proton pump inhibitor-responsive oesophageal eosinophilia have similar clinical, endoscopic and histological findings. Aliment Pharmacol Ther 2014;39(6):603–8.

22. Navarro P, Arias A, Arias-Gonzalez L, et al. Systematic review with meta-analysis: the growing incidence and prevalence of eosinophilic oesophagitis in children and adults in population-based studies. Aliment Pharmacol Ther 2019;49(9): 1116–25.

23. Dellon ES, Erichsen R, Baron JA, et al. The increasing incidence and prevalence of eosinophilic oesophagitis outpaces changes in endoscopic and biopsy practice: national population-based estimates from Denmark. Aliment Pharmacol Ther 2015;41(7):662–70.

24. Hruz P, Straumann A, Bussmann C, et al. Escalating incidence of eosinophilic esophagitis: a 20-year prospective, population-based study in Olten County, Switzerland. J Allergy Clin Immunol 2011;128(6):1349–50, e1345.

25. Prasad GA, Alexander JA, Schleck CD, et al. Epidemiology of eosinophilic esophagitis over three decades in Olmsted County, Minnesota. Clin Gastroenterol Hepatol 2009;7(10):1055–61.

26. van Rhijn BD, Verheij J, Smout AJ, et al. Rapidly increasing incidence of eosinophilic esophagitis in a large cohort. Neurogastroenterol Motil 2013;25(1): 47–52.e45.

27. Arias A, Perez-Martinez I, Tenias JM, et al. Systematic review with meta-analysis: the incidence and prevalence of eosinophilic oesophagitis in children and adults in population-based studies. Aliment Pharmacol Ther 2016;43(1):3–15.

28. de Rooij WE, Barendsen ME, Warners MJ, et al. Emerging incidence trends of eosinophilic esophagitis over 25 years: results of a nationwide register-based pathology cohort. Neurogastroenterol Motil 2021;e14072.

29. Kapel RC, Miller JK, Torres C, et al. Eosinophilic esophagitis: a prevalent disease in the United States that affects all age groups. Gastroenterology 2008;134(5): 1316–21.

30. Katzka DA. Eosinophilic esophagitis. Ann Intern Med 2020;172(9):ITC65–80.

31. Hill DA, Dudley JW, Spergel JM. The prevalence of eosinophilic esophagitis in pediatric patients with IgE-mediated food allergy. J Allergy Clin Immunol Pract 2017; 5(2):369–75.

32. Dellon ES, Gibbs WB, Fritchie KJ, et al. Clinical, endoscopic, and histologic findings distinguish eosinophilic esophagitis from gastroesophageal reflux disease. Clin Gastroenterol Hepatol 2009;7(12):1305–13, quiz 1261.

33. Straumann A, Katzka DA. Diagnosis and treatment of eosinophilic esophagitis. Gastroenterology 2018;154(2):346–59.

34. Dellon ES, Katzka DA, Collins MH, et al. Budesonide oral suspension improves symptomatic, endoscopic, and histologic parameters compared with placebo in patients with eosinophilic esophagitis. Gastroenterology 2017;152(4): 776–86.e775.

35. Sallis BF, Acar U, Hawthorne K, et al. A distinct esophageal mRNA pattern identifies eosinophilic esophagitis patients with food impactions. Front Immunol 2018; 9:2059.

36. Alexander R, Alexander JA, Ravi K, et al. Measurement of observed eating behaviors in patients with active and inactive eosinophilic esophagitis. Clin Gastroenterol Hepatol 2019;17(11):2371–3.

37. Nielsen JA, Lager DJ, Lewin M, et al. The optimal number of biopsy fragments to establish a morphologic diagnosis of eosinophilic esophagitis. Am J Gastroenterol 2014;109(4):515–20.

38. Enns R, Kazemi P, Chung W, et al. Eosinophilic esophagitis: clinical features, endoscopic findings and response to treatment. Can J Gastroenterol 2010; 24(9):547–51.
39. Rodriguez-Sanchez J, Barrio-Andres J, Nantes Castillejo O, et al. The endoscopic reference score shows modest accuracy to predict either clinical or histological activity in adult patients with eosinophilic oesophagitis. Aliment Pharmacol Ther 2017;45(2):300–9.
40. van Rhijn BD, Verheij J, Smout AJ, et al. The endoscopic reference score shows modest accuracy to predict histologic remission in adult patients with eosinophilic esophagitis. Neurogastroenterol Motil 2016;28(11):1714–22.
41. Dellon ES, Speck O, Woodward K, et al. Distribution and variability of esophageal eosinophilia in patients undergoing upper endoscopy. Mod Pathol 2015;28(3): 383–90.
42. Collins MH, Martin LJ, Alexander ES, et al. Newly developed and validated eosinophilic esophagitis histology scoring system and evidence that it outperforms peak eosinophil count for disease diagnosis and monitoring. Dis Esophagus 2017;30(3):1–8.
43. Conner JR, Kirsch R. Editorial: validating reliability of the eosinophilic oesophagitis histological scoring system (EOE-HSS)-an important first step. Aliment Pharmacol Ther 2018;47(12):1713–4.
44. Hirano I, Collins MH, Assouline-Dayan Y, et al. RPC4046, a Monoclonal Antibody Against IL13, Reduces Histologic and Endoscopic Activity in Patients With Eosinophilic Esophagitis. Gastroenterology 2019;156(3):592–603.e510.
45. Hirano I, Safroneeva E, Roumet MC, et al. Randomised clinical trial: the safety and tolerability of fluticasone propionate orally disintegrating tablets versus placebo for eosinophilic oesophagitis. Aliment Pharmacol Ther 2020.
46. Warners MJ, Ambarus CA, Bredenoord AJ, et al. Reliability of histologic assessment in patients with eosinophilic oesophagitis. Aliment Pharmacol Ther 2018; 47(7):940–50.
47. Nicodeme F, Hirano I, Chen J, et al. Esophageal distensibility as a measure of disease severity in patients with eosinophilic esophagitis. Clin Gastroenterol Hepatol 2013;11(9):1101–7.e1101.
48. Carlson DA, Hirano I, Zalewski A, et al. Improvement in esophageal distensibility in response to medical and diet therapy in eosinophilic esophagitis. Clin Transl Gastroenterol 2017;8(10):e119.
49. Barrett C, Choksi Y, Vaezi MF. Mucosal impedance: a new approach to diagnosing gastroesophageal reflux disease and eosinophilic esophagitis. Curr Gastroenterol Rep 2018;20(7):33.
50. Katzka DA, Ravi K, Geno DM, et al. Endoscopic mucosal impedance measurements correlate with eosinophilia and dilation of intercellular spaces in patients with eosinophilic esophagitis. Clin Gastroenterol Hepatol 2015;13(7): 1242–8.e1241.
51. Ates F, Yuksel ES, Higginbotham T, et al. Mucosal impedance discriminates GERD from non-GERD conditions. Gastroenterology 2015;148(2):334–43.
52. Richter JE. Eosinophilic esophagitis dilation in the community–try it–you will like it–but start low and go slow. Am J Gastroenterol 2016;111(2):214–6.
53. Singla MB, Moawad FJ. An overview of the diagnosis and management of eosinophilic esophagitis. Clin Transl Gastroenterol 2016;7:e155.
54. de Rooij WE, Dellon ES, Parker CE, et al. Pharmacotherapies for the treatment of eosinophilic esophagitis: state of the art review. Drugs 2019;79(13):1419–34.

55. Moawad FJ, Cheatham JG, DeZee KJ. Meta-analysis: the safety and efficacy of dilation in eosinophilic oesophagitis. Aliment Pharmacol Ther 2013;38(7):713–20.

56. Vazquez-Elizondo G, Ngamruengphong S, Khrisna M, et al. The outcome of patients with oesophageal eosinophilic infiltration after an eight-week trial of a proton pump inhibitor. Aliment Pharmacol Ther 2013;38:1312–9.

57. Molina-Infante J, Rivas MD, Hernandez-Alonso M, et al. Proton pump inhibitor-responsive oesophageal eosinophilia correlates with downregulation of eotaxin-3 and Th2 cytokines overexpression. Aliment Pharmacol Ther 2014;40:955–65.

58. Van Malenstein H, Farré R, Sifrim D. Esophageal dilated intercellular spaces (DIS) and nonerosive reflux disease. Am J Gastroenterol 2008;103:1021–8.

59. van Rhijn BD, Weijenborg PW, Verheij J, et al. Proton pump inhibitors partially restore mucosal integrity in patients with proton pump inhibitor-responsive esophageal eosinophilia but not eosinophilic esophagitis. Clin Gastroenterol Hepatol 2014;12(11):1815–1823 e1812.

60. Lucendo AJ, Arias Á, Molina-Infante J. Efficacy of proton pump inhibitor drugs for inducing clinical and histologic remission in patients with symptomatic esophageal eosinophilia: a systematic review and meta-analysis. Clin Gastroenterol Hepatol 2016;14:13–22.e11.

61. Rank MA, Sharaf RN, Furuta GT, et al. Technical review on the management of eosinophilic esophagitis: a report from the AGA institute and the joint task force on allergy-immunology practice parameters. Gastroenterology 2020;158(6): 1789–810.e1715.

62. Miehlke S, Hruz P, Vieth M, et al. A randomised, double-blind trial comparing budesonide formulations and dosages for short-term treatment of eosinophilic oesophagitis. Gut 2016;65(3):390–9.

63. Straumann A, Conus S, Degen L, et al. Budesonide is effective in adolescent and adult patients with active eosinophilic esophagitis. Gastroenterology 2010; 139(5):1526–37, 1537.e1521.

64. Greuter T, Bussmann C, Safroneeva E, et al. Long-term treatment of eosinophilic esophagitis with swallowed topical corticosteroids: development and evaluation of a therapeutic concept. Am J Gastroenterol 2017;112(10):1527–35.

65. Gupta SK, Vitanza JM, Collins MH. Efficacy and safety of oral budesonide suspension in pediatric patients with eosinophilic esophagitis. Clin Gastroenterol Hepatol 2015;13(1):66–76.e63.

66. Philpott H, Dellon ES. The role of maintenance therapy in eosinophilic esophagitis: who, why, and how? J Gastroenterol 2018;53(2):165–71.

67. Straumann A, Conus S, Degen L, et al. Long-term budesonide maintenance treatment is partially effective for patients with eosinophilic esophagitis. Clin Gastroenterol Hepatol 2011;9(5):400–9.e401.

68. Hsu S, Wood C, Pan Z, et al. Adrenal insufficiency in pediatric eosinophilic esophagitis patients treated with swallowed topical steroids. Pediatr Allergy Immunol Pulmonol 2017;30(3):135–40.

69. Philpott H, Dougherty MK, Reed CC, et al. Systematic review: adrenal insufficiency secondary to swallowed topical corticosteroids in eosinophilic oesophagitis. Aliment Pharmacol Ther 2018;47(8):1071–8.

70. Reed CC, Dellon ES. Eosinophilic esophagitis. Med Clin North Am 2019;103(1): 29–42.

71. Dellon ES, Sheikh A, Speck O, et al. Viscous topical is more effective than nebulized steroid therapy for patients with eosinophilic esophagitis. Gastroenterology 2012;143(2):321–4.e321.

72. Dellon ES, Woosley JT, Arrington A, et al. Efficacy of budesonide vs fluticasone for initial treatment of eosinophilic esophagitis in a randomized controlled trial. Gastroenterology 2019;157(1):65–73.e65.
73. Patel RV, Hirano I, Gonsalves N. Eosinophilic esophagitis: etiology and therapy. Annu Rev Med 2021;72:183–97.
74. Peterson KA, Byrne KR, Vinson LA, et al. Elemental diet induces histologic response in adult eosinophilic esophagitis. Am J Gastroenterol 2013;108(5):759–66.
75. Doerfler B, Bryce P, Hirano I, et al. Practical approach to implementing dietary therapy in adults with eosinophilic esophagitis: the Chicago experience. Dis Esophagus 2015;28(1):42–58.
76. Gonsalves N, Yang GY, Doerfler B, et al. Elimination diet effectively treats eosinophilic esophagitis in adults; food reintroduction identifies causative factors. Gastroenterology 2012;142(7):1451–9.e1451, quiz e1414-1455.
77. Kagalwalla AF, Shah A, Li BU, et al. Identification of specific foods responsible for inflammation in children with eosinophilic esophagitis successfully treated with empiric elimination diet. J Pediatr Gastroenterol Nutr 2011;53(2):145–9.
78. Arias A, Gonzalez-Cervera J, Tenias JM, et al. Efficacy of dietary interventions for inducing histologic remission in patients with eosinophilic esophagitis: a systematic review and meta-analysis. Gastroenterology 2014;146(7):1639–48.
79. Kagalwalla AF, Wechsler JB, Amsden K, et al. Efficacy of a 4-food elimination diet for children with eosinophilic esophagitis. Clin Gastroenterol Hepatol 2017;15(11):1698–707.e1697.
80. Kagalwalla AF, Amsden K, Shah A, et al. Cow's milk elimination: a novel dietary approach to treat eosinophilic esophagitis. J Pediatr Gastroenterol Nutr 2012;55(6):711–6.
81. Kliewer K, AS, Atkins D, et al. Efficacy of 1-food and 4-food elimination diets for pediatric eosinophilic esophagitis in a randomized multi-site study. Gastroenterology 2019;156(6):S-172.
82. Molina-Infante J, Arias A, Alcedo J, et al. Step-up empiric elimination diet for pediatric and adult eosinophilic esophagitis: the 2-4-6 study. J Allergy Clin Immunol 2018;141(4):1365–72.
83. Straumann A, Lucendo AJ, Miehlke S, et al. Budesonide orodispersible tablets maintain remission in a randomized, placebo-controlled trial of patients with eosinophilic esophagitis. Gastroenterology 2020;159(5):1672–85.e1675.
84. Schoepfer A. Treatment of eosinophilic esophagitis by dilation. Dig Dis 2014;32(1–2):130–3.
85. Alexander J. Esophageal dilation in eosinophilic esophagitis. Tech Gastrointest Endosc 2014;16(16):26–31.
86. Runge TM, Eluri S, Cotton CC, et al. Outcomes of esophageal dilation in eosinophilic esophagitis: safety, efficacy, and persistence of the fibrostenotic phenotype. Am J Gastroenterol 2016;111(2):206–13.
87. Moawad FJ, Molina-Infante J, Lucendo AJ, et al. Systematic review with meta-analysis: endoscopic dilation is highly effective and safe in children and adults with eosinophilic oesophagitis. Aliment Pharmacol Ther 2017;46(2):96–105.
88. Olivieri B, Tinazzi E, Caminati M, et al. Biologics for the treatment of allergic conditions: eosinophil disorders. Immunol Allergy Clin N Am 2020;40(4):649–65.

Functional Chest Pain and Esophageal Hypersensitivity
A Clinical Approach

Richa Bhardwaj, MBBS[a], Rita Knotts, MD, MSc[b],
Abraham Khan, MD[b],*

KEYWORDS

- Esophageal • Hypersensitivity • Functional • Heartburn • Chest pain

KEY POINTS

- Functional chest pain, functional heartburn, and reflux hypersensitivity are defined by Rome IV criteria based on symptom duration for 3 months with onset at least 6 months before and relies on results of objective diagnostic testing
- The spectrum of therapy for functional heartburn and functional chest pain should focus on patient education and pharmacologic neuromodulation, which helps to modulate neural perceptions from peripheral and central sensitization, as well as relaxation strategies and psychological interventions such as gut-directed hypnotherapy and cognitive behavioral therapy
- The treatment of reflux hypersensitivity should focus on acid suppression and selective serotonin reuptake inhibitors, along with psychogastroenterology approaches.

INTRODUCTION

Functional esophageal disorders are characterized by typical esophageal symptoms that are not explained by structural disorders, histopathology-based motor disturbances, or gastroesophageal reflux disease (GERD).[1] These disease conditions lead to significant impairment of quality of life and result in a considerable economic burden on the health care system.[2] The Rome IV criteria describe 5 distinct functional esophageal disorders that include functional chest pain, functional heartburn, reflux hypersensitivity, globus, and functional dysphagia.[3,4]

Given that these patients present with potential GERD symptoms, thoughtful consideration of all factors that may contribute to disease pathology allows for increased diagnostic accuracy and further stratification into a particular GERD phenotype. This review focuses on functional chest pain, functional heartburn, and reflux

[a] Department of Internal Medicine, Lenox Hill Hospital, 100 East 77th Street, New York, NY 10075, USA; [b] Department of Medicine, NYU Langone Health, 240 East 38th Street, 23rd Floor, New York, NY 10016, USA
* Corresponding author.
E-mail address: Abraham.khan@nyulangone.org

Gastroenterol Clin N Am 50 (2021) 843–857
https://doi.org/10.1016/j.gtc.2021.08.004
0889-8553/21/© 2021 Elsevier Inc. All rights reserved.

hypersensitivity, including the approach to diagnosis, pathogenesis, and an evidence-based approach to treatment.

DEFINITIONS

The Rome IV criteria were introduced in 2016 and are defined primarily by symptoms along with results of specific diagnostic testing. The Rome IV criteria[3] for functional chest pain, heartburn, and reflux hypersensitivity are defined as follows:

Functional Chest Pain

Functional chest pain is recurring, unexplained retrosternal chest pain of presumed esophageal origin, not explained based on reflux disease, other mucosal or motor processes, and representing pain different from heartburn with frequency at least once a week.

Functional Heartburn

Functional heartburn is defined as retrosternal burning, discomfort or pain refractory to optimal antisecretory therapy in the absence of GERD, histopathologic mucosal abnormalities, major motor disorders, or structural explanations with frequency at least twice a week.

Reflux Hypersensitivity

Patients with esophageal symptoms (heartburn or chest pain) who lack evidence of reflux on endoscopy or abnormal acid burden on reflux monitoring but show triggering of symptoms by physiologic reflux, with frequency at least twice a week.

All these disorders must have criteria fulfilled for 3 months with symptom onset at least 6 months before diagnosis (**Table 1**). Each of the disorders is characterized by an absence of a major esophageal motor disorder, eosinophilic esophagitis, and pathologic GERD as defined by ambulatory pH testing. Thus, the diagnostic evaluation for all these conditions would include upper endoscopy with histopathology assessment of esophageal biopsies, high-resolution esophageal manometry, and ambulatory reflux monitoring.

APPROACH TO DIAGNOSIS

When evaluating a patient, a thorough clinical history is crucial in elucidating the characteristics that define a particular GERD phenotype. An initial consultation should focus on clinical symptoms, known anatomic defects such as a hiatal hernia as well as comorbid conditions which may alter esophageal motility (eg, scleroderma, obesity). Particularly among patients with complaints of chest pain, an evaluation must be performed to exclude cardiac etiology before further evaluation of reflux-induced causes. An initial survey of symptom-specific anxiety, psychological comorbidity, and hypervigilance should be conducted because this may also identify therapeutic targets. Accurately characterizing esophageal symptoms is vital, especially in the early phases of management, as esophageal motility disorders such as achalasia or behavioral disorders such as rumination or supragastric belching can frequently masquerade as gastroesophageal reflux.

Guidelines recommend an 8-week proton pump inhibitor (PPI) trial for typical symptoms of GERD in the absence of alarm signs (dysphagia, odynophagia, anemia, weight loss) to assess for resolution of symptoms.[5] When unresponsive to a PPI trial, an endoscopic evaluation should be performed and can uncover objective evidence of pathologic GERD if erosive esophagitis (Los Angeles Grade C or D), Barrett's

Table 1
Defining functional chest pain, functional heartburn, and reflux hypersensitivity as per Rome IV

Diagnosis	Symptom Presentation	Need for Medication Trial	Results of Reflux Testing	Endoscopic Findings	Other Features
Functional chest pain	Retrosternal chest pain or discomfort after exclusion of cardiac causes Absence of associated esophageal symptoms such as heartburn and dysphagia		Absence of evidence that gastroesophageal reflux is cause for symptoms	Normal endoscopy	Absence of major esophageal motor disorders AND No evidence of eosinophilic esophagitis as the cause for symptoms
Functional heartburn	Burning retrosternal discomfort or pain	No symptom relief despite optimal antisecretory therapy			
Reflux hypersensitivity	Retrosternal symptoms including heartburn and chest pain		Evidence of triggering of symptoms by reflux events despite normal acid exposure on pH or pH–impedance monitoring (response to antisecretory therapy does not exclude the diagnosis)		

esophagus, or a peptic stricture is found and can rule out alternative diagnoses such as eosinophilic esophagitis, peptic ulcer disease, or mechanical obstruction.[6] When endoscopy fails to yield a diagnosis or in the setting of extraesophageal symptoms, ambulatory reflux monitoring is recommended.[5,7] Ambulatory reflux monitoring with the addition of a 48 to 96 hour wireless pH capsule can be performed during initial endoscopy to confirm the presence of abnormal esophageal acid exposure and can be a powerful addition to increase diagnostic yield.[8] Of note, patients with chest pain may perceive the capsule when attached to the esophagus, and this should be discussed before the procedure is undertaken. Combined transnasal pH-impedance testing is an additional means of ambulatory reflux monitoring and has utility in the assessment of extraesophageal symptoms or among patients who present after a recent endoscopic evaluation. Esophageal motility testing may also be performed with transnasal pH monitoring or if suspicion is high for an alternative esophageal motility disorder as an etiology of symptoms. A postprandial high-resolution manometry can be a practically useful tool to uncover rumination in a patient presenting with regurgitation mischaracterized as GERD.[9]

When performing ambulatory pH testing (wireless pH testing or pH-impedance testing) off of antisecretory therapy, esophageal acid exposure time greater than 6.0% is considered pathologic and acid exposure time less than 4.0% is considered physiologic, with borderline results between these thresholds.[6] The temporal relationship between acid reflux events and symptom perception is assessed through the Symptom Index (SI), the percentage of symptoms preceded by reflux events, and Symptom Association Probability (SAP), a statistical measure of probability. A combined SI $\geq$50% and SAP greater than 95% are considered confidently positive. Positive symptom-related indices in the setting of physiologic acid exposure can indicate the presence of reflux hypersensitivity. Negative symptom indices without pathologic acid exposure signify a diagnosis of functional heartburn or functional chest pain if other diagnostic criteria are met. **Fig. 1** shows a recommended algorithm for the evaluation of suspected GERD, while also demonstrating the method that may lead to a diagnosis of either functional heartburn, functional chest pain, or reflux hypersensitivity. Of note, a patient may qualify as having pathologic GERD with persistent symptoms on PPI, and still have a functional esophageal disorder in addition to pathologic GERD.

ETIOPATHOGENESIS

The pathophysiology of functional esophageal disorders is multifactorial, with a complex interplay between several physiologic disturbances that may include peripheral and central sensitization, altered central processing of esophageal stimuli, autonomic dysregulation, abnormal mechanophysical properties of the esophagus, psychological comorbidity, hypervigilance, and visceral hypersensitivity.[10–13] Overall, esophageal hypersensitivity is likely the primary mechanism for esophageal functional disorders and can be further categorized into allodynia and hyperalgesia.[1,14–16] Allodynia is defined as the perception of nonpainful esophageal stimuli as being painful, whereas hyperalgesia is defined as the perception of painful esophageal stimuli as being more painful than expected.[17] Stimuli leading to peripheral and central sensitization have been implicated in symptom causation with peripheral hypersensitivity occurring at sites like the esophageal mucosa while central hypersensitivity has been linked to neurons of the spinal cord dorsal horn.

Noxious mechanical, thermal, or chemical signals in the esophageal mucosa are converted to action potentials by nociceptive receptors on esophageal nerves and

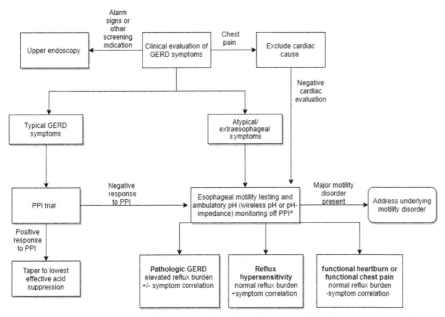

Fig. 1. A recommended algorithm in the clinical evaluation of GERD symptoms leading to definable functional esophageal disorders. PPI, proton pump inhibitor; GERD, gastroesophageal reflux disease. [a]In patients with known pathologic GERD and symptoms on PPI would recommend pH-impedance testing on PPI.

are then transmitted to the central nervous system via either spinal nerves or vagal nerves.[18] Either physiologic or noxious stimuli can act by releasing mediators such as serotonin, prostaglandins and reduce the transduction threshold of several cation channels on primary afferent myelinated (A-delta fiber) and myelinated (C fiber) neurons, resulting in the phenomenon known as peripheral hypersensitivity. The upregulation of TRPV1 receptors in response to nociceptive stimuli appear to play a central role in patients with nonerosive reflux disease (NERD) and GERD.[19–22] Another receptor, the protease-activated receptor 2 (PAR2), a G-protein-coupled receptor stimulated by proteases, has also been studied in the pathogenesis of inflammation in the gastrointestinal tract and functional GI disorders. These receptors lead to pain mediation via release of substance P in response to noxious stimuli.[21] Prostaglandin E2 (PGE2) is a mediator in both peripheral and central sensitization and mediates its effects via the prostaglandin E2 receptor-1 (EP-1) that has also been implicated in visceral hypersensitivity.[23]

Central hypersensitivity represents increased excitability of spinal neurons at the level of primary afferent neurons. This phenomenon is usually caused by repetitive firing of the afferent neurons that are triggered by release of neurotransmitters such as substance P, glutamate, and brain-derived neurotrophic factor, which further results in phosphorylation of the NMDA (N-methyl-D-aspartate) receptor. Esophageal hypersensitivity and altered pain perception are further supported by balloon distension and impedance planimetry studies that have shown evidence of lower pain threshold in patients with noncardiac chest pain and without GERD. Studies using hydrochloric acid infusion into the distal esophagus further support this concept.[24–27]

Stress has been implicated as a potential causative agent in the pathogenesis of mucosal hypersensitivity and increased perception of esophageal symptoms in patients with GERD and NERD. It has been postulated that stress may induce changes in mucosal permeability by degranulation of mast cells and redistribution of tight junctions and/or desmosomes.[28,29] Stress may also enhance the perception of heartburn through increased exposure of esophageal sensory nerve endings to gastric contents. Some smaller studies have found a correlation between increased mucosal mast cell infiltration in patients with hypersensitive esophagus and functional chest pain implicating the possible role of low-grade inflammation and immunologic alterations.[30]

Psychiatric comorbidities contribute to esophageal hypersensitivity with studies showing a role of stress and childhood adversity as potential risk factors in patients with noncardiac chest pain.[31] In addition, patients with functional chest pain have higher underlying anxiety, depression, and decreased tolerance to somatic and visceral stimuli.[32] A biopsychosocial model has been postulated that attributes the pathogenesis of functional gastrointestinal disorders (FGIDs) as an interaction between early life factors that can influence the psychosocial milieu of an individual and their gastrointestinal physiology through the brain-gut axis.[33] **Fig. 2** uses the concepts of this model and displays the variety of factors that may ultimately lead to functional esophageal disorders.

CURRENT TREATMENT EVIDENCE

Esophageal hypersensitivity, which occurs due to alterations in pain processing mechanisms and consequent disruptions in the normal brain-gut axis, remains the central pathophysiological mechanism for functional chest pain, functional heartburn, and reflux hypersensitivity. However, each of these disorders may have unique patient-specific clinical presentations, and the treatment approach is often tailored to an individual patient. Treatment options include neuromodulators, PPIs, prokinetics, gabapentinoids, complementary and alternative medicine practices, as well as psychological and behavioral interventions targeting the brain-gut axis.[3,34–36]

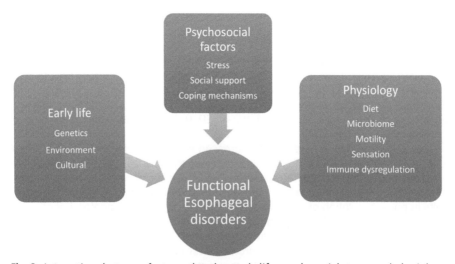

Fig. 2. Interactions between factors related to early life, psychosocial stress, and physiology as the possible pathogenesis of functional esophageal disorders.

Neuromodulators

These are often recommended as the first-line therapy for functional esophageal disorders with different categories of drugs that can be selected and tailored based on the patients underlying disease process, other comorbidities, and side effect profile. The predominant mechanism is believed to be brain-gut axis modulation via central and peripheral pathways, which allows for pain modulation and altering visceral hypersensitivity.[37,38] Drugs included in this category are tricyclic antidepressants, selective serotonin reuptake inhibitor, serotonin and norepinephrine reuptake inhibitors, and trazodone.

A systematic review by Weijenborg and colleagues that included 15 randomized controlled trials found that the esophageal pain thresholds increased from 7% to 37% after use of antidepressants and reduced functional chest pain from 18% to 67%.[39] Venlafaxine in particular has demonstrated significant symptomatic improvement in the treatment of functional chest pain.[40] Citalopram has demonstrated efficacy in the treatment of esophageal hypersensitivity in a randomized controlled study.[41] Citalopram has been shown to have diverse effects on esophageal physiology, with increased esophagogastric junction pressures, reduced transient lower esophageal sphincter (LES) relaxations and reflux events. However, it has also been associated with elevated upper esophageal sphincter pressures and globus sensation. Citalopram should thus be used cautiously in patients with globus.[42]

Park and colleagues demonstrated that the addition of low-dose amitriptyline to a conventional dose of PPI was more effective than a double-dose of PPI (70.6% vs 26.3%) in patients with functional chest pain resistant to a conventional dose of PPI treatment.[43]

An expert review by Coss-Adame and colleagues concluded that imipramine, trazodone, citalopram, sertraline, venlafaxine, and paroxetine provided symptom benefit in patients with esophageal chest pain related to esophageal hypersensitivity.[44] In a 3-week trial of imipramine, clonidine, and placebo, noncardiac chest pain decreased significantly in the imipramine group.[45] In another study by Clouse and colleagues, a 6-week trial of trazodone (100–150 mg/d) showed greater global symptom improvement ($P = .02$) compared with placebo, in patients with esophageal symptoms and contraction abnormalities.[46] In a randomized controlled trial examining patients who presented to a cardiology service with a negative cardiac evaluation, sertraline (up to 200 mg/d) for a period of 8 weeks resulted in a significant reduction in esophageal pain related to hypersensitivity when compared with placebo.[47] Keefe and colleagues studied the effects of sertraline and coping skills training (CST) in patients with noncardiac chest pain and observed that CST and sertraline either alone or in combination significantly reduced symptoms in these patients.[48]

Ostovaneh and colleagues compared omeprazole with fluoxetine in endoscopy negative patients with heartburn who failed once daily PPIs. Patients were further subgrouped based on ambulatory pH monitoring. Among patients with physiologic acid exposure, fluoxetine was found to be superior to both omeprazole and placebo with respect to percentage of heartburn-free days.[49]

Gamma-Aminobutyric Acid (GABA) Mediators

Gabapentin and pregabalin reduce visceral hypersensitivity and exert peripheral neuromodulation by affecting the signal transduction in nociceptive pathways through their action on voltage-sensitive calcium channels. Pregabalin additionally has central effects by reducing the levels of glutamate levels in the brain insula.[37] Although their actions on pain moderation and visceral hypersensitivity may justify their use in functional esophageal disorders, there is a lack of relevant clinical studies at this time.

Prokinetics

Currently, the data are very limited with regards to the use of promotility agents in the treatment of functional esophageal disorders. In a study by Rodriguez-Stanley and colleagues, tegaserod, a 5-HT4-receptor partial agonist, was found to improve the esophageal pain threshold to mechanical distention and distressing upper gastrointestinal symptoms in patients with functional heartburn.[50]

Acid Suppression

Patients with reflux hypersensitivity respond positively to acid suppression therapy as compared with other functional esophageal disorders. Rodriguez and colleagues studied the effects of the H2 blocker ranitidine on esophageal acid sensitivity in patients with functional heartburn. In a double-blind randomized crossover design, 18 patients with functional heartburn received oral ranitidine 150 mg twice a day or placebo for 7 consecutive days. After a single dose of ranitidine, esophageal pain thresholds as measured by esophageal acid infusion were increased and there was a reduction in overall pain compared with placebo, which persisted after 1 week of therapy.[51]

Watson and colleagues studied the response to omeprazole in patients with reflux symptoms with normal levels of acid reflux in a randomized placebo-controlled trial. They observed that patients with a positive SI showed a decrease in symptom frequency, severity, and consumption of antacids in comparison with placebo.[52] Hence, it is suggested that acid suppression may be considered as a possible treatment option in reflux hypersensitivity.

Antireflux Surgery

A surgical procedure at the LES should be considered cautiously in patients with reflux hypersensitivity that do not respond favorably to PPI therapy or neuromodulation. In their study on treatment outcomes in patients with reflux hypersensitivity, Patel and colleagues found that 16 of the total 53 patients underwent antireflux surgery and reported better symptom improvement compared with 37 treated medically. The surgical treatment group had lower LES basal pressures ($P = .04$), suggesting these patients may benefit more from these procedures.[53]

Theophylline

Theophylline is an adenosine receptor antagonist and relaxes smooth muscles and has visceral analgesic properties as well.[54] In their study on patients with functional chest pain, Rao and colleagues performed esophageal balloon distention using impedance planimetry. In patients with hypersensitive esophagi, intravenous theophylline was administered and balloon distension was repeated. If the hypersensitivity improved oral theophylline was prescribed for 3 months. They observed that after theophylline infusion, pain thresholds increased in 75% patients and median threshold pressures for discomfort and pain improved as well with a $P<.01$ and 7 of 8 patients reported sustained improvement in pain with oral theophylline use.[55]

In another randomized placebo-controlled study of theophylline, Rao and colleagues observed that 58% of patients with esophageal chest pain showed improvement in overall symptoms compared with 6% in the placebo group.[56]

Melatonin

Melatonin is a neurohormone related to serotonin that can exert a nociceptive effect by interaction with adrenergic, serotonergic, dopaminergic, and opioid receptors, thus affecting visceral hypersensitivity. In a study by Basu and colleagues, patients with functional heartburn were randomized to receive either melatonin, nortriptyline, or placebo at bedtime for 3 months and concluded that melatonin improved quality of life scores with fewer side effects when compared with nortriptyline.[57] Another study by Tan and colleagues found that melatonin may exert a protective effect on the esophageal epithelial barrier by suppressing the expression of myosin light chain kinase via signal transduction pathways involving ERK1/2.[58]

Complementary and Alternative Medicines

Complementary and alternative medicines (CAMs) include acupuncture, biofeedback therapy, and counseling. CAM methods that have been used for the treatment of FGIDs traditionally include acupuncture or electroacupuncture, herbal medicines, and behavioral therapies. Transcutaneous electroacupuncture (TEA) has also been proposed wherein surface electrodes are used to replace acupuncture needles. Acupuncture, electroacupuncture, and TEA have been shown to improve gastrointestinal intestinal motility and reduce visceral hypersensitivity in both human and animal models of FGID.[59] In a study by Shapiro and colleagues, patients with functional chest pain showed significant improvement in symptoms in response to biofeedback therapy.[60]

Psychogastroenterology

Behavioral therapies including cognitive behavioral therapy (CBT), hypnotherapy, relaxation exercise, and mindfulness-based therapies have been used for the treatment of a variety of FGID including functional esophageal disorders.

A Cochrane review by Kisely and colleagues that included 17 randomized controlled trials concluded that psychological treatments, especially CBT and hypnotherapy may be effective in the treatment of noncardiac chest pain although the analysis was limited because of small number of trials and heterogeneity in the studies.[61]

Hypnotherapy has been a burgeoning treatment modality in patients with FGIDs and appears to modulate brain activation patterns associated with pain processing patterns involved in the underlying pathophysiology of these disorders. Esophageal hypersensitivity and hypervigilance are 2 key factors related to the symptomatology of functional esophageal disorders and it has been proposed that hypnotherapy may affect these processes and hence impact patient response.[62] Gut-directed hypnotherapy usually involves 30- to 60-minute sessions, at weekly intervals, for a total of 6 to 12 weeks. It is a verbal intervention that uses a mental state of enhanced receptivity to suggestion in order to facilitate therapeutic psychological and physiologic changes. The goal is to induce a state of deep relaxation, so as to guide patients in exerting some control over their gut function.[63]

In a study by Keefer and colleagues, patients with functional heartburn were subjected to 7 weekly hypnotherapy sessions based on a protocol adapted from an irritable bowel syndrome hypnotherapy protocol and all participants reported improvement in their symptoms post-treatment. 50% of patients reported substantial improvement, while the rest reported slight improvement as per predefined criteria.[64] In a randomized controlled study in patients with noncardiac chest pain, hypnotherapy demonstrated reduction of global pain scores in 80% of patients compared with only a 23% response in controls.[65]

Hypnotherapy and CBT are key brain-gut psychotherapies that encompass the evolving field of psychogastroenterology and may be considered as an adjunctive treatment option for patients with functional esophageal disorders. These therapies may especially be useful in patients with inadequate response to standard medical therapy or for those with additional psychological comorbidities by facilitating coping, resilience, and self-regulation.[66] Diaphragmatic breathing is a nonpharmacological therapy that has shown benefit in patients with GERD and there is some evidence that it may have a potential role in the management of functional esophageal disorders as well.[67] Keefer and colleagues observed that in patients with noncardiac chest pain, diaphragmatic breathing and relaxation training served as an effective coping strategy in the setting of symptom flares.[68,69]

Table 2 summarizes the current evidence-based therapeutic interventions for functional chest pain, functional heartburn, and reflux hypersensitivity.

DISCUSSION

Functional chest pain, functional heartburn, and reflux hypersensitivity now have accepted definitions using Rome IV criteria, which serve to categorize patients clinically. When confronted with a patient with one of these functional esophageal disorders, it is imperative to associate a detailed clinical history, including psychosocial components, to results of diagnostic testing in order to have a proposed pathophysiology of symptoms for that individual. The categorization of patients with these disorders has changed over time, and trials assessing treatments have often included patients with several distinct functional esophageal conditions. Thus, the recommended treatments for patients with these disorders remain very personalized.

Patients with functional chest pain and functional heartburn by definition do not have active gastroesophageal reflux as the cause of symptoms. In these patients, a variety of neuromodulators, alternative medical treatments, and psychogastroenterology approaches have evidence of being valuable treatment options. This is in contrast

Table 2 Current evidence-based therapies for functional esophageal disorders; recommended doses are in mg per day	
Diagnosis	**Current Evidence-Based Treatment Options**

Functional chest pain	TCAs: Imipramine 25–50 mg
	    Amitriptyline 10–20 mg
	SNRIs: Venlafaxine 75 mg
	SSRIs: Sertraline 50–200 mg
	Trazodone: 100–150 mg
	Theophylline: 100–400 mg
	GABA mediators: gabapentin
	    up to 900 mg/d
	Psychogastroenterology/gut-brain
	    psychotherapy referral

Functional heartburn	TCAs: Imipramine 25–50 mg SSRIs: Fluoxetine 20 mg Melatonin: 6–12 mg Psychogastroenterology/gut-brain psychotherapy referral
Reflux hypersensitivity	Acid suppression SSRI: Citalopram 20 mg Antireflux surgery

Abbreviations: SNRI, serotonin and norepinephrine reuptake inhibitor; SSRI, selective serotonin reuptake inhibitor; TCA, tricyclic antidepressant.

with reflux hypersensitivity, in which the focus must be on the reflux events in conjunction with the associated esophageal hypersensitivity.

Over time, the important role of anxiety and hypervigilance in the onset of challenging esophageal symptoms has become clearer.[70,71] More clinical trials are needed, with patients strictly categorized by their Rome IV functional esophageal disorder, in order to guide practitioners further in this area. Until then, an individualized approach is recommended that combines a meticulous review of symptoms and diagnostic test results to create a personalized treatment approach. Patient preferences regarding medical, complementary, alternative, and psychogastroenterology treatment options are vital when developing a tailored treatment plan for patients with functional esophageal disorders.

CLINICS CARE POINTS

- Functional chest pain, functional heartburn, and reflux hypersensitivity must be defined by Rome IV criteria based on symptoms over specific time intervals and specific results of diagnostic testing

- Treatment approaches for functional heartburn and functional chest pain include neuromodulation, other medications targeting esophageal hypersensitivity, as well as psychogastroenterology approaches such as gut-directed hypnotherapy

- The treatment of reflux hypersensitivity should focus on both acid suppression and selective serotonin reuptake inhibitors along with psychogastroenterology approaches.

DISCLOSURE

A. Khan is a consultant for Medtronic. R. Bhardwaj and R. Knotts have nothing to disclose.

REFERENCES

1. Galmiche JP, Clouse RE, Bálint A, et al. Functional esophageal disorders. Gastroenterology 2006;130(5):1459–65.
2. Mourad G, Alwin J, Strömberg A, et al. Societal costs of non-cardiac chest pain compared with ischemic heart disease–a longitudinal study. BMC Health Serv Res 2013;13:403.
3. Aziz Q, Fass R, Gyawali CP, et al. Esophageal disorders. Gastroenterology 2016; 150(6):1368–79.
4. Schmulson MJ, Drossman DA. What is new in rome IV. J Neurogastroenterol Motil 2017;23(2):151–63.
5. Katz PO, Gerson LB, Vela MF. Guidelines for the diagnosis and management of gastroesophageal reflux disease. Am J Gastroenterol 2013;108(3):308–28.
6. Gyawali CP, Kahrilas PJ, Savarino E, et al. Modern diagnosis of GERD: the Lyon Consensus. Gut 2018;67(7):1351–62.
7. Zerbib F, Bredenoord AJ, Fass R, et al. ESNM/ANMS consensus paper: diagnosis and management of refractory gastro-esophageal reflux disease. Neurogastroenterol Motil 2021;33(4):e14075.
8. Yadlapati R, Masihi M, Gyawali CP, et al. Ambulatory reflux monitoring guides proton pump inhibitor discontinuation in patients with gastroesophageal reflux symptoms: a clinical trial. Gastroenterology 2021;160(1):174–82.e171.

9. Yadlapati R, Tye M, Roman S, et al. Postprandial high-resolution impedance manometry identifies mechanisms of nonresponse to proton pump inhibitors. Clin Gastroenterol Hepatol 2018;16(2):211–8.e211.

10. Fass R, Shibli F, Tawil J. Diagnosis and management of functional chest pain in the Rome IV era. J Neurogastroenterol Motil 2019;25(4):487–98.

11. Hachem C, Shaheen NJ. Diagnosis and management of functional heartburn. Am J Gastroenterol 2016;111(1):53–61.

12. Remes-Troche JM. The hypersensitive esophagus: pathophysiology, evaluation, and treatment options. Curr Gastroenterol Rep 2010;12(5):417–26.

13. Fass R, Dickman R. Non-cardiac chest pain: an update. Neurogastroenterol Motil 2006;18(6):408–17.

14. Farmer AD, Ruffle JK, Aziz Q. The role of esophageal hypersensitivity in functional esophageal disorders. J Clin Gastroenterol 2017;51(2):91–9.

15. Kondo T, Miwa H. The role of esophageal hypersensitivity in functional heartburn. J Clin Gastroenterol 2017;51(7):571–8.

16. Fass R, Achem S. Noncardiac chest pain: epidemiology, natural course and pathogenesis. J Neurogastroenterol Motil 2011;17:110–23.

17. Yamasaki T, Fass R. Reflux hypersensitivity: a new functional esophageal disorder. J Neurogastroenterol Motil 2017;23(4):495–503.

18. Miwa H, Kondo T, Oshima T, et al. Esophageal sensation and esophageal hypersensitivity - overview from bench to bedside. J Neurogastroenterol Motil 2010; 16(4):353–62.

19. Yang S-C, Chen C-L, Yi C-H, et al. Changes in gene expression patterns of circadian-clock, transient receptor potential vanilloid-1 and nerve growth factor in inflamed human esophagus. Sci Rep 2015;5(1):13602.

20. Du Q, Liao Q, Chen C, et al. The role of transient receptor potential vanilloid 1 in common diseases of the digestive tract and the cardiovascular and respiratory system. Front Physiol 2019;10(1064).

21. Yoshida N, Kuroda M, Suzuki T, et al. Role of nociceptors/neuropeptides in the pathogenesis of visceral hypersensitivity of nonerosive reflux disease. Dig Dis Sci 2013;58(8):2237–43.

22. Aggarwal P, Kamal AN. Reflux hypersensitivity: how to approach diagnosis and management. Curr Gastroenterol Rep 2020;22(9):42.

23. Sarkar S, Hobson AR, Hughes A, et al. The prostaglandin E2 receptor-1 (EP-1) mediates acid-induced visceral pain hypersensitivity in humans. Gastroenterology 2003;124(1):18–25.

24. Sarkar S, Aziz Q, Woolf CJ, et al. Contribution of central sensitisation to the development of non-cardiac chest pain. Lancet 2000;356(9236):1154–9.

25. Barish CF, Castell DO, Richter JE. Graded esophageal balloon distention. A new provocative test for noncardiac chest pain. Dig Dis Sci 1986;31(12):1292–8.

26. Richter JE, Barish CF, Castell DO. Abnormal sensory perception in patients with esophageal chest pain. Gastroenterology 1986;91(4):845–52.

27. Rao SS, Gregersen H, Hayek B, et al. Unexplained chest pain: the hypersensitive, hyperreactive, and poorly compliant esophagus. Ann Intern Med 1996;124(11): 950–8.

28. Farré R, De Vos R, Geboes K, et al. Critical role of stress in increased oesophageal mucosa permeability and dilated intercellular spaces. Gut 2007;56(9): 1191–7.

29. Woodland P, Shen Ooi JL, Grassi F, et al. Superficial esophageal mucosal afferent nerves may contribute to reflux hypersensitivity in nonerosive reflux disease. Gastroenterology 2017;153(5):1230–9.

30. Lee H, Chung H, Park JC, et al. Heterogeneity of mucosal mast cell infiltration in subgroups of patients with esophageal chest pain. Neurogastroenterol Motil 2014;26(6):786–93.
31. Biggs AM, Aziz Q, Tomenson B, et al. Effect of childhood adversity on health related quality of life in patients with upper abdominal or chest pain. Gut 2004; 53(2):180.
32. Farmer AD, Coen SJ, Kano M, et al. Psychophysiological responses to visceral and somatic pain in functional chest pain identify clinically relevant pain clusters. Neurogastroenterol Motil 2014;26(1):139–48.
33. Drossman DA. Functional gastrointestinal disorders: history, pathophysiology, clinical features and Rome IV. Gastroenterology 2016;150(6):1262–79.
34. George N, Abdallah J, Maradey-Romero C, et al. Review article: the current treatment of non-cardiac chest pain. Aliment Pharmacol Ther 2016;43(2):213–39.
35. Nguyen TM, Eslick GD. Systematic review: the treatment of noncardiac chest pain with antidepressants. Aliment Pharmacol Ther 2012;35(5):493–500.
36. Hershcovici T, Achem SR, Jha LK, et al. Systematic review: the treatment of noncardiac chest pain. Aliment Pharmacol Ther 2012;35(1):5–14.
37. Drossman DA, Tack J, Ford AC, et al. Neuromodulators for functional gastrointestinal disorders (Disorders of Gut-Brain Interaction): a Rome Foundation Working Team Report. Gastroenterology 2018;154(4):1140–71.e1141.
38. Sobin HW, Heinrich TW, Drossman DA. Central neuromodulators for treating functional GI disorders: a primer. Am J Gastroenterol 2017;112(5):693–702.
39. Weijenborg PW, de Schepper HS, Smout AJPM, et al. Effects of antidepressants in patients with functional esophageal disorders or gastroesophageal reflux disease: a systematic review. Clin Gastroenterol Hepatol 2015;13(2):251–9.e251.
40. Lee H, Kim JH, Min B-H, et al. Efficacy of venlafaxine for symptomatic relief in young adult patients with functional chest pain: a randomized, double-blind, placebo-controlled, crossover trial. Am J Gastroenterol 2010;105(7):1504–12.
41. Viazis N, Keyoglou A, Kanellopoulos AK, et al. Selective serotonin reuptake inhibitors for the treatment of hypersensitive esophagus: a randomized, double-blind, placebo-controlled study. Am J Gastroenterol 2012;107(11):1662–7.
42. Manolakis AC, Broers C, Geysen H, et al. Effect of citalopram on esophageal motility in healthy subjects-implications for reflux episodes, dysphagia, and globus. Neurogastroenterol Motil 2019;31(8):e13632.
43. Park SW, Lee H, Lee HJ, et al. Low-dose amitriptyline combined with proton pump inhibitor for functional chest pain. World J Gastroenterol 2013;19(30): 4958–65.
44. Coss-Adame E, Erdogan A, Rao SS. Treatment of esophageal (noncardiac) chest pain: an expert review. Clin Gastroenterol Hepatol 2014;12(8):1224–45.
45. Cannon RO, Quyyumi AA, Mincemoyer R, et al. Imipramine in patients with chest pain despite normal coronary angiograms. N Engl J Med 1994;330(20):1411–7.
46. Clouse RE, Lustman PJ, Eckert TC, et al. Low-dose trazodone for symptomatic patients with esophageal contraction abnormalities. A double-blind, placebo-controlled trial. Gastroenterology 1987;92(4):1027–36.
47. Varia I, Logue E, O'Connor C, et al. Randomized trial of sertraline in patients with unexplained chest pain of noncardiac origin. Am Heart J 2000;140(3):367–72.
48. Keefe FJ, Shelby RA, Somers TJ, et al. Effects of coping skills training and sertraline in patients with non-cardiac chest pain: a randomized controlled study. Pain 2011;152(4):730–41.
49. Ostovaneh MR, Saeidi B, Hajifathalian K, et al. Comparing omeprazole with fluoxetine for treatment of patients with heartburn and normal endoscopy who failed

once daily proton pump inhibitors: double-blind placebo-controlled trial. Neuro-gastroenterol Motil 2014;26(5):670–8.

50. Rodriguez-Stanley S, Zubaidi S, Proskin HM, et al. Effect of tegaserod on esophageal pain threshold, regurgitation, and symptom relief in patients with functional heartburn and mechanical sensitivity. Clin Gastroenterol Hepatol 2006;4(4): 442–50.

51. Rodriguez-Stanley S, Ciociola AA, Zubaidi S, et al. A single dose of ranitidine 150 mg modulates oesophageal acid sensitivity in patients with functional heartburn. Aliment Pharmacol Ther 2004;20(9):975–82.

52. Watson RG, Tham TC, Johnston BT, et al. Double blind cross-over placebo controlled study of omeprazole in the treatment of patients with reflux symptoms and physiological levels of acid reflux–the "sensitive oesophagus. Gut 1997; 40(5):587–90.

53. Patel A, Sayuk GS, Gyawali CP. Prevalence, characteristics, and treatment outcomes of reflux hypersensitivity detected on pH-impedance monitoring. Neuro-gastroenterol Motil 2016;28(9):1382–90.

54. Achem SR. New frontiers for the treatment of noncardiac chest pain: the adenosine receptors. Am J Gastroenterol 2007;102(5):939–41.

55. Rao SS, Mudipalli RS, Mujica V, et al. An open-label trial of theophylline for functional chest pain. Dig Dis Sci 2002;47(12):2763–8.

56. Rao SS, Mudipalli RS, Remes-Troche JM, et al. Theophylline improves esophageal chest pain–a randomized, placebo-controlled study. Am J Gastroenterol 2007;102(5):930–8.

57. Basu PP, Hempole H, Krishnaswamy N, et al. The effect of melatonin in functional heartburn: a randomized, placebo-controlled clinical trial. Open J Gastroenterol 2014;04(02):6.

58. Tan J, Wang Y, Xia Y, et al. Melatonin protects the esophageal epithelial barrier by suppressing the transcription, expression and activity of myosin light chain kinase through ERK1/2 signal transduction. Cell Physiol Biochem 2014;34(6): 2117–27.

59. Chen JDZ, Yin J, Takahashi T, et al. Complementary and alternative therapies for functional gastrointestinal diseases. Evid Based Complement Alternat Med 2015; 2015:138645.

60. Shapiro M, Shanani R, Taback H, et al. Functional chest pain responds to biofeedback treatment but functional heartburn does not: what is the difference? Eur J Gastroenterol Hepatol 2012;24(6):708–14.

61. Kisely SR, Campbell LA, Yelland MJ, et al. Psychological interventions for symptomatic management of non-specific chest pain in patients with normal coronary anatomy. Cochrane Database Syst Rev 2015;2015(6):Cd004101.

62. Riehl ME, Keefer L. Hypnotherapy for esophageal disorders. Am J Clin Hypn 2015;58(1):22–33.

63. Vasant DH, Whorwell PJ. Gut-focused hypnotherapy for functional gastrointestinal disorders: evidence-base, practical aspects, and the manchester protocol. Neurogastroenterol Motil 2019;31(8):e13573.

64. Riehl ME, Pandolfino JE, Palsson OS, et al. Feasibility and acceptability of esophageal-directed hypnotherapy for functional heartburn. Dis Esophagus 2016;29(5):490–6.

65. Jones H, Cooper P, Miller V, et al. Treatment of non-cardiac chest pain: a controlled trial of hypnotherapy. Gut 2006;55(10):1403–8.

66. Keefer L, Palsson OS, Pandolfino JE. Best practice update: incorporating psychogastroenterology into management of digestive disorders. Gastroenterology 2018;154(5):1249–57.
67. Ong AM, Chua LT, Khor CJ, et al. Diaphragmatic breathing reduces belching and proton pump inhibitor refractory gastroesophageal reflux symptoms. Clin Gastroenterol Hepatol 2018;16(3):407–16.e402.
68. Riehl ME, Kinsinger S, Kahrilas PJ, et al. Role of a health psychologist in the management of functional esophageal complaints. Dis Esophagus 2015;28(5): 428–36.
69. Halland M, Bharucha AE, Crowell MD, et al. Effects of diaphragmatic breathing on the pathophysiology and treatment of upright gastroesophageal reflux: a randomized controlled trial. Am J Gastroenterol 2021;116(1):86–94.
70. Carlson DA, Gyawali CP, Roman S, et al. Esophageal hypervigilance and visceral anxiety are contributors to symptom severity among patients evaluated with high-resolution esophageal manometry. Am J Gastroenterol 2020;115(3):367–75.
71. Taft TH, Guadagnoli L, Carlson DA, et al. Validation of the short-form esophageal hypervigilance and anxiety scale. Clin Gastroenterol Hepatol 2021; S0016-5085(16):00223–7.

Gastroesophageal Reflux Disease and the Patient with Obesity

Yewande Alimi, MD, MHS[a], Dan E. Azagury, MD[b,*]

KEYWORDS

- GERD • Sleeve gastrectomy • Roux-en-Y gastric bypass • Fundoplication • Obesity

KEY POINTS

- Patients with obesity who present with GERD with BMI 30 to 35 should be considered for laparoscopic Roux-en-Y gastric bypass. Alternatively, they can be offered medical weight loss followed by laparoscopic fundoplication or magnetic sphincter augmentation.
- In patients with objective evidence of GERD with obesity (BMI > 35) Roux-en-Y gastric bypass should be considered the gold standard for attaining weight loss management and reflux resolution.
- Patients who present following metabolic surgery, specifically laparoscopic sleeve gastrectomy, with reflux disease, who fail to resolve with medical therapy, should be offered conversion to Roux-en-Y gastric bypass.

INTRODUCTION AND DEFINITIONS

Obesity is defined as having a body mass index (BMI), calculated as the weight in kilograms divided by height in meters squared, greater than 30. Gastroesophageal reflux disease (GERD) is characterized by heartburn and/or regurgitation and is commonly associated with obesity. This phenomenon's pathophysiology has been well described previously but centers around increased intra-abdominal pressures associated with patients with BMI greater than 30. The increase in obesity has dovetailed with an increase of patients with GERD; this is likely secondary to mechanical, behavioral, and neurohormonal factors that are related to being overweight and likely explain the increased prevalence. This review is centered on the epidemiology, management, and algorithm that the authors use to approach patients with obesity and concomitant GERD. The authors discuss their approach to the patient with obesity who presents

[a] Department of Surgery, Stanford University School of Medicine, 3800 Reservoir Rd NW, Washington, DC 20007, USA; [b] Department of Surgery, Stanford University School of Medicine, 300 Pasteur Drive, H3680H, Stanford, CA 94305-5655, USA
* Corresponding author.
E-mail address: dazagury@stanford.edu
Twitter: @yewandealimiMD (Y.A.); @dazagury (D.E.A.)

Gastroenterol Clin N Am 50 (2021) 859–870
https://doi.org/10.1016/j.gtc.2021.08.010
0889-8553/21/© 2021 Elsevier Inc. All rights reserved.

with reflux, in addition to those undergoing bariatric surgery, as well as the various operations used to manage metabolic disease and patients with obesity, with particular attention to those patients with an associated diagnosis of GERD, as well as managing reflux disease after various surgical interventions used in the management of metabolic disease.

Epidemiology

According to the National Health and Nutrition Examination Survey (NHANES) longitudinal study of obesity in the United States, the prevalence of patients with obesity has increased among adults from the era of 1999 to 2000 to 2017 to 2018 from 30.5% to 42.4%, with some predictions that this could reach as high as 50%.[1] These rates remain markedly elevated compared with data from 2003 to 2004 with obesity prevalence at that time being 32.9%. Similar to the trend seen in obesity, GERD in the US population has continued to increase. In a recent meta-analysis of 79 studies from more than 36 countries, the overall prevalence of GERD in adults was found to be 13.3%, with higher rates on average seen in South Asia (22.1%) and the overall lowest rates in North America (15.4%). However, a meta-analysis of 22 studies found the prevalence of GERD to be 22.1% in patients with obesity, compared with 14.2% in patients without obesity.[2] These data were corroborated by Eusubi and colleagues[3] who demonstrated that obesity was associated with a 1.7 times increased odds of GERD (odds ratio, 1.73; 95% confidence interval, 1.46–2.06). Similarly, Ruhl and Everhart[4] in evaluating more than 12,000 participants in the NHANES found that with every 5 increase in BMI there was a 1.2 increased risk of GERD. Although the increased prevalence of GERD in patients with obesity is noted to be multifactorial, prior evidence suggests that this association is related to increased intra-abdominal pressure, higher prevalence of hiatal hernias (HHs), a higher gradient of abdominal to thoracic pressure, increased production of bile and pancreatic enzymes, and increased levels of estrogen, all postulated in the pathophysiology of GERD associated with patients with obesity.[2,5–8] Nilsson and colleagues[8] found that with every unit increase in BMI, there was an increase in reflux symptoms. More specifically, there is evidence of esophagitis associated with increased central obesity and HHs and that obesity was significantly associated with these conditions. Pandolfino and colleagues[9] reported that patients with obesity have a pressure gradient present along the esophagogastric junction that supports the development of a HH. El-Serag and colleagues[10] found that obesity was a significant risk factor in those with severe esophagitis, and this was independent of the presence of a HH. In addition, patients with obesity have an increased prevalence of esophageal dysmotility, even in the absence of symptoms. Common abnormal findings include hypercontractile esophagus, nonspecific motility disorders, and a hypotensive lower esophageal sphincter.[11] These findings are particularly worthwhile noting because we further discuss the management of surgical intervention in patients with obesity and GERD.

Surgical Management: Nissen Fundoplication

The management of GERD has evolved. First-line therapy includes medical therapy and lifestyle modifications. There have been conflicting data regarding weight loss and resolution of reflux symptoms. A Norwegian qualitative survey study of 44,997 subjects, HUNT 3, found a dose-dependent reduction of reflux symptoms in relation to weight loss.[12] These results were corroborated by the prospective study by Singh and colleagues[13] that evaluated 332 adults with obesity enrolled in a structured weight loss program who had a mean weight loss of 13 kg. In this cohort, the prevalence of GERD symptoms reduced from 37% to 15% with most patients experiencing a reduction in GERD symptom scores. However, others have reported no change in GERD symptoms following significant weight loss.[14,15] Medical weight loss approaches have been demonstrated to achieve as high as 10% total body weight loss, but a meta-analysis of behavioral weight loss programs demonstrates only an average weight loss of 4% compared with 1% in controls.[11,16,17] Although encouraged medical weight loss (lifestyle modification, exercise, and pharmaceutical agents where indicated) may be of benefit, surgical approaches to weight loss with more durable effects may also be indicated in patients with obesity with associated GERD.

In patients in whom medical therapy is not tolerated or is ineffective, laparoscopic Nissen fundoplication with cruroplasty is the mainstay of management. In our practice, patients with objective markers of GERD, that is, esophagitis, evidence of Barrett's transformation, elevated DeMeester score, or increased time with elevated acid exposure who fail medical management may require surgical intervention. Fundoplication is an effective management of GERD in patients with BMIs less than 30, with multiple studies and meta-analyses demonstrating that 90% of patients have resolution of symptoms.[11] However, in patients with obesity who have undergone fundoplication, recurrence rates have been reported as high as 31%.[18] Morgenthal and colleagues[19] demonstrated that BMI less than 35 was an important factor in successful outcomes following fundoplication after 10-year follow-up. The increased recurrence rate of GERD in patients with obesity following laparoscopic fundoplication requires that a careful and thoughtful algorithm be applied. Akimoto and colleagues[20] demonstrated that patients with obesity were more often found to have disrupted or herniated fundoplications compared with controls. Although some have reported similar outcomes in patients with obesity compared with normal weight controls undergoing laparoscopic antireflux surgery,[21,22] we still favor weight loss and avoidance of fundoplication in patients with obesity.

Patients with obesity who present with a BMI less than 30 to 32, without other significant obesity-associated comorbidities, are counseled regarding weight loss before surgical intervention. In these patients, we offer medical weight loss strategies to include behavioral modifications as advised through registered dieticians, pharmaceutical interventions where indicated, and a healthy exercise regimen. With successful weight loss, in these patients, we offer surgical fundoplication ± cruroplasty, with 360° versus 270° partial wrap dependent on esophageal motility.

Surgical Management: Gastric Bypass

Patients who present with obesity with a BMI 30 to 35 require careful forethought beyond standard pursuit of Nissen fundoplication with cruroplasty and undergo an extensive workup. We typically discuss both options with patients: medical weight loss + Nissen and laparoscopic Roux-en-Y gastric bypass (LRYGB). Depending on patient preference, comorbidities, prior abdominal surgeries, age, and size of HH we typically attempt medical weight loss in patients with BMI 30 to 32 and attempt to obtain insurance approval for LRYGB for patients with BMI greater than 33.

For patients who present with a BMI greater than 35 we routinely recommend LRYGB. In this patient cohort who meet National Institutes of Health criteria for surgical management of their obesity and are amenable to bypass surgery, we process them through our surgical weight loss program to manage both their reflux disease and their obesity-related comorbidities. Although routine preoperative endoscopy is a matter of debate, evaluation for HH via upper endoscopy or upper gastrointestinal contrast study is routine in our practice. Che and colleagues[23] in evaluating 181 patients undergoing bariatric surgery found that nearly 40% of patients had an HH.[24] DuPree and colleagues[25] in evaluating patients in the Bariatric Outcomes Longitudinal

Database (BOLD), a retrospective review of a prospectively maintained cohort, found that up to 45% of patients undergoing bariatric surgery undergoing sleeve gastrectomy and 50% of patients undergoing Roux-en-Y gastric bypass (RYGB) had preoperative GERD. In patients with preoperative history of GERD-like symptoms, we rely on upper endoscopy for evaluation of HH as well as for evaluation of esophagitis. Several series evaluating preoperative bariatric patients identified that up to 34% of patients have esophagitis and up to 6% have evidence of Barrett's transformation.[24] Based on expert consensus, Barrett's esophagus is an absolute contraindication for laparoscopic sleeve gastrectomy (LSG),[26] and in patients with these findings preoperatively we counsel toward LRYGB.

Historically, RYGB has been used as a standalone reflux procedure. RYGB comprised about 20% of bariatric surgery in 2018.[27] A prospective study by Braghetto and colleagues,[28] in evaluating bariatric surgical procedures, found that gastric bypass was the most effective at reducing symptoms of GERD.[25] Specifically, the physiologic considerations of the LRYGB in construction of a small gastric pouch of 15 to 30 mL results in low acid production. In addition, with the use of a Roux limb that measures at least 100 cm, there is reduced exposure to the esophagus of biliopancreatic secretions.[29] In Pallati and colleagues'[30] evaluation of GERD symptoms following bariatric surgical procedures in the BOLD patient cohort, GERD symptom improvement was the highest in the LRGYB cohort with almost 60% of patients showing improvement of symptoms. Mechanisms suggested for reduction of GERD symptoms in those undergoing LRYGB include greater weight reduction, as well as decreased gastric secretions in the proximal pouch.[30] Frezza and colleagues[31] corroborated these findings and mechanistic suggestions including elimination of acid production in the gastric pouch and weight loss in their 3-year study after LRYGB in which they found a significant reduction of reported heartburn from 87% to 22% ($P < .001$). In addition to symptom resolution depicted in these studies, LRYGB has also been shown to improve objective benchmarks of reflux disease. Mandalossoo and colleagues[32] found a significant decrease in total acid exposure in patients before and after RYGB (5.1% vs 1.1%, $P = .0002$). In addition to the resolution of GERD symptoms, LRYGB provides management of patient's metabolic comorbidities, and it is for these reasons that in patients who present with obesity with significant concomitant GERD, we recommend LRYGB.

Surgical Management: Nissen Versus Gastric Bypass

Nissen fundoplication is a mainstay approach for treating longstanding GERD. However, data regarding the management GERD in patients with obesity with fundoplication versus gastric bypass are mixed. Winslow and colleagues[21] found in their evaluation of 505 patients undergoing laparoscopic antireflux surgery (LARS) to include Nissen and Toupet fundoplications that although operative time was longer in patients with obesity, complication and anatomic failures were similar in both cohorts in the long term with an average follow-up time of 35 months. Albeit with shorter mean follow-up time (14.7 months), Luketina and colleagues[33] found similar outcomes in those undergoing LARS with obesity. The investigators describe similar Gastrointestinal Quality of Life Index (GIQLI) scores, symptom grading, esophageal manometry, and multichannel intraluminal impedance monitoring in patients with obesity compared with those without.[33] However, others report alternative conclusions. Patterson and colleagues[34] demonstrated that both LARS and LRYGB are effective at reducing the symptoms of heartburn; however, they concluded that LRYGB provides additional health benefits in patients with obesity. Perez and colleagues[35] in evaluating 224 patients undergoing antireflux surgery (laparoscopic Nissen fundoplication and

Belsey Mark IV) found increased recurrence in patients with obesity when compared with patients with normal BMI (31% vs 4.5%, $P < .0001$). The investigators similarly found a significant difference in recurrence when comparing overweight patients with those with obesity (31.3 vs 8.0, $P < .001$).[35] In addition to the resolution of GERD symptoms, patients with obesity undergoing LRYGB also benefit from quality-of-life improvements and resolution of obesity-related comorbidities, traits not associated with fundoplication.[36]

In patients who have had failed fundoplications and present with refractory GERD, we approach this in a similar diagnostic manner. In most of these patients, barium esophagram is highly elucidative and demonstrates a slip or recurrent HH. In these patients with failed fundoplications we recommend conversion to RYGB. Although technically tedious, laparoscopic conversion of a Nissen or Toupet fundoplication to RYGB is a feasible salvage operation for patients with obesity with recurrent GERD. Kellogg and colleagues[37] in their evaluation of 11 patients undergoing conversion had 100% symptom resolution and 78% objective resolution of GERD. Most of their patients were found to have wrap disruption $\pm$ herniation.[37] Short-term data regarding fundoplication in patients with obesity demonstrate equivalence, whereas long-term data suggest that LRYGB offers a more durable resolution of GERD symptoms. Multiple studies have reported improvement of GERD symptoms following LRYGB, and given this it is generally widely accepted for the management of GERD in patients with obesity.[38,39] Our approach to patients with obesity and concomitant GERD is depicted in **Fig. 1**.

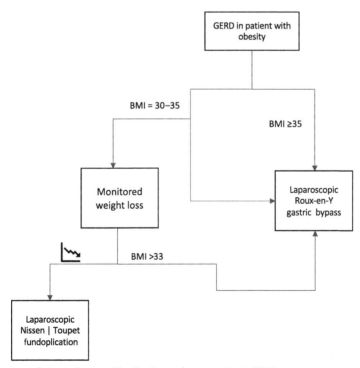

Fig. 1. Approach to patients with obesity and concomitant GERD.

Surgical Management: Sleeve Gastrectomy

In recent times, bariatric surgical procedures for the management of metabolic disease have been increasing. In 2018, the American Society for Metabolic and Bariatric Surgery Numbers Taskforce reported that more than 250,000 bariatric surgical procedures were performed, an increase of almost 11%. The most prominent surgical intervention for metabolic disease in the United States at this time has increasingly become the LSG, with as much as 60% of bariatric surgeries being performed in 2016 being a sleeve gastrectomy.[27]

A thorough preoperative evaluation is necessary because de novo occurrence of GERD following sleeve gastrectomy has been reported.[40] In the BOLD cohort, 8.6% of patients developed de novo symptoms of GERD following LSG, whereas 84.1% of patients with preoperative GERD continued to have symptoms.[25,41] These findings have been corroborated in other studies as well. In a systematic review of GERD following LSG, Oor and colleagues[42] found a pooled incidence of de novo GERD following LSG of 20%, with some reports as high as 34.9%. In 2020, this was corroborated by Yueng and colleagues[43] in their systematic review and meta-analysis in which they found a de novo reflux rate of 23%. Raj and colleagues[44] found in asymptomatic patients that the incidence of GERD following LSG was as high as 67%, with mean DeMeester score elevation of more than 30 points ($P = .006$). Notably, Thereaux and colleagues[40] found that preoperative pH levels were not predictive of development of postoperative GERD in patients undergoing LSG. In a larger randomized trial, at 5-year follow-up, the Swiss Multicenter Bypass or Sleeve Study (SM-BOSS) found worsening of GERD-related morbidity following LSG when compared with LRGYB. This worsening was demonstrated by elevated de novo GERD in LSG (32 vs 11%) and lower remission of reflux symptoms (25% vs 60%), when compared with LRYGB.[45] There are a multitude of proposed mechanisms that result in GERD following LSG. These include anatomic factors such as decreased lower esophageal sphincter resting pressure, increased intragastric pressure, tubular sleeve with inferior pouch, an incompetent pylorus, and a concomitant presence of HH. Some technical aspects reported include stapling near the angle of His, narrowing the sleeve, dissection of the phrenoesophageal ligament, and narrowing the incisura angularis leading to dilation of the fundus.[38] Himpens and colleagues in their evaluation of 53 patients undergoing LSG identify a bimodal distribution of reflux symptoms following LSG. The first peak was noted during the first year following LSG. The investigators attribute this peak to the widening of the angle of His, decreased LES pressure due to the resection of the gastric sling fibers, and overall decreased gastric compliance. This peak resolved in this cohort before the third postoperative year. A second peak was noted later on (greater than 7 years), and this was attributed to development of a neofundus, weight gain, as well as the recurrence or development of a HH.[46]

Data for concomitant hiatal hernia repair (HHR) are mixed; however, most reports find that concomitant repair results in favorable or similar postoperative GERD symptoms. Fifteen percent of the Sheppard and colleagues'[47] cohort of 378 patients undergoing LSG had a significant HH requiring repair. In this cohort there was no significant difference in reflux rates between patients with and without HH, and similarly no differences in those who had their HH repaired compared with those who did not.[47] However, Soricelli and colleagues[48] similarly compared patients undergoing LSG alone and those with concomitant HHR, and they found the de novo prevalence of GERD symptoms following LSG alone was as high as 23% compared with 0% in those undergoing concomitant repair. In 2011, the International Sleeve Gastrectomy Expert Panel Consensus based on more than 12,000 case experiences recommended the best practice in several areas as it related to GERD. Notably, more than 80% of experts recommend aggressive identification of HH intraoperatively as well as repair if one is found.[26] Based on these data and consensus guidelines, we routinely repair HHs if found preoperatively or during LSG. Attention to technical detail points highlighted by Daes and colleagues[49] including avoidance of relative narrowing at the junction of the vertical and horizontal parts of the sleeve, twisting of the sleeve, dilation of the fundus, and repair of HHs helps to decrease GERD following LSG.

Gastroesophageal Reflux Disease After Sleeve Gastrectomy: Revisional Surgery for Reflux in Patients with Obesity

In patients presenting with GERD following bariatric surgery, we begin as we do in the general population with medical therapy. In addition to this, we explore objective studies to document GERD including endoscopy, barium esophagram, pH studies, and manometry. These studies serve a dual purpose because they both assist in documenting GERD while also helping delineate possible causes. Objective data including DeMeester scores and acid exposure to document the presence of reflux and barium esophagram and endoscopy to evaluate for esophagitis, HHs, and anatomic anomalies can be helpful in guiding the next steps.

In patients who have had LSG who present with reflux refractory to medical management, we recommend conversion to LRYGB. Although there are reported endoscopic as well as alternate operative approaches to management of GERD, in our clinical practice and based on reports to date, conversion to LRYGB remains the mainstay. In Guan and colleagues'[50] systematic review of revisional surgery after LSG, in patients with at least 5 years of follow-up the need for revision for GERD was 3%. Langer and colleagues[51] in evaluating 73 patients who underwent conversion to LRYGB for refractory reflux found that 100% of patients had resolution of symptoms and were successfully able to wean off proton pump inhibitors. Similarly, Lim and colleagues[52] in a small cohort of patients undergoing conversion for reflux demonstrated resolution of erosive esophagitis in 85% of patients and complete resolution of GERD symptoms. These data were also corroborated by Quezada and colleagues[53] in their evaluation of 16 patients who underwent conversion to RYGB for GERD and had more than 90% symptom resolution. Although evidence remains small, conversion of LSG to RYGB is safe, feasible, and effective in the resolution of GERD symptoms following LSG.[53–55] Our algorithmic approach is detailed in **Fig. 2**.

Additional Considerations

Although adjustable gastric bands (AGB) have evolved into rather a historical procedure due to their complication profile with only 2816 bands performed in 2016 (3.4%),[27] the bariatric patient with a previously placed gastric band with subsequent GERD and/or dysphagia is a common consultation. As it relates to GERD, the AGB has been associated with esophageal motor dysfunction and esophageal dilation.[56] Ardili-Hani and colleagues[56] found mixed results as it related to GERD following AGB, with 4 of 13 studies reporting improved GERD by pH testing and 3 of 13 studied reporting worsening GERD by similar metrics. Notably, those patients with significant GERD symptoms following AGB had notable preoperative motor dysfunction.[56] In a systematic review of patients undergoing AGB, de Jong and colleagues[57] concluded that while patients in the short term had a reduction of GERD symptoms and pH levels, a nonnegligible number of patients had worsening or newly developed esophagitis and reflux symptoms during long term follow up. Shen and colleagues[58] found in their 2015 systematic review of 17 studies evaluating AGB with greater than 10-year follow-

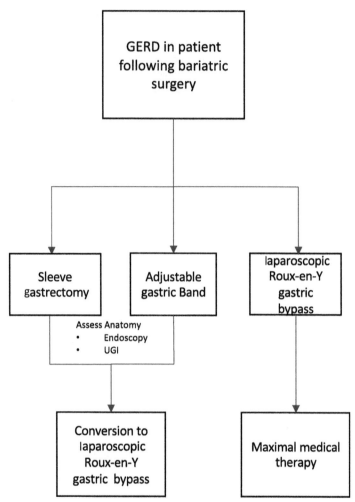

Fig. 2. GERD in patient following bariatric surgery.

up that reflux esophagitis occurred 5% of the time and as high as 28.8% of the time in some studies. It is for these reasons that many providers still placing AGB defer it in patients with reflux.

Other procedures considered in patients with obesity with concomitant GERD have been described. These procedures include Stretta (Mederi Therapeutics Inc.; Norwalk, CT), the use of magnetic sphincter augmentation at the time of sleeve gastrectomy or RYGB, and the MUSE system. There remains a paucity of data as it relates to these modalities for the management of GERD following bariatric surgery. Stretta has been proposed as a strategy for management of GERD in patients with obesity following sleeve gastrectomy or in those who have previously undergone fundoplication; however, the current data do not support its regular use.[59] It is our suggestion that these patients be discussed in a multidisciplinary forum (gastroenterology, interventional endoscopy, foregut and bariatric surgery) for consensus on the ideal approach because these cases often require individualized management.

CLINICS CARE POINTS

- When patients present at BMI greater than 35, consider monitored medical weight loss as strategy to get them to their goal weight of less than 30.
- Patients with GERD and a BMI greater than 35 should be considered for RYGB as first-line surgical therapy.
- Postoperative sleeve patients who present with GERD should be evaluated with upper gastrointestinal series and endoscopy to evaluate for mucosal-based disease (ie, Barrett's, esophagitis) and to evaluate the anatomy of the sleeve.
- Patients with obesity who present with slipped Nissen fundoplications can be safely converted to LRYGB, but should have a through preoperative evaluation before initiation operative intervention.

DISCLOSURE

The authors have no relevant disclosures.

REFERENCES

1. Hales CM. Prevalence of Obesity and Severe Obesity Among Adults: United States, 2017–2018. NCHS Data Brief 2020;(360):8.
2. Maret-Ouda J, Markar SR, Lagergren J. Gastroesophageal Reflux Disease: A Review. J Am Med Assoc 2020;324(24):2536.
3. Eusebi LH, Ratnakumaran R, Yuan Y, et al. Global prevalence of, and risk factors for, gastro-oesophageal reflux symptoms: a meta-analysis. Gut 2018;67(3): 430–40.
4. Ruhl CE, Everhart JE. Overweight, but not high dietary fat intake, increases risk of gastroesophageal reflux disease hospitalization: the NHANES I Epidemiologic Followup Study. First National Health and Nutrition Examination Survey. Annals of Epidemiology. 1999 Oct;9(7):424-35.
5. Murray L, Johnston B, Lane A, et al. Relationship between body mass and gastro-oesophageal reflux symptoms: The Bristol Helicobacter Project. Int J Epidemiol 2003;32(4):645–50.
6. Foster A, Richards WO, McDowell J, et al. Gastrointestinal symptoms are more intense in morbidly obese patients. Surg Endosc 2003;17(11):1766–8.
7. Kaltehbach T, Crockett S, Gerson L. Are Lifestyle Measures Effective in Patients with Gastroesophageal Reflux Disease? An Evidence-Based Approach. Gastrointest Endosc 2005;61(5):AB134.
8. Nilsson M, Johnsen R, Ye W, et al. Obesity and Estrogen as Risk Factors for Gastroesophageal Reflux Symptoms. J Am Med Assoc 2003;290(1):66.
9. Pandolfino JE, El–Serag HB, Zhang Q, et al. Obesity: A Challenge to Esophagogastric Junction Integrity. Gastroenterology 2006;130(3):639–49.
10. El-Serag HB, Sweet S, Winchester CC, et al. Update on the epidemiology of gastro-oesophageal reflux disease: a systematic review. Gut 2014;63(6):871–80.
11. Duke MC, Farrell TM. Surgery for Gastroesophageal Reflux Disease in the Morbidly Obese Patient. J Laparoendoscopic Adv Surg Tech 2017;27(1):12–8.
12. Chang P, Friedenberg F. Obesity and GERD. Gastroenterol Clin North Am 2014; 43(1):161–73.

13. Singh M, Lee J, Gupta N, et al. Weight loss can lead to resolution of gastroesophageal reflux disease symptoms: A prospective intervention trial. Obesity 2013; 21(2):284–90. https://doi.org/10.1002/oby.20279.
14. Kjellin A, Ramel S, Rössner S, et al. Gastroesophageal Reflux in Obese Patients Is Not Reduced by Weight Reduction. Scand J Gastroenterol 1996;31(11): 1047–51.
15. Frederiksen G, Johansson J, Neither FS. Low-calorie Diet nor Vertical Banded Gastroplasty Influence Gastro-oesophageal Reflux in Morbidly Obese Patients. Eur J Surg 2000;166(4):296–300.
16. Jensen MD, Ryan DH, Apovian CM, et al. 2013 AHA/ACC/TOS Guideline for the Management of Overweight and Obesity in Adults. J Am Coll Cardiol 2014; 63(25):2985–3023.
17. LeBlanc ES, O'Connor E, Whitlock EP, et al. Effectiveness of Primary Care–Relevant Treatments for Obesity in Adults: A Systematic Evidence Review for the U.S. Preventive Services Task Force. Ann Intern Med 2011;155(7):434.
18. Perez AR, Moncure AC, Rattner DW. Obesity adversely affects the outcome of antireflux operations. Surg Endosc 2001;15(9):986–9.
19. Morgenthal CB, Lin E, Shane MD, et al. Who will fail laparoscopic Nissen fundoplication? Preoperative prediction of long-term outcomes. Surg Endosc 2007; 21(11):1978–84.
20. Akimoto S, Nandipati KC, Kapoor H, et al. Association of Body Mass Index (BMI) with Patterns of Fundoplication Failure: Insights Gained. J Gastrointest Surg 2015;19(11):1943–8.
21. Winslow ER, Frisella MM, Soper NJ, et al. Obesity does not adversely affect the outcome of laparoscopic antireflux surgery (LARS). Surg Endosc 2003;17(12): 2003–11.
22. Telem DA, Altieri M, Gracia G, et al. Perioperative outcome of esophageal fundoplication for gastroesophageal reflux disease in obese and morbidly obese patients. The Am J Surg 2014;208(2):163–8.
23. Che F, Nguyen B, Cohen A, et al. Prevalence of hiatal hernia in the morbidly obese. Surg Obes Relat Dis 2013;9(6):920–4.
24. Guzman-Pruneda FA, Brethauer SA. Gastroesophageal Reflux After Sleeve Gastrectomy. J Gastrointest Surg 2021;25(2):542–50.
25. DuPree CE, Blair K, Steele SR, et al. Laparoscopic sleeve gastrectomy in patients with preexisting gastroesophageal reflux disease: a national analysis. JAMA Surg 2014;149(4):328–34.
26. Rosenthal RJ. International Sleeve Gastrectomy Expert Panel Consensus Statement: best practice guidelines based on experience of >12,000 cases. Surg Obes Relat Dis 2012;8(1):8–19.
27. English WJ, DeMaria EJ, Brethauer SA, et al. American Society for Metabolic and Bariatric Surgery estimation of metabolic and bariatric procedures performed in the United States in 2016. Surg Obes Relat Dis 2018;14(3):259–63.
28. Braghetto I, Korn O, Csendes A, et al. Laparoscopic Treatment of Obese Patients with Gastroesophageal Reflux Disease and Barrett's Esophagus: a Prospective Study. OBES SURG 2012;22(5):764–72. https://doi.org/10.1007/s11695-011-0531-x.
29. Prachand VN, Alverdy JC. Gastroesophageal reflux disease and severe obesity: Fundoplication or bariatric surgery? World J Gastroenterol 2010;16(30):3757–61.
30. Pallati PK, Shaligram A, Shostrom VK, et al. Improvement in gastroesophageal reflux disease symptoms after various bariatric procedures: Review of the Bariatric Outcomes Longitudinal Database. Surg Obes Relat Dis 2014;10(3):502–7.

31. Frezza EE, Ikramuddin S, Gourash W, et al. Symptomatic improvement in gastro-esophageal reflux disease (GERD) following laparoscopic Roux-en-Y gastric bypass. Surg Endosc 2002;16(7):1027–31.
32. Madalosso CAS, Gurski RR, Callegari-Jacques SM, et al. The Impact of Gastric Bypass on Gastroesophageal Reflux Disease in Morbidly Obese Patients. Ann Surg 2016;263(1):110–6.
33. Luketina R-R, Koch OO, Köhler G, et al. Obesity does not affect the outcome of laparoscopic antireflux surgery. Surg Endosc 2015;29(6):1327–33.
34. Patterson EJ, Davis DG, Khajanchee Y, et al. Comparison of objective outcomes following laparoscopic Nissen fundoplication versus laparoscopic gastric bypass in the morbidly obese with heartburn. Surg Endosc 2003;17(10):1561–5.
35. Perez AR, Moncure AC, Rattner DW. Obesity adversely affects the outcome of antireflux operations. Surg Endosc 2001;15(9):986–9.
36. Varela JE, Hinojosa MW, Nguyen NT. Laparoscopic fundoplication compared with laparoscopic gastric bypass in morbidly obese patients with gastroesophageal reflux disease. Surg Obes Relat Dis 2009;5(2):139–43.
37. Kellogg TA, Andrade R, Maddaus M, et al. Anatomic findings and outcomes after antireflux procedures in morbidly obese patients undergoing laparoscopic conversion to Roux-en-Y gastric bypass. Surg Obes Relat Dis 2007;3(1):52–7 [discussion 58-59].
38. Altieri MS, Pryor AD. Gastroesophageal Reflux Disease After Bariatric Procedures. Surg Clin North Am 2015;95(3):579–91.
39. Nau P, Jackson HT, Aryaie A, et al. Surgical management of gastroesophageal reflux disease in the obese patient. Surg Endosc 2020;34(1):450–7.
40. Thereaux J, Barsamian C, Bretault M, et al. pH monitoring of gastro-oesophageal reflux before and after laparoscopic sleeve gastrectomy. Br J Surg 2016;103(4):399–406.
41. Fass OZ, Mashimo H. The Effect of Bariatric Surgery and Endoscopic Procedures on Gastroesophageal Reflux Disease. J Neurogastroenterol Motil 2021;27(1):35–45.
42. Oor JE, Roks DJ, Ünlü Ç, et al. Laparoscopic sleeve gastrectomy and gastro-esophageal reflux disease: a systematic review and meta-analysis. The Am J Surg 2016;211(1):250–67.
43. Yeung KTD, Penney N, Ashrafian L, et al. Does Sleeve Gastrectomy Expose the Distal Esophagus to Severe Reflux?: A Systematic Review and Meta-analysis. Ann Surg 2020;271(2):257–65.
44. Raj PP, Bhattacharya S, Misra S, et al. Gastroesophageal reflux–related physiologic changes after sleeve gastrectomy and Roux-en-Y gastric bypass: a prospective comparative study. Surg Obes Relat Dis 2019;15(8):1261–9.
45. Peterli R, Wölnerhanssen BK, Peters T, et al. Effect of Laparoscopic Sleeve Gastrectomy vs Laparoscopic Roux-en-Y Gastric Bypass on Weight Loss in Patients With Morbid Obesity: The SM-BOSS Randomized Clinical Trial. J Am Med Assoc 2018;319(3):255.
46. Himpens J, Dobbeleir J, Peeters G. Long-term Results of Laparoscopic Sleeve Gastrectomy for Obesity. Ann Surg 2010;252(2):319–24.
47. Sheppard CE, Sadowski DC, de Gara CJ, et al. Rates of Reflux Before and After Laparoscopic Sleeve Gastrectomy for Severe Obesity. OBES SURG 2015;25(5):763–8.
48. Soricelli E, Casella G, Rizzello M, et al. Initial Experience with Laparoscopic Crural Closure in the Management of Hiatal Hernia in Obese Patients Undergoing Sleeve Gastrectomy. OBES SURG 2010;20(8):1149–53.

49. Daes J, Jimenez ME, Said N, et al. Improvement of Gastroesophageal Reflux Symptoms After Standardized Laparoscopic Sleeve Gastrectomy. OBES SURG 2014;24(4):536–40.

50. Guan B, Chong TH, Peng J, et al. Mid-long-term Revisional Surgery After Sleeve Gastrectomy: a Systematic Review and Meta-analysis. OBES SURG 2019;29(6): 1965–75.

51. Langer FB, Bohdjalian A, Shakeri-Leidenmühler S, et al. Conversion from Sleeve Gastrectomy to Roux-en-Y Gastric Bypass—Indications and Outcome. OBES SURG 2010;20(7):835–40.

52. Lim CH, Lee PC, Lim E, et al. Resolution of Erosive Esophagitis After Conversion from Vertical Sleeve Gastrectomy to Roux-en-Y Gastric Bypass. OBES SURG 2020;30(12):4751–9.

53. Quezada N, Hernández J, Pérez G, et al. Laparoscopic sleeve gastrectomy conversion to Roux-en-Y gastric bypass: experience in 50 patients after 1 to 3 years of follow-up. Surg Obes Relat Dis 2016;12(8):1611–5.

54. Iannelli A, Debs T, Martini F, et al. Laparoscopic conversion of sleeve gastrectomy to Roux-en-Y gastric bypass: indications and preliminary results. Surg Obes Relat Dis 2016;12(8):1533–8.

55. Landreneau JP, Strong AT, Rodriguez JH, et al. Conversion of Sleeve Gastrectomy to Roux-en-Y Gastric Bypass. OBES SURG 2018;28(12):3843–50.

56. Ardila-Hani A, Soffer EE. Review article: the impact of bariatric surgery on gastrointestinal motility. Aliment Pharmacol Ther 2011;34(8):825–31.

57. Jong JRD, Besselink MGH, Ramshorst BV, et al. Effects of adjustable gastric banding on gastroesophageal reflux and esophageal motility: a systematic review. Obes Rev 2010;11(4):297–305.

58. Shen X, Zhang X, Bi J, et al. Long-term complications requiring reoperations after laparoscopic adjustable gastric banding: a systematic review. Surg Obes Relat Dis 2015;11(4):956–64.

59. Khidir N, Angrisani L, Al-Qahtani J, et al. Initial Experience of Endoscopic Radiofrequency Waves Delivery to the Lower Esophageal Sphincter (Stretta Procedure) on Symptomatic Gastroesophageal Reflux Disease Post-Sleeve Gastrectomy. OBES SURG 2018;28(10):3125–30.

How to Understand and Treat Laryngopharyngeal Reflux

Grace Snow, MD, Shumon I. Dhar, MD, Lee M. Akst, MD*

KEYWORDS

- Laryngopharyngeal reflux • Extraesophageal reflux • Reflux laryngitis

KEY POINTS

- Laryngopharyngeal reflux (LPR) is typically diagnosed using a combination of history and physical examination with endoscopy, response to a trial of medication, and objective reflux testing.
- Proton pump inhibitors taken twice daily for at least 2 to 3 months are often used in the empiric treatment of presumed LPR.
- If presumed LPR does not respond to empiric therapy, pH testing with or without impedance, as well as evaluation for nonreflux etiologies of patient complaints, should be considered.

INTRODUCTION

Laryngopharyngeal reflux (LPR), also known as extraesophageal reflux, refers to reflux of gastric and/or duodenal contents beyond the esophagus into the larynx and pharynx. Common symptoms of LPR include globus pharyngeus, throat clearing, dysphonia, cough, sore throat, and excessive phlegm.[1,2] The diagnosis of LPR remains controversial, as there is no gold standard for conclusive identification of this condition. The nonspecific complaints associated with LPR and the uncertain diagnostic criteria for LPR have created a situation in which, for many patients, LPR is overdiagnosed and overtreated. This article will review approaches to the diagnosis and management of LPR, including issues of cost, patient safety, and evaluation for nonreflux etiologies of patient complaints.

HISTORY AND EPIDEMIOLOGY

Since the early 1990s, the clinical entity of LPR has become widely recognized. Research by Koufman[3] demonstrated that many patients with nonspecific complaints

Division of Laryngology, Department of Otolaryngology–Head & Neck Surgery, Johns Hopkins University School of Medicine, 601 North Caroline Street, 6th Floor, Baltimore, MD 21287, USA
* Corresponding author.
E-mail address: Lakst1@jhmi.edu

Gastroenterol Clin N Am 50 (2021) 871–884
https://doi.org/10.1016/j.gtc.2021.08.002
0889-8553/21/© 2021 Elsevier Inc. All rights reserved.
gastro.theclinics.com

such as hoarseness, cough, and throat clearing had abnormal esophageal pH studies, even in the absence of classic heartburn and regurgitation symptoms, and that acid and pepsin can induce laryngeal damage in an animal model if there is prior mucosal injury. Survey data suggest that symptoms consistent with possible LPR affect 20% to 60% of the US population, and only, about 1/3 of patients suspected of having LPR experience classic gastroesophageal reflux disease (GERD) symptoms such as heartburn and regurgitation.[4–6]

PATHOPHYSIOLOGY OF LARYNGOPHARYNGEAL REFLUX

LPR can exist in the absence of GERD symptoms as laryngeal mucosa has different susceptibility to injury than gastric or esophageal mucosa. Laryngeal epithelial cells contain pepsin receptors, and it is thought that reflux events and/or consumption of acidic foods and beverages can reactivate tissue-bound pepsin within the larynx and pharynx.[7–9] Acid and pepsin can directly cause laryngeal mucosal injury and can trigger chronic cough or throat clearing leading to further laryngeal irritation.[10] Additionally, the esophagus is able to clear refluxate through peristalsis, and carbonic anhydrase in esophageal mucosa may buffer acidic reflux. These tissue defense mechanisms are not present in the larynx. These differences in tissue susceptibility of the larynx and pharynx compared with the esophagus may explain why some patients experience symptoms of LPR even in the absence of GERD symptoms.

DIAGNOSIS OF LARYNGOPHARYNGEAL REFLUX
Patient-Reported Measures

In clinical practice, the presence of multiple symptoms such as hoarseness, throat clearing, excessive mucus, dysphagia, coughing, and globus pharyngeus is thought to be suggestive of LPR. Although each symptom individually may have a number of causes other than reflux, the aggregate of multiple different symptoms into a "composite" score may better reflect the presence of reflux. The Reflux Symptom Index (RSI) published by Belafsky and colleagues[11] is a nine-item questionnaire for patients to report symptoms suggestive of LPR, and an RSI greater than 13 is considered to be abnormal (**Table 1**).[11] However, hoarseness, cough, globus pharyngeus, and throat clearing can occur for reasons other than LPR, and the RSI has only a moderate sensitivity and low specificity for LPR.[12–15] While clinical history can suggest LPR, a definitive diagnosis cannot be made solely through history.

Physical Examination/Laryngoscopy

Laryngopharyngeal examination can be used in the workup of possible LPR, both to evaluate for nonreflux etiologies of patient complaints and also possibly to identify signs of reflux—though laryngoscopy cannot be used to diagnose LPR definitively. The Reflux Finding Score (RFS) is a scoring system to evaluate the presence or absence of findings on laryngoscopy that may be associated with LPR (**Table 2**).[16] An RFS greater than 7 is considered to be abnormal. The RFS does not have a high specificity for LPR, as physical examination findings that are included in the RFS can also be found in patients who do not have LPR.[17] Furthermore, the interrater and intrarater reliability of the RFS is poor.[18] As with symptoms, a definitive diagnosis of LPR cannot be made based on examination findings on laryngoscopy.

Although LPR cannot be reliably diagnosed by examination findings on laryngoscopy, visualization of the larynx is helpful in ruling out alternate etiologies of laryngopharyngeal complaints. In particular, the American Academy of Otolaryngology–Head and Neck Surgery clinical practice guidelines recommend that patients with

Table 1						
The reflux symptom index						
Within the Last Month, How Did the Following Problems Affect You? *Circle the Appropriate Response*	**0 = No Problem** **5 = Severe Problem**					
1. Hoarseness or a problem with your voice	0	1	2	3	4	5
2. Clearing your throat	0	1	2	3	4	5
3. Excess throat mucus or postnasal drip	0	1	2	3	4	5
4. Difficulty swallowing food, liquids, or pills	0	1	2	3	4	5
5. Coughing after you ate or after lying down	0	1	2	3	4	5
6. Breathing difficulties or choking episodes	0	1	2	3	4	5
7. Troublesome or annoying cough	0	1	2	3	4	5
8. Sensations of something sticking in your throat or a lump in your throat	0	1	2	3	4	5
9. Heartburn, chest pain, indigestion, or stomach acid coming up	0	1	2	3	4	5
	TOTAL:					

A questionnaire for patients to report symptoms suggestive of LPR. A score greater than 13 is considered abnormal.

From Belafsky PC, Postma GN, Koufman JA. Validity and reliability of the reflux symptom index (RSI). J Voice. 2002;16(2):274-277. https://doi.org/10.1016/s0892-1997(02)00097-8; with permission.

hoarseness lasting for ≥ 4 weeks should undergo laryngoscopy for further evaluation.[19] One study of 132 patients referred to academic laryngology practices for presumed LPR found that 64% of the patients had a different final diagnosis than LPR, and the most of these alternative pathologies were diagnosed using laryngeal stroboscopy, an examination used to visualize vocal cord vibration, structure, and motion.[20] Visualization of the larynx using laryngoscopy or stroboscopy is important in patients with suspected LPR to exclude other laryngeal disorders, including laryngeal cancer.

Empiric Treatment with Proton Pump Inhibitor

Empiric treatment with proton pump inhibitor (PPI) is often prescribed to patients with suspected LPR, with the thought that improvement in LPR symptoms with PPI treatment can confirm the diagnosis of LPR, while lack of improvement with PPI can refute

Table 2				
The reflux finding score				
Laryngeal Finding	**Scoring (Points)**			
Subglottic edema	Absent (0)		Present (2)	
Ventricular obliteration	Partial (2)		Complete (4)	
Erythema/hyperemia	Arytenoids only (2)		Diffuse (4)	
Vocal fold edema	Mild (1)	Moderate (2	Severe (3)	Polypoid (4)
Diffuse laryngeal edema	Mild (1)	Moderate (2)	Severe (3)	Obstructive (4)
Posterior commissure hypertrophy	Mild (1)	Moderate (2)	Severe (3)	Obstructive (4)
Granuloma/granulation tissue	Absent (0)		Present (2)	
Thick endolaryngeal mucus	Absent (0)		Present (2)	

A scoring system to assess laryngeal findings that can be associated with LPR.[16] A score greater than 7 is considered abnormal.

From Belafsky PC, Postma GN, Koufman JA. The validity and reliability of the reflux finding score (RFS). Laryngoscope. 2001;111(8):1313-1317. https://doi.org/10.1097/00005537-200108000-00001; with permission.

the diagnosis of LPR. Empiric trials of antireflux therapy are associated with some drawbacks such as cost and side effects but remain a popular approach for pragmatic reasons. The American College of Gastroenterology recommends an empiric trial of PPI in patients with LPR who also have typical symptoms of GERD.[21] However, the most patients with LPR symptoms do not have heartburn or regurgitation.[4–6]

Depending on the criteria that are used to diagnose LPR, PPIs do not always show superiority compared with placebo in addressing presumed LPR complaints. A systematic review of empiric PPI treatment for LPR symptoms casts some doubt on whether response to empiric PPI treatment can be used to diagnose LPR.[22] The fourteen uncontrolled studies included in this systematic review demonstrated a statistically significant improvement in LPR symptoms with once or twice daily PPI, but none of the six randomized, controlled trials demonstrated statistically significant differences in frequency or severity of symptoms with twice daily PPI for 8 to 16 weeks compared with placebo.[22] A more recent randomized, controlled trial did not demonstrate a statistically significant difference between twice daily PPI and placebo after 6 weeks of treatment but did demonstrate a statistically significant improvement in RSI and RFS at 3 months compared with placebo.[23] Although twice daily PPI for at least 2 months may lead to symptomatic improvement in many patients with LPR symptoms, there is also a high rate of symptomatic improvement with placebo. Furthermore, a lack of response to PPI does not differentiate between patients who do not actually have LPR and patients who have LPR that is refractory to the treatment regimen. Empiric treatment of presumed LPR with PPI can be more convenient for patients than up-front objective reflux testing, but if an empiric trial of PPI is attempted and a patient does not respond, further workup should be initiated.[24]

Objective pH/Impedance Testing

PH testing with or without impedance can be used as a more objective method of diagnosing LPR before starting antireflux therapy and has the benefit of avoiding unnecessary medications in patients who do not actually have LPR. This testing is also useful in patients with suspected LPR who have not had improvement after an empiric trial of therapy. The American College of Gastroenterology recommends consideration of ambulatory reflux testing before a PPI trial in patients with LPR symptoms who do not have typical GERD symptoms; this is a conditional recommendation with a low level of evidence, given the relative lack of evidence for PPI benefit in the absence of traditional heartburn and concerns for PPI side effects.[21]

PH testing with or without impedance is complicated for isolated LPR because the normative values for pharyngeal reflux events are not as well established as they are for distal esophageal reflux events. However, comparisons between asymptomatic individuals and patients with LPR suggest that even one pharyngeal reflux event in a 24 hour period may be abnormal.[25,26] Several different types of diagnostic tests are available (**Table 3**). Dual pH probe with multichannel intraluminal impedance can be used to detect acidic and nonacidic reflux events in the distal esophagus and the proximal esophagus/hypopharynx. The proximal pH sensor can be placed at or just distal to the upper esophageal sphincter rather than in the pharynx to prevent drying, and catheters with variable lengths between the proximal and distal probe are available, as the location of the proximal probe will vary depending on the individual length of the esophagus if the distal probe is placed at 5 cm above the lower esophageal sphincter.[27,28] Dual pH/impedance testing before a trial of PPI in patients with LPR may result in cost savings as unnecessary trials of PPI in patients who do not have pathologic acid reflux can be avoided.[29]

Table 3
Diagnostic testing for gastroesophageal and laryngopharyngeal reflux

Test	Description	Pros	Cons
Dual pH probe with multichannel intraluminal impedance	Catheter placed through nose using manometry to identify the lower esophageal sphincter. Measures distal esophageal and proximal esophageal or pharyngeal pH and impedance.	Provides data on acid and nonacid reflux in the distal and proximal esophagus	Catheter is visible externally protruding from the nose and can be uncomfortable. Variable position of proximal pH probe based on length of esophageal necessitating availability various catheter sizes
Single pH probe with multichannel intraluminal impedance	Catheter placed through nose using manometry to identify the lower esophageal sphincter. Measures distal esophageal pH and impedance.	Provides data on acid and nonacid reflux in the distal esophagus	Catheter is visible externally, single pH probe, only measures distal esophageal pH
Wireless Bravo pH probe	Capsule placed during endoscopy, attached to esophageal mucosa.	Not visible externally, greater patient tolerability	Does not measure nonacid reflux, measures only esophageal and not pharyngeal reflux Limited studies and normative data available on proximal esophageal placement of the probe
Restech pharyngeal pH probe	Oropharyngeal probe attached to a catheter placed through the nose. LED light can be visualized in the oropharynx.	Measures pharyngeal acid reflux, less susceptible to drying	Does not measure nonacid reflux or esophageal reflux
PepsinCheck or PepTest salivary pepsin test	Salivary samples are collected by the patient at predefined times or during symptomatic periods	High patient tolerability, lower cost	Optimal cutoff value to maximize sensitivity and specificity is not fully defined

Wireless Bravo pH probes (Medtronic, Sunnyvale, CA, USA) can be used to diagnose esophageal acid reflux but cannot measure nonacidic reflux. Some patients may find the wireless probe preferable to pH/impedance, as the wireless probe is endoscopically placed in the esophagus, while the wired pH/impedance catheter is placed transnasally, and the end of the catheter is visible externally for the duration of the test. Wireless probes are typically placed in the lower esophagus, and studies are limited regarding the tolerability and normative data for placement of these probes in the upper esophagus in order to diagnose LPR.[30,31]

The Restech pharyngeal pH probe (Respiratory Technology Corp., Houston, TX, USA) is placed in the pharynx for direct measurement of LPR rather than GERD. It is designed to resist drying but does not measure nonacidic reflux.[32] A pH lower than 5.0 in the supine position and 5.5. in the upright position is considered abnormal, and a Ryan composite score greater than 6.8 in the supine position or greater than 9.4 in the upright position is considered abnormal.[32] A study of simultaneous pharyngeal and esophageal pH testing demonstrated that 23% of patients with normal esophageal acid exposure had abnormal pharyngeal acid exposure.[33] The situation could occur in patients who have a small number of reflux events but a high proportion of reflux events reaching the pharynx. Patients who had pharyngeal pH testing before starting treatment for LPR appear to have greater adherence to lifestyle modifications and medications and a greater improvement in symptoms compared with patients who had empiric PPI treatment.[34]

As described earlier, there are several methods for performing pH testing with or without impedance to evaluate LPR. These tests provide objective data on esophageal or pharyngeal acid exposure, and impedance testing also provides information on nonacid reflux. This testing can be useful in patients whose LPR symptoms do not improve with empiric PPI treatment. Some physicians also use pH testing before starting medication for LPR, particularly in patients who do not have classic GERD symptoms. This approach has the benefit of decreasing medication overuse but is less convenient and less tolerable for patients.

Salivary Pepsin Detection

The detection of pepsin in the saliva has been proposed as a means to diagnose LPR, as the presence of pepsin in the saliva provides evidence that reflux into the oral cavity has occurred.[35] PepsinCheck (in the United States) or PepTest (outside of the United States) are commercially available tests that provide qualitative and quantitative measures of oral salivary pepsin and can be purchased directly by the consumer (RD Biomed Limited). Detection of salivary pepsin is less expensive than dual pH/impedance. The manufacturer defines a positive test result as $\geq$ 16 ng/mL; however, the optimal cutoff value to maximize sensitivity and specificity is still being defined.[35] Salivary pepsin detection is noninvasive and may become a useful quantitative test for LPR, but additional research is needed to determine how to use this test in a clinically meaningful way.

IMPORTANCE OF TREATING LARYNGOPHARYNGEAL REFLUX ECONOMICALLY

The evaluation and treatment of LPR may incur higher economic costs compared with the treatment of GERD. This is because of the difficulties associated with diagnosing LPR and the fact that symptoms of LPR can overlap with other laryngopharyngeal complaints, so multiple specialist visits and procedures may be needed to reach a diagnosis. Francis and colleagues[36] estimated the cost of care for presumed LPR to be 5.6 times higher than that for typical GERD and found that only 54% of patients with LPR symptoms reported improvement with the treatment they received. Patient satisfaction with treatment of presumed LPR remains low, despite the amount of money being spent. PPI treatment appears to be less effective in controlling LPR symptoms than it is at controlling heartburn, and this may be because many patients presumed to have LPR may actually have a different etiology of their symptoms.[37–39] Patients with LPR symptoms who also have typical GERD symptoms appear to be more likely to respond to PPI, which is logical given that these patients would be more likely to have reflux if they are having GERD symptoms. These findings highlight the importance of an appropriate workup to confirm the diagnosis of LPR and exclude alternative laryngeal diagnoses in patients with symptoms presumed to be related to LPR who do not have classic GERD symptoms.[17,31]

PRACTICE PATTERNS, GUIDELINES, AND TREATMENT OPTIONS FOR LARYNGOPHARYNGEAL REFLUX

PPIs are generally considered to be the mainstay of treatment for LPR. However, some patients wish to avoid long-term PPI use, particularly as there is increasing recognition of the long-term side effects of PPI.[40] Several additional treatment options are available, including diet and lifestyle modifications, histamine receptor blockers, alginates, and surgical or endoscopic treatment options to address the lower esophageal sphincter.

Proton Pump Inhibitor

PPIs have been considered the main treatment of LPR since the early 2000s.[6,41] The dosage and duration of treatment vary widely among studies.[42] A systematic review of treatment of LPR that included 76 studies and over 6000 patients found that a variety of different PPIs were prescribed once or twice daily for anywhere from 4 to 24 weeks, with an efficacy ranging from 18% to 87%.[43] The wide variation in efficacy with PPI treatment and the lack of difference between PPI and placebo in some studies may reflect the fact that many studies of LPR include patients diagnosed based on RSI and RFS, which do not have a high specificity for LPR—inclusion of nonreflux patients in the study cohort would erode any therapeutic advantage of PPI over placebo.[1,12,17,18,22]

Twice daily PPI may be superior to once daily PPI in the treatment of LPR. A prospective cohort study comparing twice daily PPI with once daily PPI in patients with signs and symptoms of LPR showed a higher response rate with twice daily PPI compared with once daily PPI, and 54% of the patients who did not respond to once daily PPI had symptomatic improvement after an additional 8 weeks of twice daily PPI.[44] At least a 2 to 3-month trial of PPI is considered to be optimal in order to allow laryngeal mucosal injury to heal.[1,6]

Although many patients with LPR will have symptomatic improvement with PPI, patients with predominantly nonacid or mixed reflux may have symptoms that are refractory to PPI.[10,45–47] Furthermore, potential long-term side effects of PPI are increasingly recognized, including increased fracture risk, cardiovascular events, nutritional deficiencies, and increased risk of infections such as pneumonia and *Clostridium difficile*.[40]

In spite of the long-term side effects, PPI remains a popular treatment option for LPR. Variable dosages and durations of treatment are used, but treatment twice daily for at least 2 to 3 months may lead to greater symptom improvement than shorter or lower-dose treatment regimens.

Lifestyle and Dietary Approaches

Lifestyle and dietary changes are commonly recommended in the treatment of LPR, as these interventions are inexpensive and there is no risk of medication side effects.[43] A systematic review of lifestyle and dietary changes in patients with GERD has demonstrated that weight loss and tobacco smoking cessation can decrease reflux symptoms, and elevation of the head of bed and avoidance of late evening meals within 2 hours of bedtime can decrease esophageal acid exposure time.[48] By extension, these interventions are often recommended in patients with LPR symptoms as well.

While the data regarding dietary changes in the treatment of LPR are less conclusive, some studies suggest that a dietary approach to controlling LPR symptoms can be effective. Initial studies by Koufman[49] and Koufman and Johnston[50] suggested that a low acid diet and alkaline water (pH 8.8) could benefit reflux patients. A more recent study retrospectively compared patients treated with esomeprazole twice daily or dexlansoprazole daily to patients who were instructed to follow a diet consisting of alkaline water (pH > 8.0) and a 90% to 95% plant-based diet. Both groups were instructed to avoid coffee, tea, chocolate, soda, greasy, fried, fatty and spicy foods, and alcohol. After 6 weeks of treatment, both groups showed improvement in RSI, and there was not a greater improvement in RSI in the group treated with PPI compared witth the group treated with dietary change alone.[51] However, patients adhering to a very restrictive diet may lose weight as a result of the diet, and weight loss could account for the improvement in LPR symptoms.[52] Lifestyle and dietary changes appear to be safe and effective for some patients with LPR symptoms, although patient adherence can be a limitation.

Alginates

Alginates are gaining popularity as a treatment for LPR as they appear to have some efficacy without significant side effects. Alginate-containing compounds are derived from algae and form a mechanical antireflux barrier within the stomach when taken after meals. For patients with GERD symptoms, a systematic review of 2095 subjects in 14 studies demonstrated that alginates are more effective than placebo or antacids and appear to be less effective than PPI or histamine-2 blockers, although this was not statistically significant.[53] In a randomized, controlled trial of liquid alginate suspension (Gaviscon Advance, GlaxoSmithKline) four times daily after meals and at bedtime in patients with LPR symptoms, patients treated with alginate had a significant improvement in RSI and RFS compared with the control group who received no treatment.[54] Another trial did not demonstrate any additional improvement in LPR symptoms in patients who took alginate with a PPI compared with those who took only alginate.[55] Alginates appear to improve LPR symptoms compared with placebo and are safe and well tolerated.[40,54]

Histamine-2 Receptor Antagonists

Histamine-2 (H2) receptor antagonists such as ranitidine and famotidine are sometimes used for patients with LPR who wish to avoid or decrease their dose of PPIs. H2 receptor antagonists are used in the treatment of mild-to-moderate GERD but are known to be less effective than PPIs in the treatment of GERD and erosive esophagitis.[21,56,57] Therefore, it can be extrapolated that H2 receptor antagonists would be less effective in the treatment of LPR as well. Tachyphylaxis or tolerance to the effects of H2 receptor antagonists can occur within 1 to 2 weeks of treatment, which can limit the long-term effectiveness of these medications.[58] Although H2 receptor antagonists are an option for the treatment of LPR, they appear to be less effective than PPIs.

Surgical and Endoscopic Treatment Options

Surgical and endoscopic treatment options for LPR appear to be beneficial in a carefully selected patient population. Laparoscopic Nissen fundoplication is a surgical treatment option for long-term therapy in patients with GERD.[21] Patients with LPR that is refractory to PPI who are demonstrated to have pathologic reflux using dual pH/impedance appear to demonstrate improvement in LPR symptoms after Nissen, as do patients with LPR symptoms who have a type 1 hiatal hernia.[59–61]

Transoral incisionless fundoplication (TIF) is an endoscopic procedure that is an alternative to a traditional Nissen and can be performed with a concurrent laparoscopic hiatal hernia repair in patients with a hiatal hernia greater than 2 cm.[62,63] TIF appears to be more effective than PPI in controlling regurgitation and extraesophageal/LPR symptoms, with results that are sustained at 5 years post-TIF.[58,64] There has been a significant amount of research and device improvements over the past decade, leading to greater acceptance of these procedures.[21,58,63–65]

Other procedural treatment options for reflux, such as Stretta radiofrequency lower esophageal sphincter augmentation (Respiratory Technology Corp., Houston, TX, USA), and Linx magnetic esophageal sphincter augmentation (Torax Medical, Inc., Shoreview, MN, USA) also exist but are not currently well studied in patients with LPR.[66,67]

Most patients with LPR will be able to gain symptomatic relief with more conservative measures, but carefully selected patients with LPR may benefit from endoscopic or surgical reflux treatment.

SUMMARY

Awareness of LPR has increased among patients and physicians over the past few decades. The nonspecific symptoms of LPR and the frequent use of empiric trials of PPI in patients with suspected LPR have led to some patients being treated for LPR when they may actually have an alternate diagnosis. This has led to increased cost to patients and increased risk of medication side effects. Empiric PPI trial is a pragmatic approach that can be convenient for patients, but if patients do not experience symptomatic relief, then additional workup should be performed. Patients with symptoms refractory to PPI may have nonacid or mixed reflux or may have a diagnosis other than LPR. PH testing with or without impedance can provide more objective data on esophageal and pharyngeal reflux. Workup for alternative laryngeal etiologies of symptoms with laryngoscopy or stroboscopy should also be performed. Instead of an empiric trial of PPI, some patients and clinicians prefer to begin with objective testing for acid reflux in order to avoid the use of medications unnecessarily.

PPIs are commonly used to treat LPR and are effective for many patients. Twice daily dosing for at least 2 to 3 months is often used. Lifestyle and dietary changes can be effective as well if patients are able to adhere to them. Other treatment options include alginates, H2 blockers, and surgical or endoscopic treatment options.

CLINICS CARE POINTS

- Symptoms consistent with possible laryngopharyngeal reflux (LPR) affect 20% to 60% of the US population, and only, 1/3 of patients suspected of having LPR have classic GERD symptoms.
- LPR cannot be definitively diagnosed solely by history or laryngoscopy.

- If a patient with suspected LPR is treated with an empiric trial of proton pump inhibitor (PPI) and does not have symptomatic improvement after 2 to 3 months of twice daily dosing, additional workup should be performed, such as pH testing with or without impedance, and laryngoscopy, or stroboscopy to assess for an alternate cause of symptoms.

- Up-front pH testing with or without impedance before a trial of PPI is another option for the diagnosis of LPR.

- PPIs and diet and lifestyle modifications are the mainstay of treatment for patients with LPR

- Other treatment options include alginates, H2 receptor antagonists, and surgical or endoscopic treatment options.

DISCLOSURE

The authors have nothing to disclose

REFERENCES

1. Lechien JR, Akst LM, Hamdan AL, et al. Evaluation and management of laryngopharyngeal reflux disease: state of the art review. Otolaryngol Neck Surg 2019; 160(5):762–82.
2. Book DT, Rhee JS, Toohill RJ, et al. Perspectives in laryngopharyngeal reflux: an international survey. Laryngoscope 2002;112(8):1399–406.
3. Koufman JA. The otolaryngologic manifestations of gastroesophageal reflux disease (GERD): a clinical investigation of 225 patients using ambulatory 24-hour pH monitoring and an experimental investigation of the role of acid and pepsin in the development of laryngeal injury. Laryngoscope 1991;101(4 Pt 2 Suppl 53):1–78.
4. Connor NP, Palazzi-Churas KLP, Cohen SB, et al. Symptoms of extraesophageal reflux in a community-dwelling sample. J Voice 2007;21(2):189–202.
5. Reulbach TR, Belafsky PC, Blalock PD, et al. Occult laryngeal pathology in a community-based cohort. Otolaryngol Head Neck Surg 2001;124(4):448–50.
6. Koufman JA, Aviv JE, Casiano RR, et al. Laryngopharyngeal reflux: position statement of the committee on speech, voice, and swallowing disorders of the American Academy of Otolaryngology-Head and Neck Surgery. Otolaryngol Head Neck Surg 2002;127(1):32–5.
7. Johnston N, Wells CW, Blumin JH, et al. Receptor-mediated uptake of pepsin by laryngeal epithelial cells. Ann Otol Rhinol Laryngol 2007;116(12):934–8.
8. Johnston N, Wells CW, Samuels TL, et al. Pepsin in nonacidic refluxate can damage hypopharyngeal epithelial cells. Ann Otol Rhinol Laryngol 2009;118(9): 677–85.
9. Samuels TL, Johnston N. Pepsin as a causal agent of inflammation during nonacidic reflux. Otolaryngol Head Neck Surg 2009;141(5):559–63.
10. Johnston N, Wells CW, Samuels TL, et al. Rationale for targeting pepsin in the treatment of reflux disease. Ann Otol Rhinol Laryngol 2010;119(8):547–58.
11. Belafsky PC, Postma GN, Koufman JA. Validity and reliability of the reflux symptom index (RSI). J Voice 2002;16(2):274–7.
12. DeVore EK, Chan WW, Shin JJ, et al. Does the reflux symptom index predict increased pharyngeal events on HEMII-pH testing and correlate with general quality of life? J Voice 2019. https://doi.org/10.1016/j.jvoice.2019.11.019.

13. Schneider SL, Clary MS, Fink DS, et al. Voice therapy associated with a decrease in the reflux symptoms index in patients with voice complaints. Laryngoscope 2019;129(5):1169–73.

14. Patel AK, Mildenhall NR, Kim W, et al. Symptom overlap between laryngopharyngeal reflux and glottic insufficiency in vocal fold atrophy patients. Ann Otol Rhinol Laryngol 2014;123(4):265–70.

15. Kavookjian H, Irwin T, Garnett JD, et al. The reflux symptom index and symptom overlap in dysphonic patients. Laryngoscope 2020;130(11):2631–6.

16. Belafsky PC, Postma GN, Koufman JA. The validity and reliability of the reflux finding score (RFS). Laryngoscope 2001;111(8):1313–7.

17. Hicks DM, Ours TM, Abelson TI, et al. The prevalence of hypopharynx findings associated with gastroesophageal reflux in normal volunteers. J Voice 2002; 16(4):564–79.

18. Branski RC, Bhattacharyya N, Shapiro J. The reliability of the assessment of endoscopic laryngeal findings associated with laryngopharyngeal reflux disease. Laryngoscope 2002;112(6):1019–24.

19. Stachler RJ, Francis DO, Schwartz SR, et al. Clinical practice guideline: hoarseness (dysphonia) (update). Otolaryngol Head Neck Surg 2018;158(1_suppl): S1–42.

20. Fritz MA, Persky MJ, Fang Y, et al. The accuracy of the laryngopharyngeal reflux diagnosis: utility of the stroboscopic exam. Otolaryngol Head Neck Surg 2016; 155(4):629–34.

21. Katz PO, Gerson LB, Vela MF. Guidelines for the diagnosis and management of gastroesophageal reflux disease. Am J Gastroenterol 2013;108(3):308–28.

22. Karkos PD, Wilson JA. Empiric treatment of laryngopharyngeal reflux with proton pump inhibitors: a systematic review. Laryngoscope 2006;116(1):144–8.

23. Reichel O, Dressel H, Wiederänders K, et al. Double-blind, placebo-controlled trial with esomeprazole for symptoms and signs associated with laryngopharyngeal reflux. Otolaryngol Head Neck Surg 2008;139(3):414–20.

24. Lechien JR, Bock JM, Carroll TL, et al. Is empirical treatment a reasonable strategy for laryngopharyngeal reflux? A contemporary review. Clin Otolaryngol 2020; 45(4):450–8.

25. Maldonado A, Diederich L, Castell DO, et al. Laryngopharyngeal reflux identified using a new catheter design: defining normal values and excluding artifacts. Laryngoscope 2003;113(2):349–55.

26. Hoppo T, Sanz AF, Nason KS, et al. How much pharyngeal exposure is "normal"? Normative data for laryngopharyngeal reflux events using hypopharyngeal multichannel intraluminal impedance (HMII). J Gastrointest Surg 2012;16(1):16–24 [discussion 24–5].

27. Cumpston EC, Blumin JH, Bock JM. Dual pH with multichannel intraluminal impedance testing in the evaluation of subjective laryngopharyngeal reflux symptoms. Otolaryngol Neck Surg 2016;155(6):1014–20.

28. Borges LF, Chan WW, Carroll TL. Dual pH probes without proximal esophageal and pharyngeal impedance may be deficient in diagnosing LPR. J Voice 2019; 33(5):697–703.

29. Carroll TL, Werner A, Nahikian K, et al. Rethinking the laryngopharyngeal reflux treatment algorithm: Evaluating an alternate empiric dosing regimen and considering up-front, pH-impedance, and manometry testing to minimize cost in treating suspect laryngopharyngeal reflux disease. Laryngoscope 2017;127(Suppl 6): S1–13.

30. Friedman M, Schalch P, Vidyasagar R, et al. Wireless upper esophageal monitoring for laryngopharyngeal reflux (LPR). Otolaryngol Neck Surg 2007;137(3): 471–6.

31. Dhillon VK, Akst LM. How to approach laryngopharyngeal reflux: an otolaryngology perspective. Curr Gastroenterol Rep 2016;18(8):44.

32. Ayazi S, Lipham JC, Hagen JA, et al. A new technique for measurement of pharyngeal pH: normal values and discriminating pH threshold. J Gastrointest Surg 2009;13(8):1422–9.

33. Fuchs HF, Müller DT, Berlth F, et al. Simultaneous laryngopharyngeal pH monitoring (Restech) and conventional esophageal pH monitoring-correlation using a large patient cohort of more than 100 patients with suspected gastroesophageal reflux disease. Dis Esophagus 2018;31(10). https://doi.org/10.1093/dote/doy018.

34. Friedman M, Maley A, Kelley K, et al. Impact of pH monitoring on laryngopharyngeal reflux treatment: improved compliance and symptom resolution. Otolaryngol Head Neck Surg 2011;144(4):558–62.

35. Zhang M, Chia C, Stanley C, et al. Diagnostic utility of salivary pepsin as compared with 24-hour dual ph/impedance probe in laryngopharyngeal reflux. Otolaryngol Neck Surg 2021;164(2):375–80.

36. Francis DO, Rymer JA, Slaughter JC, et al. High economic burden of caring for patients with suspected extraesophageal reflux. Am J Gastroenterol 2013; 108(6):905–11.

37. Chan WW, Chiou E, Obstein KL, et al. The efficacy of proton pump inhibitors for the treatment of asthma in adults: a meta-analysis. Arch Intern Med 2011;171(7): 620–9.

38. Qadeer MA, Phillips CO, Lopez AR, et al. Proton pump inhibitor therapy for suspected GERD-related chronic laryngitis: a meta-analysis of randomized controlled trials. Am J Gastroenterol 2006;101(11):2646–54.

39. Steward DL, Wilson KM, Kelly DH, et al. Proton pump inhibitor therapy for chronic laryngo-pharyngitis: a randomized placebo-control trial. Otolaryngol Head Neck Surg 2004;131(4):342–50.

40. Reimer C. Safety of long-term PPI therapy. Best Pract Res Clin Gastroenterol 2013;27(3):443–54.

41. Ford CN. Evaluation and management of laryngopharyngeal reflux. JAMA 2005; 294(12):1534–40.

42. Lechien JR, Allen JE, Barillari MR, et al. Management of laryngopharyngeal reflux around the world: an international study. Laryngoscope 2020. https://doi.org/10.1002/lary.29270.

43. Lechien JR, Mouawad F, Barillari MR, et al. Treatment of laryngopharyngeal reflux disease: a systematic review. World J Clin Cases 2019;7(19):2995–3011.

44. Park W, Hicks DM, Khandwala F, et al. Laryngopharyngeal reflux: prospective cohort study evaluating optimal dose of proton-pump inhibitor therapy and pretherapy predictors of response. Laryngoscope 2005;115(7):1230–8.

45. Tutuian R, Mainie I, Agrawal A, et al. Nonacid reflux in patients with chronic cough on acid-suppressive therapy. Chest 2006;130(2):386–91.

46. Martinucci I, de Bortoli N, Savarino E, et al. Optimal treatment of laryngopharyngeal reflux disease. Ther Adv Chronic Dis 2013;4(6):287–301.

47. Johnston N, Ondrey F, Rosen R, et al. Airway reflux: airway reflux. Ann N Y Acad Sci 2016;1381(1):5–13.

48. Ness-Jensen E, Hveem K, El-Serag H, et al. Lifestyle intervention in gastroesophageal reflux disease. Clin Gastroenterol Hepatol 2016;14(2):175–82.e1-3.

49. Koufman JA. Low-acid diet for recalcitrant laryngopharyngeal reflux: therapeutic benefits and their implications. Ann Otol Rhinol Laryngol 2011;120(5):281–7.

50. Koufman JA, Johnston N. Potential benefits of pH 8.8 alkaline drinking water as an adjunct in the treatment of reflux disease. Ann Otol Rhinol Laryngol 2012; 121(7):431–4.

51. Zalvan CH, Hu S, Greenberg B, et al. A comparison of alkaline water and mediterranean diet vs proton pump inhibition for treatment of laryngopharyngeal reflux. JAMA Otolaryngol Head Neck Surg 2017;143(10):1023–9.

52. Kavitt RT. Dietary modifications in the treatment of laryngopharyngeal reflux-will "an apple a day" keep the laryngopharyngeal reflux away? JAMA Otolaryngol Head Neck Surg 2017;143(10):1030–1.

53. Leiman DA, Riff BP, Morgan S, et al. Alginate therapy is effective treatment for GERD symptoms: a systematic review and meta-analysis. Dis Esophagus 2017;30(5):1–9.

54. McGlashan JA, Johnstone LM, Sykes J, et al. The value of a liquid alginate suspension (Gaviscon Advance) in the management of laryngopharyngeal reflux. Eur Arch Otorhinolaryngol 2009;266(2):243–51.

55. Wilkie MD, Fraser HM, Raja H. Gaviscon® Advance alone versus co-prescription of Gaviscon® Advance and proton pump inhibitors in the treatment of laryngopharyngeal reflux. Eur Arch Otorhinolaryngol 2018;275(10):2515–21.

56. Chiba N, De Gara CJ, Wilkinson JM, et al. Speed of healing and symptom relief in grade II to IV gastroesophageal reflux disease: a meta-analysis. Gastroenterology 1997;112(6):1798–810.

57. Wang W-H, Huang J-Q, Zheng G-F, et al. Head-to-head comparison of H2-receptor antagonists and proton pump inhibitors in the treatment of erosive esophagitis: a meta-analysis. World J Gastroenterol 2005;11(26):4067–77.

58. Trad KS, Barnes WE, Simoni G, et al. Transoral incisionless fundoplication effective in eliminating GERD symptoms in partial responders to proton pump inhibitor therapy at 6 months: the TEMPO Randomized Clinical Trial. Surg Innov 2015; 22(1):26–40.

59. Carroll TL, Nahikian K, Asban A, et al. Nissen fundoplication for laryngopharyngeal reflux after patient selection using dual pH, full column impedance testing: a pilot study. Ann Otol Rhinol Laryngol 2016;125(9):722–8.

60. Park A, Weltz AS, Sanford Z, et al. Laparoscopic antireflux surgery (LARS) is highly effective in the treatment of select patients with chronic cough. Surgery 2019;166(1):34–40.

61. Zhang C, Hu Z-W, Yan C, et al. Nissen fundoplication vs proton pump inhibitors for laryngopharyngeal reflux based on pH-monitoring and symptom-scale. World J Gastroenterol 2017;23(19):3546–55.

62. Sami Trad K. Transoral incisionless fundoplication: current status. Curr Opin Gastroenterol 2016;32(4):338–43.

63. Ihde GM, Pena C, Scitern C, et al. pH scores in hiatal repair with transoral incisionless fundoplication. JSLS 2019;23(1). e2018.00087.

64. Trad KS, Barnes WE, Prevou ER, et al. The TEMPO trial at 5 years: transoral fundoplication (TIF 2.0) Is safe, durable, and cost-effective. Surg Innov 2018;25(2): 149–57.

65. Testoni PA, Vailati C, Testoni S, et al. Transoral incisionless fundoplication (TIF 2.0) with EsophyX for gastroesophageal reflux disease: long-term results and findings affecting outcome. Surg Endosc 2012;26(5):1425–35.

66. Noar MD, Squires P, Kahn S. Tu1232 LPR and LPR-GERD subtypes of reflux respond to sphincter targeted endoluminal gerd therapy. Gastrointest Endosc 2017;85(5):AB594–5.

67. Skubleny D, Switzer NJ, Dang J, et al. LINX® magnetic esophageal sphincter augmentation versus Nissen fundoplication for gastroesophageal reflux disease: a systematic review and meta-analysis. Surg Endosc 2017;31(8):3078–84.

Making Sense of Nonachalasia Esophageal Motor Disorders

Benjamin D. Rogers, MD[a,b], C. Prakash Gyawali, MD, MRCP[a],*

KEYWORDS

- Absent contractility • Hypercontractile disorder • Distal esophageal spasm
- Ineffective esophageal motility

KEY POINTS

- Achalasia spectrum disorders are diagnosed using high resolution manometry (HRM), but non-achalasia motor disorders can also be identified in symptomatic patients undergoing esophageal investigation.
- Ancillary HRM maneuvers (multiple rapid swallows, rapid drink challenge, solid swallows) identify smooth muscle contraction reserve and unveil obstructive motor physiology, which can guide management.
- Impedance topographs superimposed on HRM, barium radiography and functional lumen imaging probe studies can augment the clinical value of HRM in non-achalasia motor disorders.
- Non-achalasia motor disorders do not always explain esophageal symptoms, and the clinical context needs to be considered in determining clinical relevance and management options.

INTRODUCTION

The transition from conventional manometry to high-resolution manometry (HRM) began in the 1990s.[1] A key feature of HRM is the increased numbers of esophageal pressure recording sites, which are spaced no more than 1 cm apart on an esophageal manometry catheter. New software programs fill in best-fit data between the recorded pressures, further improving resolution of pressure phenomena, and set the stage for spatiotemporal displays of esophageal peristalsis. The resulting 3D topographic plots of a test swallow, with time along the x-axis, esophageal length along the y-axis, and

[a] Division of Gastroenterology, Washington University School of Medicine, 660 South Euclid Avenue, Campus Box 8124, St Louis, MO 63110, USA; [b] Division of Gastroenterology, Hepatology, and Nutrition, University of Louisville School of Medicine, 550 South Preston Street, Louisville, KY 40202, USA
* Corresponding author.
E-mail address: cprakash@wustl.edu

Gastroenterol Clin N Am 50 (2021) 885–903
https://doi.org/10.1016/j.gtc.2021.08.003
0889-8553/21/© 2021 Elsevier Inc. All rights reserved.
gastro.theclinics.com

pressure amplitude displayed as concentric color isobars along the z-axis, are termed Clouse plots in honor of the late Ray Clouse who conceived and pioneered the technology.[2]

Manometry is frequently used in the evaluation of transit symptoms, particularly dysphagia, not explained on endoscopy and/or contrast radiography, or when a motor disorder is suspected on these tests. Chief among the clinical advantages of HRM over conventional manometry is the diagnosis and classification of achalasia and its subtypes.[3] Now in its fourth iteration, the Chicago classification (CCv4.0) characterizes achalasia as elevated median integrated relaxation pressure (IRP) and no normal esophageal body peristalsis.[3] Panesophageal pressurization or spastic (premature) distal esophageal contractions in ≥20% of swallows define types 2 and 3 achalasia, respectively.[3] However, notwithstanding IRP thresholds, achalasia needs to be considered when esophageal peristalsis uniformly fails in the context of suggestive symptoms because therapeutics can successfully improve achalasia symptoms, and adequate recognition is paramount to appropriate management.[4,5]

The Chicago classification has evolved as new data have shed light on which manometric findings are of clinical relevance. The entire spectrum of nonachalasia esophageal motor disorders, from hypomotile to spastic and hypermotile disorders (**Table 1**), has undergone changes since the first Chicago Classification was published.[3,6–8] The most important of these entities remains esophagogastric junction outflow obstruction (EGJOO), a heterogenous motor pattern that only occasionally requires invasive management in the context of demonstrable obstruction on alternate testing. Hypermotility disorders, including hypercontractile esophagus and distal esophageal spasm (DES), can present with transit or perceptive symptoms but are sometimes encountered in the context of reflux; therefore, these disorders also require independent confirmation of an obstructive pattern before invasive management. Ineffective esophageal motility (IEM) criteria are now refined and made more stringent, but association with symptoms remains poor. The Chicago classification further nods to the central role of the EGJ, whether it be hypotensive or hypertensive, by specifically outlining metrics of tone and morphology, despite not including specific EGJ diagnoses in the main CC 4.0 algorithm. This review will describe motor disorders that do not fulfill criteria for achalasia and discuss how to approach these disorders in the clinical setting.

MOTILITY DISORDERS OF THE ESOPHAGOGASTRIC JUNCTION

The esophagogastric junction is a complex structure that is comprised of the intrinsic lower esophageal sphincter (LES) and muscle fibers from the right and left crura of the diaphragm.[9] In health, the LES and CD are superimposed, creating a structural and mechanical barrier between the esophageal and gastric lumens that participates in prevention of gastroesophageal reflux.[10] The LES relaxes during swallow-induced primary peristalsis and with secondary peristalsis, allowing passage of esophageal contents into the stomach. Abnormal relaxation of the LES creates an obstructive process that can overlap with structural EGJ obstruction, leading to retention of ingested food and resulting in dysphagia. Manometric pressure measurements are not discriminative between obstruction from abnormal LES relaxation and structural EGJ obstruction, which is a primary reason why HRM is typically performed after structural etiologies are excluded using endoscopy or barium radiography.

ESOPHAGOGASTRIC JUNCTION OUTFLOW OBSTRUCTION

As the category was introduced in the second iteration of the Chicago Classification,[7] EGJOO has generated significant confusion and debate regarding diagnostic criteria

Table 1			
Nonachalasia esophageal motor disorders			
	Esophagogastric Junction	Esophageal Body	Other
Hypomotility disorders, potential for reflux physiology	Hypotensive EGJ Abnormal EGJ morphology	Absent contractility Ineffective esophageal motility	Supragastric belching Rumination
Hypermotility disorders, potential for obstructive physiology	EGJ outflow obstruction Hypertensive LES	Distal esophageal spasm Hypercontractile esophagus	

and management. The fact that 5% of asymptomatic volunteers meet criteria for EGJOO[11] and that many diagnoses of EGJOO are not clinically relevant[5] underscores the importance of segregating this motor pattern from achalasia to ensure intervention is targeted and performed only when necessary. The hallmark of EGJOO is elevated median IRP in the presence of adequate esophageal body peristalsis[3] (**Fig. 1**). In large series, EGJOO accounts for 2% to 8% of HRM studies performed in tertiary care motility centers and includes diverse etiologies, such as achalasia, pseudoachalasia, strictures, obstructing hernias, and eosinophilic esophagitis.[12–15] Opioid use has also been reported as an etiologic mechanism for EGJOO.[16] When an achalasia-like pattern is diagnosed using alternative testing, especially a timed upright barium swallow, as many as 75% benefit from treatments designed to disrupt LES function.[12] Other EGJOO patients do not progress symptomatically, and 19% to 52% are reported to improve despite no specific management.[12,14] The heterogeneity of EGJOO can make the distinction from achalasia clinically challenging.

The latest version of the Chicago Classification considers all manometric EGJOO to be inconclusive (**Table 2**) because healthy asymptomatic individuals may fulfill criteria for EGJOO,[11] and many patients with EGJOO do not require specific management.[12] Consequently, additional evaluation is always needed to confirm obstructive features before invasive management.[3] Clinically relevant symptoms, especially dysphagia or noncardiac chest pain,[15] should be present for additional evaluation to be undertaken. Furthermore, manometry should not be used in isolation when making management decisions, and confirmation of obstruction with additional modalities such as timed upright barium esophagography or functional lumen imaging probe (FLIP) should be obtained.[17,18]

To deal with the heterotypic nature of this disorder, CCv4.0 describes 3 EGJOO subtypes: (1) EGJOO with hypercontractile features; (2) EGJOO with no evidence of disordered peristalsis; and (3) artifactual rise in IRP.[3] This definition also requires IRP elevation in both the primary and secondary (upright) positions, with upright IRP greater than 12 mm Hg defining obstruction.[19] Manometric evidence for true obstruction is supported by obstructive features on rapid drink challenge (RDC),[20] during solid test meal,[21] or after administration of amyl nitrite.[22]

The strategy outlined in CCv4.0 ensures proper identification of the subset of patients who have achalasia-like characteristics,[23] reserving invasive management for patients with conclusive outflow obstruction on multiple testing modalities. Although some options for the medical management of EGJOO are emerging,[24] to date, no evidence exists to support pharmacologic intervention.[25] There is no evidence supporting the use of calcium channel blockers or nitrates in EGJOO. The limited evidence available suggests that injection of botulinum toxin may resolve symptoms in some patients,[26] although predicting responders remains challenging. Additionally, in a

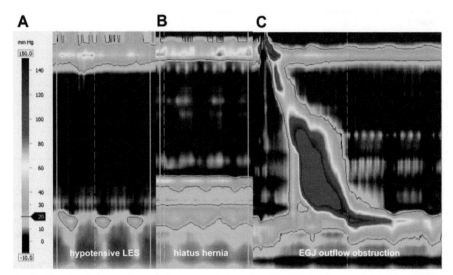

Fig. 1. Abnormalities at the esophagogastric junction (EGJ). (*A*) Hypotensive EGJ, with diaphragmatic crural contraction visible only during inspiration. (*B*) Abnormal EGJ morphology with a hiatus hernia, manifesting as a separation between the intrinsic lower esophageal sphincter (LES) and the diaphragmatic crura. (*C*) EGJ outflow obstruction, with intact esophageal body peristalsis, and abnormal EGJ relaxation with compartmentalization of intrabolus pressure between the contraction front and the EGJ.

subset of patients with distal esophageal spasm (DES), jackhammer esophagus, or EGJOO, per oral endoscopic myotomy (POEM) was found to be efficacious,[27] and separate reports exist supporting the use of Heller myotomy (HM). Taken together, these findings suggest that for appropriately identified patients, a botulinum toxin injection trial may be used to identify individuals in whom definitive intervention could be of value.

ABNORMAL ESOPHAGOGASTRIC JUNCTION TONE AND MORPHOLOGY

Although gastroesophageal reflux primarily occurs during transient LES relaxations (TLESR), basal LES pressure and tone impact EGJ compliance, and a weak EGJ barrier as well as abnormal morphology are important components of reflux pathophysiology[28] (**Fig. 1**). At the most basic level, reduced resting LES pressures have been associated with reflux disease, linking reduced mechanical barrier function to clinically relevant reflux.[29] Structural disruption in the form of a hiatus hernia is known to adversely affect EGJ barrier function and contribute to abnormal reflux burden,[30] both by reducing LES pressure and by increasing TLESR frequency. A hypertensive EGJ barrier has unclear clinical implications in the absence of abnormal LES relaxation or obstruction but could be a marker for a structural process such as a paraesophageal hernia.[31]

Both traditional and novel HRM metrics have been used to evaluate EGJ barrier function at baseline, measured during a 30-second period of quiet rest without swallows or artifacts.[32] Pressure-based traditional EGJ and LES metrics consist of end-expiratory LES pressure, representing intrinsic resting LES pressure at the end of respiration with a relaxed diaphragm, and basal LES pressure, measured during mid-respiration that takes both LES and crural diaphragmatic contributions into

Table 2
High-resolution manometry criteria for nonachalasia motor disorders

	Conclusive Diagnosis	Inconclusive Criteria	Other Relevant Actionable Findings
Disorders of esophagogastric junction (EGJ) function			
Hypotensive EGJ	Basal LES pressure <10 mm Hg End-expiratory LES pressure <5 mm Hg	EGJ-CI<25 mm Hg.cm.s	Abnormal reflux burden on ambulatory reflux monitoring
Abnormal EGJ morphology	Separation between LES and CD		Hiatus hernia on endoscopy, barium studies Abnormal reflux burden on ambulatory reflux monitoring
EGJ outflow obstruction		IRP>upper limit of normal with normal esophageal body peristalsis	Obstructive features on RDC, solid swallows Abnormal barium study Abnormal FLIP
Hypertensive LES		Basal LES pressure >35 mm Hg End-expiratory LES pressure >25 mm Hg	Obstructive features on RDC, solid swallows Abnormal barium study Abnormal FLIP
Disorders of esophageal body peristalsis			
Absent contractility	100% failed peristalsis with normal IRP	Borderline IRP	Abnormal reflux burden on ambulatory reflux monitoring Esophageal dilation on barium studies
Ineffective esophageal motility	>70% ineffective swallows; ≥50% failed swallows with normal IRP	50%–70% ineffective swallows	Absent contraction reserve on multiple rapid swallows; abnormal reflux burden on ambulatory reflux monitoring
Hypercontractile esophagus	>20% hypercontractile swallows (DCI >8000 mm Hg.cm.s) with normal IRP in patients with compatible symptoms	Hypercontractile features in asymptomatic patients or without compatible symptoms	Obstructive features on RDC, solid swallows Abnormal barium study Abnormal FLIP

(continued on next page)

	Conclusive Diagnosis	Inconclusive Criteria	Other Relevant Actionable Findings
Table 2 (*continued*)			
	(dysphagia, chest pain)		
Distal esophageal spasm	>20% premature swallows (DL<4.5 s) with normal IRP in patients with compatible symptoms (dysphagia, chest pain)	Premature swallows in asymptomatic patients or without compatible symptoms	Obstructive features on RDC, solid swallows Abnormal barium study Abnormal FLIP

consideration.[9,33] EGJ contractile integral (EGJ-CI) is calculated using a distal contractile integral-like tool across the EGJ over three respiratory cycles and corrected for respiration (see **Table 2**).

EGJ hypomotility is defined as low EGJ resting tone, when end expiratory LES pressure is less than 5 mm Hg,[34] basal LES pressure is less than 10 mm Hg, or EGJ-CI is less than 39 to 47 mm Hg.cm,[35–37] based on studies performed using conventional manometry in healthy volunteers and gastroesophageal reflux disease (GERD) patients (see **Table 2**). A large multicenter normative HRM study reported 5th percentile values of end-expiratory LES pressure to be 2 mm Hg, and basal LES pressure to be 7 to 11 mm Hg, based on the HRM system.[33] There are limited data suggesting that a low EGJ-CI associates with abnormal reflux burden on pH-impedance monitoring with modest performance characteristics[35,38] and could predict response to medical management of GERD.[37] However, newer normative data demonstrate that the spectrum of normal EGJ-CI values is broad (median 35–57 mm Hg.cm depending on HRM system, range 7–122 mm Hg.cm)[33] and overlaps considerably with values previously documented in individuals with reflux,[33,39] suggesting that EGJ-CI cannot function as a stand-alone metric defining abnormal barrier function in GERD. Novel metrics on standard HRM and 3D EGJ assessment using a special 3D HRM catheter have added to our understanding of the physiologic interrelationships between LES and crural diaphragm (CD). Although not available commercially, 3D HRM provides more detailed structural EGJ analysis, demonstrating significant asymmetry in the EGJ barrier, and implicating CD contribution to be perhaps the most important factor in EGJ barrier function.[40,41]

The relationship between LES and CD defines EGJ morphologic integrity (type 1 EGJ) or lack thereof (type 2 and 3 EGJ).[42] Separation between the intrinsic LES and CD identifies the presence of a hiatus hernia, with less than 3 cm separation indicating type 2 and ≥3 cm indicating type 3 EGJ[3,8] (see **Table 2**). HRM has better performance characteristics in detection of hiatus hernia than endoscopy or barium radiography and is more accurate in measuring hernia size in sliding hiatus hernias,[43] thus making HRM a useful presurgical tool. The presence of a hiatus hernia (type 2 or 3 EGJ) has been associated with greater reflux severity, increased rates of Barrett's esophagus, and impaired LES function.[44,45] High rates of patients with proven GERD and Barrett's esophagus also have a hiatus hernia,[45,46] while a hiatus hernia is uncommon in asymptomatic volunteers.[33] Furthermore, as the distance between the LES and CD increase, so does esophageal reflux burden.[47] The presence of both hypotensive EGJ and a hiatus hernia is synergistic rather than just additive in predicting elevated esophageal reflux burden.[44,46,48]

Dynamic maneuvers can be used during HRM to elucidate adequacy of EGJ barrier function. By having the patient raise their leg or by placing an abdominal binder across the abdomen, intraabdominal pressures can be elevated artificially, and EGJ barrier can be stressed to assess its ability to contain intraabdominal pressure within the abdominal compartment.[49,50] Type 3 EGJ is consistently associated with an incompetent EGJ barrier on straight leg raise maneuver.[51] Increase in intrathoracic pressures concurrent with intra-abdominal pressures during straight leg raise can associate with abnormal reflux burden on reflux monitoring.[49] However, the straight leg raise as a provocative maneuver has not been extensively studied, and outcome studies are lacking.

At the opposite end of the spectrum, HRM occasionally demonstrates a hypertensive EGJ but with adequate relaxation in the postswallow period. Unlike individuals with hypotensive EGD, the clinical significance of a hypertensive EGJ at baseline is less clear. Two variants are reported: elevated resting EGJ pressures and exaggerated LES after contraction. In the modern era, hypertensive LES pressures should raise suspicion for opioid-induced esophageal dysfunction or changes secondary to obesity, in the appropriate clinical setting.[52] The presence of a paraesophageal hernia has been reported to be associated with a hypertensive LES.[31] Exaggerated LES after contraction may be isolated or associated with hypercontractile esophagus; the latter has been included as a part of distal contractile integral (DCI) calculation in the hypercontractile spectrum of disorders.[3] Therapeutic intervention needs to be targeted at specific etiologies identified, and the mere presence of a hypertensive EGJ may not be sufficient to initiate therapy of any kind.

MOTILITY DISORDERS OF THE ESOPHAGEAL BODY

As outlined in the Chicago classification algorithm, the first aim of manometric evaluation is to ensure that there is no obstruction at the level of the LES. Once adequate LES relaxation and absence of EGJ obstruction are confirmed, esophageal body peristalsis is analyzed for disorders of esophageal body motor function (see **Table 2**). The Chicago Classification includes disorders of both decreased and increased esophageal body peristaltic vigor[3] (**Figs. 2** and **3**). Where adequate esophageal contraction is absent in all test swallows, absent contractility is diagnosed. New IEM criteria are more stringent and require greater than 70% ineffective swallows or ≥50% failed swallows,[3] and fragmented swallows are now included under the IEM umbrella although formerly considered a separate entity (see **Fig. 2**). On the spastic disorder spectrum, jackhammer esophagus is now considered a specific subset of hypercontractile esophagus. Presence of ≥20% premature contractions fulfills criteria for DES, although this is a very rare condition and overlaps with type 3 achalasia (see **Fig. 3**). Individual disorders are discussed in the following paragraphs.

ABSENT CONTRACTILITY

Absent contractility is an extreme degree of esophageal body hypomotility with normal LES relaxation, sometimes encountered in the context of smooth muscle fibrosis in collagen vascular disorders such as scleroderma, where a hypotensive EGJ can coexist.[53] While the prevalence of absent contractility may be as high as 40% to 44% in patients with systemic sclerosis,[53] the condition is not synonymous with collagen vascular disorders, and the mechanism is most often idiopathic. Absent contractility can be seen in the context of GERD, with prevalence of approximately

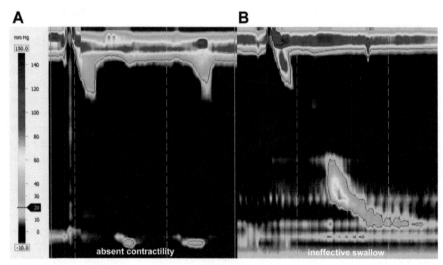

Fig. 2. Hypomotile esophageal body motor patterns. (*A*) Absent contractility, with no peristalsis in the esophageal body, and normal relaxation of the lower esophageal sphincter (LES). (*B*) Ineffective swallow, with low esophageal body contraction vigor, and a long break in peristaltic integrity between the skeletal muscle and smooth muscle contraction segments, with a normally relaxing LES.

3% in prefundoplication patients[54] and extremely high esophageal reflux burden on ambulatory reflux monitoring.[55] Absent contractility is extremely rare in healthy asymptomatic volunteers, seen in less than 1%.[11] Importantly, an absent contractility pattern may be due to achalasia in the presence of compatible symptoms (dysphagia, weight loss) even with a normal IRP.[5] Therefore, IRP greater than 10 mm Hg using the Medtronic system should be considered potentially consistent with obstruction, and confirmatory testing using timed upright barium study or FLIP study should be considered.[4]

There is no specific management targeting absent contractility. As discussed previously, achalasia and/or obstructive processes should be sought when dysphagia is prominent, where relief of obstruction will improve dysphagia. Where relevant, coexisting reflux needs to be aggressively managed. Volume regurgitation may rarely require a partial fundoplication.[56]

INEFFECTIVE ESOPHAGEAL MOTILITY

The criteria for a motor diagnosis of IEM have undergone several changes because this category was first introduced into conventional esophageal manometry over two decades ago.[57] Earlier Chicago Classification criteria of $\geq$50% ineffective swallows was determined to be nonspecific and too broad, while failed swallows had better relevance at this threshold in predicting abnormal bolus transit and abnormal reflux burden.[58–60] Fragmented peristalsis was a relatively infrequent diagnosis, although greater than 70% fragmented swallows was associated with abnormal reflux burden.[59] These concepts were incorporated into the new IEM criteria proposed by CCv4.0.[3] Ineffective swallows, under CCv4.0, include failed swallows (DCI<100 mm Hg.cm.s), weak swallows (DCI 100–450 mm Hg.cm.s), and fragmented swallows (DCI>450 mm Hg.cm.s with >5 cm peristaltic breaks using a 20 mm Hg peristaltic

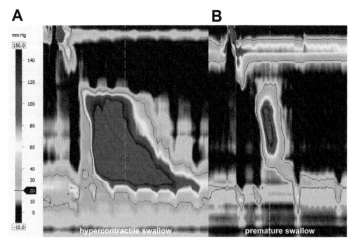

Fig. 3. Hypermotile esophageal body motor patterns. (*A*) Hypercontractile swallow, with exaggerated esophageal body contraction vigor (DCI>8000 mm Hg.cm.s) and merged smooth muscle contraction segments, and a normally relaxing lower esophageal sphincter (LES). (*B*) Premature swallow, with a rather vertical esophageal body contraction sequence (distal latency <4.5 seconds) and a normally relaxing LES.

contour tool).[3] IEM definitions have been made more stringent, and the diagnosis of IEM requires greater than 70% ineffective swallows (from 50% threshold) or $\geq$50% failed swallows.[3]

The peristaltic threshold for adequate bolus transit without proximal escape was determined to be 30 mm Hg based on concurrent conventional manometry and barium radiography.[61] The HRM correlate of this threshold was determined to be a DCI of 450 mm Hg.cm.s by comparing peristaltic amplitude to DCI values,[62] which has been used in determining the criteria for ineffective swallows. However, HRM studies on healthy asymptomatic volunteers have suggested that the 5th percentile DCI value in health is lower, perhaps 200 to 300 mm Hg.cm.s, based on the HRM system used.[11] Proportion of ineffective swallows of greater than 70% has been demonstrated to be more clinically relevant in predicting abnormal esophageal reflux burden, particularly supine acid exposure, than lesser proportions or normal manometry.[55,63,64] Additionally, recent studies have demonstrated that failed swallows and swallows with long breaks (>5 cm) are more likely to be associated with abnormal bolus transit[58,60,65] and higher esophageal reflux burden[59] than intact or weak swallows. These findings were the basis for the change in IEM diagnostic criteria in CCv4.0.

The HRM identification of IEM represents a motor pattern that does not necessarily bear a direct relationship with symptoms or the clinical scenario being investigated. In fact, IEM can be encountered in healthy asymptomatic individuals: As many as 15% of healthy volunteers fulfilled CCv3.0 criteria, which decreased to 10% when the more stringent CCv4.0 criteria were used.[11] The proportion of IEM diagnoses increases progressively with increasing severity of GERD phenotypes, with lower proportions in NERD and significantly higher proportions in erosive esophagitis and Barrett's esophagus.[66]

Adjunctive manometric tests can be used to better understand the clinical relevance of IEM. The simplest of these is multiple rapid swallows (MRS), where the patient is rapidly administered 5 swallows in 2-mL increments.[67,68] During the swallows, peristalsis is temporarily inhibited, followed by a peristaltic wave with higher contraction vigor than single swallows, which indicates presence of contraction reserve.[68] Contraction reserve on MRS has been shown to correlate with acid burden[55] and may identify subsets of IEM that may not lead to postfundoplication dysphagia[68,69] or IEM that improves over time.[70] Thus, when IEM is identified in the context of reflux evaluation, or when assessing esophageal peristalsis before antireflux surgery, performing MRS during HRM may have a prognostic value. Transit symptoms such as dysphagia are not well explained by IEM, and dysphagia perception does not correlate well with abnormal bolus transit on HRM with impedance.[71] Therefore, in patients with dysphagia, adjunctive HRM maneuvers could include RDC, where 100 to 200 mL of water is administered through a straw in the sitting position.[72,73] This test has the potential to demonstrate latent obstruction at the EGJ. Solid swallows and solid test meals have the potential to demonstrate both contraction reserve and latent obstruction.[21] The combination of impedance with HRM (high-resolution impedance manometry [HRIM]) provides assessment of bolus transit,[74,75] and recent advances allow quantification of bolus presence. By measuring impedance bolus presence before and after esophageal peristalsis using a dedicated software program, esophageal impedance integral can be calculated that describes normal and abnormal bolus transit.[65]

There is no specific treatment available for the IEM pattern, nor is such management necessary. Instead, associated symptomatic conditions are managed using standard treatment paradigms.[56,76] For instance, standard management can be offered when GERD is present,[77] although there may be concern for postfundoplication dysphagia if a standard fundoplication is performed in the absence of contraction reserve. Dysphagia symptoms need evaluation for a structural etiology, using not just HRM maneuvers but also barium studies and FLIP when indicated. In the absence of a structural mechanism, good swallow technique, eating while upright, and pushing food through with liquids are recommended.[76] An IEM pattern remains compatible with a functional esophageal disorder, which may improve with targeted symptomatic therapy.[78]

HYPERCONTRACTILE ESOPHAGUS

Exaggerated or hypertensive esophageal body peristalsis was first identified on conventional manometry as "nutcracker esophagus," which was diagnosed when distal esophageal contraction amplitudes exceeded 180 mm Hg.[79] Using HRM, esophageal contraction vigor assessment with DCI allowed assessment of not just contraction amplitudes but also the length of the contracting segment and the duration of contraction.[80,81] Formal CCv4.0 definition requires DCI greater than 8000 mm Hg.cm.s in 2 or more swallows,[3,7] a threshold that is reached in only 0.2% of healthy asymptomatic volunteers.[11] Careful inspection must also be undertaken regarding pattern and location of increased contraction vigor, specifically in determining whether LES after contraction should be included in DCI calculations and to what extent the LES is involved, although including the LES in the DCI calculation does not necessarily increase the clinical relevance of the disorder.[82] Jackhammer esophagus, previously a category unto itself, is now a subset within the broader category of hypercontractile esophagus, where prolonged, repetitive, and chaotic contraction peaks are seen in the esophageal body.[83,84]

Hypercontractile esophagus encompasses a heterogeneous group of disorders where manometric findings must be considered in the context of symptoms and clinical presentation.[3] Although a diagnosis of hypercontractile esophagus requires that no obstruction is present, hypercontractility can be associated with or a consequence of distal obstructive processes.[85,86] Recent evidence suggests that esophageal body hypercontractility and incomplete LES relaxation may share a common pathophysiologic mechanism[87] as both demonstrate increased excitation from cholinergic input and abnormal inhibition.[88,89] Hypercontractile esophagus, with or without abnormal LES relaxation, has also been demonstrated in the context of eosinophilic smooth muscle inflammation, which brings eosinophilic disorders into the etiopathogenesis of obstructive and hypercontractile esophageal disorders.[90,91] These findings suggest that latent obstruction needs to be elicited even when standard HRM demonstrates normal IRP values, especially when dysphagia is a presenting symptom. The Chicago Classification outlines the use of RDC and solid swallows in HRM protocols, which can provide adjunctive evidence for obstruction when 10 standard supine swallows are inconclusive.[88] As with primary disorders of the EGJ, where diagnosis is not definitive, adjunctive testing using timed upright barium esophagogram, FLIP, or test meal ingestion during HRM can help to clarify presence or absence of obstruction.

Hypercontractile esophageal peristalsis may also be an epiphenomenon seen with esophageal hypersensitivity,[92] and studies have demonstrated higher esophageal body contraction vigor and contraction wave abnormalities in patients with increased esophageal perception.[93–95] Hypercontractile esophagus may also be identified in the context of reflux disease,[96,97] and acid can provoke exaggerated esophageal contraction as well as atypical chest pain.[93,98] Finally, hypercontractile esophagus has been reported in chronic opiate users.[16]

As clinical presentations and the mechanisms underlying hypercontractile esophagus are diverse, nuanced management is required, primarily focused on the clinical presentation. Typical GERD management options can be initiated when reflux symptoms are reported, using invasive esophageal testing to document GERD when necessary.[77] Esophageal hypersensitivity, functional esophageal disorders, as well as psychiatric comorbidity may need to be addressed with perceptive symptoms such as atypical chest pain.[78,99] Concurrent eosinophilic disorders may require management directed at esophageal eosinophilia, motor obstruction, or both.[91] Calcium channel blockers, nitrates, and phosphodiesterase inhibitors have been studied with mixed outcomes.[100–102] For dysphagia predominant presentations, botulinum toxin injection may provide temporary symptom benefit in some but not all patients.[103,104] Tailored myotomy using an endoscopic approach (POEM) has the potential to provide symptomatic benefit of dysphagia better than a short myotomy through an abdominal approach (HM).[27,105,106]

DISTAL ESOPHAGEAL SPASM

While DES was initially characterized by simultaneous esophageal body contraction on conventional manometry,[79] HRM criteria use distal latency to measure timing of esophageal peristalsis and require 2 or more swallows to have distal latency less than 4.5 seconds.[3,8] However, where obstructive processes are present at the distal esophagus, pressurization between proximal smooth muscle segments and the EGJ can be confused for spastic esophageal peristalsis.[8] As adequate management is predicated upon localization of disordered contraction segments, differentiating between the DES and pressurization is imperative. As currently diagnosed, symptomatic DES is extremely rare in clinical practice, but a DES pattern can be encountered in 4% of healthy asymptomatic volunteers.[11] As an entity, DES is the result of inadequate inhibition at the distal esophagus,[107] which can be demonstrated as contraction during expected deglutitive inhibition during the MRS maneuver. As DES can be associated with latent obstruction despite a normal IRP when the presentation is dysphagia, and as normal IRP is the only criterion that distinguishes DES from type 3 achalasia, it is imperative that obstruction is carefully evaluated, using provocative HRM maneuvers such as RDC and solid swallows, barium radiography, and perhaps FLIP.[108] This motor disorder is also encountered in chronic opioid users and in presentations of atypical chest pain.[16] Therefore, clinically relevant symptoms such as dysphagia or noncardiac chest pain should be present before considering DES requiring management.

Management paradigms follow similar principles as for hypercontractile esophagus. Concurrent GERD needs appropriate management,[77] and perceptive symptoms, psychological comorbidities, and functional disorders are treated using standard approaches.[78,99] The value of smooth muscle relaxants remains unclear, and these approaches are not consistently effective. Achalasia spectrum disorders should always be considered when spastic esophageal contractions are seen, and the ultimate management of patients, in the appropriate clinical scenario, may involve surgical disruption of the obstructive segment.[109,110] In this context, tailored POEM has been demonstrated to be of value in small series.[27,106]

OTHER DISORDERS

HRM is increasingly used in the evaluation of nondysphagia symptoms, and thus, a broad spectrum of foregut disorders may manifest as motor findings that are not characterized by the Chicago Classification. The forceful injection or sucking of air into the esophagus with or without immediate eructation characterizes supragastric belching and aerophagia.[111] Similarly, the characteristic "r" waves of rumination have been well categorized on HRM and HRIM.[112] These behavioral disorders are better identified during postprandial monitoring after a standardized test meal[111,113,114] or on pH-impedance monitoring.[115,116] Management of both supragastric belching and rumination syndrome involves behavioral approaches, including diaphragmatic breathing and cognitive/behavioral therapy.

Although not part of the CCv4.0 algorithm, HRM can also provide valuable information on upper esophageal sphincter (UES) function. Inadequate UES relaxation can sometimes be related to structural defects, such as cricopharyngeal bars and webs, which presents on HRM as compartmentalization proximal to UES as well as elevated postswallow UES residual pressures.[117] Alternatively, decreased or absent striated muscle segments in the proximal esophagus have been correlated to skeletal muscle disorders such as muscular dystrophy, myasthenia gravis, or polymyositis.[117] A standardized diagnostic algorithm has not been established for UES and proximal esophageal skeletal muscle disorders.

SUMMARY

Three decades of research has allowed for the establishment of HRM as an established tool in the evaluation of esophageal symptoms, as well as fortification and sharpening of the Chicago classification. Although the diagnosis of achalasia is a crucial function for HRM, the clinical applications extend beyond achalasia spectrum disorders. The astute clinician has much to gain from a properly performed HRM study, and the expanded protocol proposed by CCv4.0 provides additional tools to aid in the conclusive diagnosis of both obstructive and nonobstructive nonachalasia motor disorders. The use of complementary diagnostic tools such as the timed upright barium swallow and FLIP adds to the value of esophageal investigation in planning management.

CLINICS CARE POINTS

- Ancillary measures during high resolution manometry add value to further clarification of non-achalasia motor disorders.
- Esophagogastric junction outflow obstruction (EGJOO) is a heterogenous disorder with etiologies that range from artifact to achalasia variant.
- Clarification of EGJOO requires confirmation with an alternate test, typically barium esophagography or functional lumen imaging probe.
- Ineffective esophageal motility (IEM) is a motility pattern that may not associate with symptoms, although prolonged reflux clearance and abnormal bolus transit may be consequences.
- Distal esophageal spasm and hypercontractile esophagus are relevant, actionable diagnoses only in the presence of dysphagia and/or chest pain.

DISCLOSURE

C.P. Gyawali has received honoraria for consulting from Medtronic, Diversatek, Takeda, Ironwood, and Quintiles. B.D. Rogers has no disclosures. No conflicts of interest exist.

REFERENCES

1. Clouse RE, Prakash C. Topographic esophageal manometry: an emerging clinical and investigative approach. Dig Dis 2000;18:64–74.
2. Gyawali CP. High resolution manometry: the Ray Clouse legacy. Neurogastroenterol Motil 2012;24(Suppl 1):2–4.
3. Yadlapati R, Kahrilas PJ, Fox MR, et al. Esophageal motility disorders on high-resolution manometry: Chicago classification version 4.0((c)). Neurogastroenterol Motil 2021;33:e14058.
4. Lin Z, Kahrilas PJ, Roman S, et al. Refining the criterion for an abnormal integrated relaxation pressure in esophageal pressure topography based on the pattern of esophageal contractility using a classification and regression tree model. Neurogastroenterol Motil 2012;24:e356–63.
5. Ponds FA, Bredenoord AJ, Kessing BF, et al. Esophagogastric junction distensibility identifies achalasia subgroup with manometrically normal esophagogastric junction relaxation. Neurogastroenterol Motil 2017;29:e12908.
6. Kahrilas PJ, Ghosh SK, Pandolfino JE. Esophageal motility disorders in terms of pressure topography: The Chicago Classification. J Clin Gastroenterol 2008;42:627–35.
7. Bredenoord AJ, Fox M, Kahrilas PJ, et al. Chicago classification criteria of esophageal motility disorders defined in high resolution esophageal pressure topography. Neurogastroenterol Motil 2012;24(Suppl 1):57–65.
8. Kahrilas PJ, Bredenoord AJ, Fox M, et al. The Chicago Classification of esophageal motility disorders, v3.0. Neurogastroenterol Motil 2015;27:160–74.
9. Mittal RK, Balaban DH. The esophagogastric junction. N Engl J Med 1997;336:924–32.
10. Goldani HA, Fernandes MI, Vicente YA, et al. Lower esophageal sphincter reacts against intraabdominal pressure in children with symptoms of gastroesophageal reflux. Dig Dis Sci 2002;47:2544–8.

11. Rengarajan A, Rogers BD, Wong Z, et al. High-resolution manometry thresholds and motor patterns among asymptomatic individuals. Clin Gastroenterol Hepatol 2020 (in press).

12. van Hoeij FB, Smout AJ, Bredenoord AJ. Characterization of idiopathic esophagogastric junction outflow obstruction. Neurogastroenterol Motil 2015;27:1310–6.

13. Biasutto D, Mion F, Garros A, et al. Rapid drink challenge test during esophageal high resolution manometry in patients with esophago-gastric junction outflow obstruction. Neurogastroenterol Motil 2018;30:e13293.

14. Perez-Fernandez MT, Santander C, Marinero A, et al. Characterization and follow-up of esophagogastric junction outflow obstruction detected by high resolution manometry. Neurogastroenterol Motil 2016;28:116–26.

15. Okeke FC, Raja S, Lynch KL, et al. What is the clinical significance of esophagogastric junction outflow obstruction? evaluation of 60 patients at a tertiary referral center. Neurogastroenterol Motil 2017;29:e13061.

16. Ratuapli SK, Crowell MD, DiBaise JK, et al. Opioid-Induced Esophageal Dysfunction (OIED) in patients on chronic opioids. Am J Gastroenterol 2015;110:979–84.

17. Triggs JR, Carlson DA, Beveridge C, et al. Functional luminal imaging probe panometry identifies achalasia-type esophagogastric junction outflow obstruction. Clin Gastroenterol Hepatol 2020;18(10):2209–17.

18. Blonski W, Kumar A, Feldman J, et al. Timed barium swallow: diagnostic role and predictive value in untreated achalasia, esophagogastric junction outflow obstruction, and non-achalasia dysphagia. Am J Gastroenterol 2018;113:196–203.

19. Triggs JR, Carlson DA, Beveridge C, et al. Upright integrated relaxation pressure facilitates characterization of esophagogastric junction outflow obstruction. Clin Gastroenterol Hepatol 2019;17(11):2218–26.e2.

20. Woodland P, Gabieta-Sonmez S, Arguero J, et al. 200 mL rapid drink challenge during high-resolution manometry best predicts objective esophagogastric junction obstruction and correlates with symptom severity. J Neurogastroenterol Motil 2018;24:410–4.

21. Ang D, Misselwitz B, Hollenstein M, et al. Diagnostic yield of high-resolution manometry with a solid test meal for clinically relevant, symptomatic oesophageal motility disorders: serial diagnostic study. Lancet Gastroenterol Hepatol 2017;2:654–61.

22. Babaei A, Shad S, Szabo A, et al. Pharmacologic interrogation of patients with esophagogastric junction outflow obstruction using amyl nitrite. Neurogastroenterol Motil 2019;31(9):e13668.

23. Kahrilas PJ, Katzka D, Richter JE. Clinical practice update: the use of per-oral endoscopic myotomy in achalasia: expert review and best practice advice from the AGA Institute. Gastroenterology 2017;153:1205–11.

24. Ihara E, Muta K, Fukaura K, et al. Diagnosis and treatment strategy of achalasia subtypes and esophagogastric junction outflow obstruction based on high-resolution manometry. Digestion 2017;95:29–35.

25. Samo S, Qayed E. Esophagogastric junction outflow obstruction: where are we now in diagnosis and management? World J Gastroenterol 2019;25:411–7.

26. Clayton SB, Patel R, Richter JE. Functional and anatomic esophagogastic junction outflow obstruction: manometry, timed barium esophagram findings, and treatment outcomes. Clin Gastroenterol Hepatol 2016;14:907–11.

27. Khashab MA, Familiari P, Draganov PV, et al. Peroral endoscopic myotomy is effective and safe in non-achalasia esophageal motility disorders: an international multicenter study. Endosc Int Open 2018;6:E1031–6.

28. Dodds WJ, Dent J, Hogan WJ, et al. Mechanisms of gastroesophageal reflux in patients with reflux esophagitis. N Engl J Med 1982;307:1547–52.
29. Castell DO, Murray JA, Tutuian R, et al. Review article: the pathophysiology of gastro-oesophageal reflux disease - oesophageal manifestations. Aliment Pharmacol Ther 2004;20(Suppl 9):14–25.
30. Kahrilas PJ, Lin S, Chen J, et al. The effect of hiatus hernia on gastro-oesophageal junction pressure. Gut 1999;44:476–82.
31. Rengarajan A, Arguero J, Yazaki E, et al. High-resolution manometry features of paraesophageal hernia. Neurogastroenterol Motil 2020;32:e13947.
32. Gyawali CP, Patel A. Esophageal motor function: technical aspects of manometry. Gastrointest Endosc Clin N Am 2014;24:527–43.
33. Rogers BD, Rengarajan A, Abrahao L, et al. Esophagogastric junction morphology and contractile integral on high-resolution manometry in asymptomatic healthy volunteers: an international multicenter study. Neurogastroenterol Motil 2020;33:e14009.
34. Pandolfino JE, Kahrilas PJ, American Gastroenterological Association. AGA technical review on the clinical use of esophageal manometry. Gastroenterology 2005;128:209–24.
35. Gor P, Li Y, Munigala S, et al. Interrogation of esophagogastric junction barrier function using the esophagogastric junction contractile integral: an observational cohort study. Dis Esophagus 2016;29:820–8.
36. Jasper D, Freitas-Queiroz N, Hollenstein M, et al. Prolonged measurement improves the assessment of the barrier function of the esophago-gastric junction by high-resolution manometry. Neurogastroenterol Motil 2017;29:e12925.
37. Nicodeme F, Pipa-Muniz M, Khanna K, et al. Quantifying esophagogastric junction contractility with a novel HRM topographic metric, the EGJ-Contractile Integral: normative values and preliminary evaluation in PPI non-responders. Neurogastroenterol Motil 2014;26:353–60.
38. Tolone S, de Cassan C, de Bortoli N, et al. Esophagogastric junction morphology is associated with a positive impedance-pH monitoring in patients with GERD. Neurogastroenterol Motil 2015;27:1175–82.
39. Gyawali CP, Kahrilas PJ, Savarino E, et al. Modern diagnosis of GERD: the Lyon Consensus. Gut 2018;67:1351–62.
40. Kwiatek MA, Pandolfino JE, Kahrilas PJ. 3D-High resolution manometry of the esophagogastric junction. Neurogastroenterol Motil 2011;23:e461–9.
41. Lin Z, Xiao Y, Li Y, et al. Novel 3D high-resolution manometry metrics for quantifying esophagogastric junction contractility. Neurogastroenterol Motil 2017;29:e13054.
42. Pandolfino JE, Kim H, Ghosh SK, et al. High-resolution manometry of the EGJ: an analysis of crural diaphragm function in GERD. Am J Gastroenterol 2007;102:1056–63.
43. Tolone S, Savarino E, Zaninotto G, et al. High-resolution manometry is superior to endoscopy and radiology in assessing and grading sliding hiatal hernia: a comparison with surgical in vivo evaluation. United European Gastroenterol J 2018;6:981–9.
44. Jones MP, Sloan SS, Rabine JC, et al. Hiatal hernia size is the dominant determinant of esophagitis presence and severity in gastroesophageal reflux disease. Am J Gastroenterol 2001;96:1711–7.
45. Cameron AJ. Barrett's esophagus: prevalence and size of hiatal hernia. Am J Gastroenterol 1999;94:2054–9.

46. Rengarajan A, Gyawali CP. High-resolution manometry can characterize esophagogastric junction morphology and predict esophageal reflux burden. J Clin Gastroenterol 2020;54(1):22–7.
47. Schlottmann F, Andolfi C, Herbella FA, et al. GERD: presence and size of hiatal hernia influence clinical presentation, esophageal function, reflux profile, and degree of mucosal injury. Am Surg 2018;84:978–82.
48. Sloan S, Kahrilas PJ. Impairment of esophageal emptying with hiatal hernia. Gastroenterology 1991;100:596–605.
49. Rogers BD, Rengarajan A, Ali IA, et al. Straight leg raise metrics on high-resolution manometry associate with esophageal reflux burden. Neurogastroenterol Motil 2020;32(12):e13929.
50. Mitchell DR, Derakhshan MH, Wirz AA, et al. Abdominal compression by waist belt aggravates gastroesophageal reflux, primarily by impairing esophageal clearance. Gastroenterology 2017;152:1881–8.
51. Rogers B, Hasak S, Hansalia V, et al. Trans-esophagogastric junction pressure gradients during straight leg raise maneuver on high-resolution manometry associate with large hiatus hernias. Neurogastroenterol Motil 2020;32:e13836.
52. Kraichely RE, Arora AS, Murray JA. Opiate-induced oesophageal dysmotility. Aliment Pharmacol Ther 2010;31:601–6.
53. Carlson DA, Crowell MD, Kimmel JN, et al. Loss of peristaltic reserve, determined by multiple rapid swallows, is the most frequent esophageal motility abnormality in patients with systemic sclerosis. Clin Gastroenterol Hepatol 2016; 14(10):1502–6.
54. Chan WW, Haroian LR, Gyawali CP. Value of preoperative esophageal function studies before laparoscopic antireflux surgery. Surg Endosc 2011;25:2943–9.
55. Quader F, Rogers B, Sievers T, et al. Contraction reserve with ineffective esophageal motility on esophageal high-resolution manometry is associated with lower acid exposure times compared with absent contraction reserve. Am J Gastroenterol 2020;115:1981–8.
56. Gyawali CP, Zerbib F, Bhatia S, et al. Chicago classification update (V4.0): technical review on diagnostic criteria for ineffective esophageal motility and absent contractility. Neurogastroenterol Motil 2021;33:e14134.
57. Leite LP, Johnston BT, Barrett J, et al. Ineffective esophageal motility (IEM): the primary finding in patients with nonspecific esophageal motility disorder. Dig Dis Sci 1997;42:1859–65.
58. Jain A, Baker JR, Chen JW. In ineffective esophageal motility, failed swallows are more functionally relevant than weak swallows. Neurogastroenterol Motil 2018;30:e13297.
59. Rogers BD, Rengarajan A, Mauro A, et al. Fragmented and failed swallows on esophageal high-resolution manometry associate with abnormal reflux burden better than weak swallows. Neurogastroenterol Motil 2020;32(2):e13736.
60. Zerbib F, Marin I, Cisternas D, et al. Ineffective esophageal motility and bolus clearance. A study with combined high-resolution manometry and impedance in asymptomatic controls and patients. Neurogastroenterol Motil 2020;32: e13876.
61. Kahrilas PJ, Dodds WJ, Hogan WJ. Effect of peristaltic dysfunction on esophageal volume clearance. Gastroenterology 1988;94:73–80.
62. Xiao Y, Kahrilas PJ, Kwasny MJ, et al. High-resolution manometry correlates of ineffective esophageal motility. Am J Gastroenterol 2012;107:1647–54.
63. Simren M, Silny J, Holloway R, et al. Relevance of ineffective oesophageal motility during oesophageal acid clearance. Gut 2003;52:784–90.

64. Fornari F, Blondeau K, Durand L, et al. Relevance of mild ineffective oesophageal motility (IOM) and potential pharmacological reversibility of severe IOM in patients with gastro-oesophageal reflux disease. Aliment Pharmacol Ther 2007;26:1345–54.

65. Rogers BD, Cisternas D, Rengarajan A, et al. Breaks in peristaltic integrity predict abnormal esophageal bolus clearance better than contraction vigor or residual pressure at the esophagogastric junction. Neurogastroenterol Motil 2021;e14141 (in press).

66. Savarino E, Gemignani L, Pohl D, et al. Oesophageal motility and bolus transit abnormalities increase in parallel with the severity of gastro-oesophageal reflux disease. Aliment Pharmacol Ther 2011;34:476–86.

67. Fornari F, Bravi I, Penagini R, et al. Multiple rapid swallowing: a complementary test during standard oesophageal manometry. Neurogastroenterol Motil 2009; 21:718.e41.

68. Shaker A, Stoikes N, Drapekin J, et al. Multiple rapid swallow responses during esophageal high-resolution manometry reflect esophageal body peristaltic reserve. Am J Gastroenterol 2013;108:1706–12.

69. Hasak S, Brunt LM, Wang D, et al. Clinical characteristics and outcomes of patients with postfundoplication dysphagia. Clin Gastroenterol Hepatol 2019;17: 1982–90.

70. Mello MD, Shriver AR, Li Y, et al. Ineffective esophageal motility phenotypes following fundoplication in gastroesophageal reflux disease. Neurogastroenterol Motil 2016;28:292–8.

71. Lazarescu A, Karamanolis G, Aprile L, et al. Perception of dysphagia: lack of correlation with objective measurements of esophageal function. Neurogastroenterol Motil 2010;22:1292–7, e336-7.

72. Ang D, Hollenstein M, Misselwitz B, et al. Rapid drink challenge in high-resolution manometry: an adjunctive test for detection of esophageal motility disorders. Neurogastroenterol Motil 2017;29:e12902.

73. Marin I, Serra J. Patterns of esophageal pressure responses to a rapid drink challenge test in patients with esophageal motility disorders. Neurogastroenterol Motil 2016;28:543–53.

74. Cho YK, Lipowska AM, Nicodeme F, et al. Assessing bolus retention in achalasia using high-resolution manometry with impedance: a comparator study with timed barium esophagram. Am J Gastroenterol 2014;109:829–35.

75. Bulsiewicz WJ, Kahrilas PJ, Kwiatek MA, et al. Esophageal pressure topography criteria indicative of incomplete bolus clearance: a study using high-resolution impedance manometry. Am J Gastroenterol 2009;104:2721–8.

76. Gyawali CP, Sifrim D, Carlson DA, et al. Ineffective esophageal motility: concepts, future directions, and conclusions from the Stanford 2018 symposium. Neurogastroenterol Motil 2019;31:e13584.

77. Gyawali CP, Fass R. Management of gastroesophageal reflux disease. Gastroenterology 2018;154:302–18.

78. Aziz Q, Fass R, Gyawali CP, et al. Functional esophageal disorders. Gastroenterology 2016;150:1368–79.

79. Spechler SJ, Castell DO. Classification of oesophageal motility abnormalities. Gut 2001;49:145–51.

80. Ghosh SK, Pandolfino JE, Zhang Q, et al. Quantifying esophageal peristalsis with high-resolution manometry: a study of 75 asymptomatic volunteers. Am J Physiol Gastrointest Liver Physiol 2006;290:G988–97.

81. Roman S, Pandolfino JE, Chen J, et al. Phenotypes and clinical context of hyper-contractility in high-resolution esophageal pressure topography (EPT). Am J Gastroenterol 2012;107:37–45.

82. Carlson DA, Kahrilas PJ, Tye M, et al. High-resolution manometry assessment of the lower esophageal sphincter after-contraction: normative values and clinical correlation. Neurogastroenterol Motil 2018;30:e13156.

83. Xiao Y, Carlson DA, Lin Z, et al. Jackhammer esophagus: assessing the balance between prepeak and postpeak contractile integral. Neurogastroenterol Motil 2018;30:e13262.

84. Xiao Y, Carlson DA, Lin Z, et al. Chaotic peak propagation in patients with Jack-hammer esophagus. Neurogastroenterol Motil 2020;32:e13725.

85. de Bortoli N, Gyawali PC, Roman S, et al. Hypercontractile esophagus from pathophysiology to management: proceedings of the pisa symposium. Am J Gastroenterol 2021;116:263–73.

86. Gyawali CP, Kushnir VM. High-resolution manometric characteristics help differ-entiate types of distal esophageal obstruction in patients with peristalsis. Neuro-gastroenterol Motil 2011;23:502.e7.

87. Herregods TV, Smout AJ, Ooi JL, et al. Jackhammer esophagus: observations on a European cohort. Neurogastroenterol Motil 2017;29:e12975.

88. Mauro A, Quader F, Tolone S, et al. Provocative testing in patients with jack-hammer esophagus: evidence for altered neural control. Am J Physiol Gastroint-est Liver Physiol 2019;316:G397–403.

89. Quader F, Mauro A, Savarino E, et al. Jackhammer esophagus with and without esophagogastric junction outflow obstruction demonstrates altered neural con-trol resembling type 3 achalasia. Neurogastroenterol Motil 2019;31(9):e13678.

90. Korsapati H, Babaei A, Bhargava V, et al. Dysfunction of the longitudinal mus-cles of the oesophagus in eosinophilic oesophagitis. Gut 2009;58:1056–62.

91. Ghisa M, Laserra G, Marabotto E, et al. Achalasia and obstructive motor disor-ders are not uncommon in patients with eosinophilic esophagitis. Clin Gastroen-terol Hepatol 2021;19(8):1554–63.

92. Borjesson M, Pilhall M, Eliasson T, et al. Esophageal visceral pain sensitivity: ef-fects of TENS and correlation with manometric findings. Dig Dis Sci 1998;43:1621–8.

93. Kushnir VM, Prakash Gyawali C. High resolution manometry patterns distinguish acid sensitivity in non-cardiac chest pain. Neurogastroenterol Motil 2011;23:1066–72.

94. Richter JE, Barish CF, Castell DO. Abnormal sensory perception in patients with esophageal chest pain. Gastroenterology 1986;91:845–52.

95. Winslow ER, Clouse RE, Desai KM, et al. Influence of spastic motor disorders of the esophageal body on outcomes from laparoscopic antireflux surgery. Surg Endosc 2003;17:738–45.

96. Mallet AL, Ropert A, Bouguen G, et al. Prevalence and characteristics of acid gastro-oesophageal reflux disease in Jackhammer oesophagus. Dig Liver Dis 2016;48:1136–41.

97. Kristo I, Schwameis K, Maschke S, et al. Phenotypes of Jackhammer esoph-agus in patients with typical symptoms of gastroesophageal reflux disease responsive to proton pump inhibitors. Sci Rep 2018;8:9949.

98. Crozier RE, Glick ME, Gibb SP, et al. Acid-provoked esophageal spasm as a cause of noncardiac chest pain. Am J Gastroenterol 1991;86:1576–80.

99. Fass R, Zerbib F, Gyawali CP. AGA clinical practice update on functional heart-burn: expert review. Gastroenterology 2020;158:2286–93.

100. Yoshida K, Furuta K, Adachi K, et al. Effects of anti-hypertensive drugs on esophageal body contraction. World J Gastroenterol 2010;16:987–91.
101. Bortolotti M, Mari C, Lopilato C, et al. Effects of sildenafil on esophageal motility of patients with idiopathic achalasia. Gastroenterology 2000;118:253–7.
102. Eherer AJ, Schwetz I, Hammer HF, et al. Effect of sildenafil on oesophageal motor function in healthy subjects and patients with oesophageal motor disorders. Gut 2002;50:758–64.
103. Marjoux S, Brochard C, Roman S, et al. Botulinum toxin injection for hypercontractile or spastic esophageal motility disorders: may high-resolution manometry help to select cases? Dis Esophagus 2015;28:735–41.
104. Mion F, Marjoux S, Subtil F, et al. Botulinum toxin for the treatment of hypercontractile esophagus: results of a double-blind randomized sham-controlled study. Neurogastroenterol Motil 2019;31:e13587.
105. Khan MA, Kumbhari V, Ngamruengphong S, et al. Is POEM the answer for management of spastic esophageal disorders? A systematic review and meta-analysis. Dig Dis Sci 2017;62:35–44.
106. Khashab MA, Messallam AA, Onimaru M, et al. International multicenter experience with peroral endoscopic myotomy for the treatment of spastic esophageal disorders refractory to medical therapy (with video). Gastrointest Endosc 2015; 81:1170–7.
107. Behar J, Biancani P. Pathogenesis of simultaneous esophageal contractions in patients with motility disorders. Gastroenterology 1993;105:111–8.
108. Roman S, Hebbard G, Jung KW, et al. Chicago classification update (v4.0): technical review on diagnostic criteria for distal esophageal spasm. Neurogastroenterol Motil 2021;33(5):e14119.
109. Schlottmann F, Shaheen NJ, Madanick RD, et al. The role of Heller myotomy and POEM for nonachalasia motility disorders. Dis Esophagus 2017;30:1–5.
110. Sugihara Y, Sakae H, Hamada K, et al. Peroral endoscopic myotomy is an effective treatment for diffuse esophageal spasm. Clin Case Rep 2020;8:927–8.
111. Kessing BF, Bredenoord AJ, Smout AJ. Mechanisms of gastric and supragastric belching: a study using concurrent high-resolution manometry and impedance monitoring. Neurogastroenterol Motil 2012;24:e573–9.
112. Rosen R, Rodriguez L, Nurko S. Pediatric rumination subtypes: a study using high-resolution esophageal manometry with impedance. Neurogastroenterol Motil 2017;29:e12998.
113. Yadlapati R, Tye M, Roman S, et al. Postprandial high-resolution impedance manometry identifies mechanisms of nonresponse to proton pump inhibitors. Clin Gastroenterol Hepatol 2018;16:211–218 e1.
114. Kessing BF, Bredenoord AJ, Smout AJ. Objective manometric criteria for the rumination syndrome. Am J Gastroenterol 2014;109:52–9.
115. Kessing BF, Bredenoord AJ, Smout AJ. The pathophysiology, diagnosis and treatment of excessive belching symptoms. Am J Gastroenterol 2014;109: 1196–203 (Quiz) 1204.
116. Kessing BF, Bredenoord AJ, Velosa M, et al. Supragastric belches are the main determinants of troublesome belching symptoms in patients with gastro-oesophageal reflux disease. Aliment Pharmacol Ther 2012;35:1073–9.
117. Wang YT, Yazaki E, Sifrim D. High-resolution manometry: esophageal disorders not addressed by the "Chicago Classification". J Neurogastroenterol Motil 2012; 18:365–72.

Scleroderma and the Esophagus

Nitin K. Ahuja, MD[a], John O. Clarke, MD[b],*

KEYWORDS

- Scleroderma • Dysphagia • Aperistalsis • Sjogren • Lupus • Fibromyalgia
- Ehler-Danlos • Myositis

KEY POINTS

- Esophageal involvement is seen in greater than 90% of patients with scleroderma and is often considered to be the classic gastrointestinal manifestation of scleroderma.
- Symptoms are related to dysmotility and include heartburn, regurgitation, and dysphagia.
- Given the high prevalence of esophageal involvement with scleroderma, empiric treatment is a very reasonable approach, with diagnostic studies reserved for select patients.
- Other connective tissue disorders, including mixed connective tissue disease, myositis, Sjogren syndrome, systemic lupus erythematosus, fibromyalgia, and Ehlers-Danlos syndrome, may also have esophageal manifestations, which are less prevalent and more varied than in scleroderma.

INTRODUCTION

The gastrointestinal (GI) tract is the second largest organ system in the body (other than the skin) and is commonly affected by many systemic disorders. Systemic sclerosis (SSc), or scleroderma, is the classic rheumatologic disorder with esophageal manifestations, although numerous others can have significant esophageal involvement as well. This article highlights scleroderma in particular and then focuses to a lesser extent on other key connective tissue disorders, including mixed connective tissue disease (MCTD), myositis, Sjogren syndrome (SS), systemic lupus erythematosus (SLE), fibromyalgia (FM), and Ehlers-Danlos syndrome (EDS).

SYSTEMIC SCLEROSIS (SCLERODERMA)

SSc is an autoimmune disorder characterized by vasculopathy, progressive fibrosis of the skin, and internal organ dysfunction. The GI tract is the most frequently involved

[a] Division of Gastroenterology and Hepatology, University of Pennsylvania, 3400 Civic Center Boulevard 7 South Pavilion, Philadelphia, PA 19104, USA; [b] Division of Gastroenterology and Hepatology, Stanford University School of Medicine, 430 Broadway Street, Pavilion C, 3rd Floor, C-343, Redwood City, CA 94063-6341, USA
* Corresponding author.
E-mail address: john.clarke@stanford.edu

internal organ system, and SSc can affect any region therein.[1] Esophageal involvement is highly prevalent and is often viewed as the classic GI SSc manifestation, reported in more than 90% of SSc patients via both pathology[2] and symptom assessment.[3] Symptoms are related to dysmotility and commonly consist of dysphagia, heartburn, and regurgitation. Complications include esophageal stricture formation, Barrett's esophagus, bleeding, and aspiration.

Pathogenesis

The pathogenesis of dysfunction is still not entirely clear, and several potential mechanisms have been described. Sjogren[4] proposed a progression of GI SSc involvement composed of 3 distinct steps: (1) vascular damage, (2) neurogenic impairment, and (3) replacement of normal smooth muscle by fibrosis and atrophy. However, this model remains speculative and to a certain extent controversial, because causal progression has never been demonstrated, and other competing theories exist. Autoantibodies directed against enteric neurons have been identified in a subset of patients with SSc,[5] as have antimuscarinic antibodies.[6] Responsiveness of the lower esophageal sphincter (LES) to exogenously administered methacholine, but not pharmacologic administration of agents acting via cholinergic neurons, supports the concept of a neurologic defect. Autonomic dysfunction has also been posited as a potential mechanism.[7] Interestingly, there are contradictory data with regard to whether esophageal fibrosis is even present in patients with advanced disease. On one hand, a study using endoscopic ultrasound in patients with SSc revealed significant esophageal thickening as compared with unaffected controls[8]; however, in contrast, an autopsy study evaluating the esophagi of 74 patients with SSc showed significant atrophy (94% of patients) but no evidence of abnormal fibrosis.[2] More recently, Taroni and colleagues[9,10] reported on proliferative and inflammatory molecular gene expression subsets in SSc, suggesting that the pathogenesis of SSc may stem from distinct disease subsets rather than a single homogeneous process, with immune activation posited as a major driver of disease.

Clinical Manifestations

The vast majority of SSc patients relate clinical symptoms attributable to esophageal dysmotility, including heartburn, regurgitation, and dysphagia.[1] Gastroesophageal reflux is of particular concern because of multiple contributing mechanisms, including peristaltic dysfunction, decreased LES pressure, delayed gastric emptying, autonomic dysfunction, sicca syndrome (seen in 20% of patients), and often an associated hiatal hernia.[11,12] Just as important as the loss of the LES as an antireflux barrier is the loss of native reflux clearance mechanisms like secondary peristalsis and salivary bicarbonate secretion. Medications used to treat other manifestations of SSc, including phosphodiesterase inhibitors and calcium channel blockers, can further impair LES function and may worsen reflux.

Dysphagia is related to decreased or absent peristalsis. Despite the degree of objective dysmotility, dysphagia is generally mild and intermittent owing to the ability of gravity to facilitate bolus transit. Many patients, up to 40% in some series, are asymptomatic despite well-documented esophageal dysmotility.[13–16] Symptoms can intensify in the context of a stricture. Compensatory behavioral strategies include assuming an upright posture after meals and use of liquids between swallowing of solid food.

Esophageal dysmotility and reflux in the context of SSc may be associated with significant complications. Stricture formation is particularly prevalent and has a variety of potential causes, including reflux, pill-induced injury, and candidiasis. The prevalence of SSc-related esophageal strictures has been estimated to be as high as 29%, and an SSc diagnosis is associated with an odds ratio of approximately 12 for stricture formation.[17,18] Although reflux is thought to be the classic precipitant, Candida esophagitis is also worth noting. Patients with SSc have multiple risk factors for candidiasis, including chronic acid suppression, antibiotic administration, esophageal dysmotility, and immunosuppression. One study reported Candida colonization/infection rates of 15% with strictures associated in all cases.[19] The prevalence of Barrett's esophagus has been reported to be as high as 37%,[20] although several investigators have reported significantly rates,[17,19] and it is not yet clear whether the prevalence of Barrett's esophagus or esophageal cancer in SSc exceeds that of the general public.[21] Most of these data predate the widespread use of proton pump inhibitors (PPI), suggesting that they may be overestimates.

Gastrointestinal and Pulmonary Relationship

The relationship between reflux and pulmonary disease in SSc is controversial. Reflux can theoretically lead to pulmonary disease through microaspiration, leading to direct injury, or via vagal stimulation resulting in bronchoconstriction. Conversely, pulmonary disease may exacerbate reflux because of alterations in esophageal/gastric pressure dynamics, use of medications that lower LES pressure (in particular, bronchodilators and sildenafil), and hernia formation. The vast majority of studies addressing this relationship have shown a correlation between esophageal reflux and SSc lung disease.[22–28] This finding has not been universal,[29] but given the preponderance of evidence, the relationship between reflux and pulmonary disease in SSc appears consistent and likely genuine. Causality has not been established, however, and there are no data at present to prove that treatment of reflux in patients with SSc has any effect on long-term pulmonary function.[30]

Diagnostic Considerations

Patients with typical reflux symptoms in the context of SSc should be treated empirically given the high prevalence of esophageal involvement; however, diagnostic evaluation is required for atypical symptoms, significant dysphagia, or symptoms refractory to therapy. Multiple diagnostic modalities exist to evaluate esophageal function and disease in symptomatic patients. Traditionally, a barium esophagram was the initial test of choice for symptomatic SSc patients, as it could provide a rough evaluation of both structure and function.[31,32] However, fluoroscopy is less sensitive than endoscopy for detection of esophagitis and does not allow therapeutic interventions, such as dilation. Similarly, fluoroscopy is less sensitive than manometry for detection of dysmotility. Although fluoroscopy still has a role in evaluation of the symptomatic patient with SSc, that role has become more nuanced, and most authorities do not recommend it as the initial test of choice in the absence of severe dysphagia.[11,24] In contrast, endoscopy should be considered a first-line study in patients presenting with esophageal symptoms related to SSc. Esophagitis has been reported in 32% to 77% of SSc patients undergoing endoscopy; however, multiple studies have shown that symptoms do not necessarily correlate with esophageal injury and that even SSc patients with no symptoms can have significant esophageal damage.[18,19,25,33–36] As detailed above, Candida and Barrett's esophagus are additional clinical concerns that cannot be detected reliably without endoscopy. Endoscopy also allows for dilation should a stricture be identified. For these reasons, some authorities recommend early endoscopy for all patients diagnosed with SSc[36]; there are no guidelines to support that position, however, and the decision to pursue endoscopy needs to be individualized.

Esophageal manometry is considered the gold standard for assessment of esophageal motility in patients with SSc; manometric abnormalities are detected in up to 90% of patients, even in the absence of symptoms.[37–41] Typical findings include loss of contractile reserve, low-contraction amplitudes in the distal esophagus, and, in more advanced cases, aperistalsis with a hypotensive LES. Classically, esophageal contractile forces are maintained in the proximal esophagus, whereas the upper esophageal sphincter is uninvolved. Of note, although some authorities recommend early manometry for SSc patients, there are no data to show that early manometry necessarily impacts long-term outcomes, nor are manometric findings pathognomonic for a diagnosis of SSc. The Functional Lumen Imaging Probe has also recently been used as a means to assess esophageal function in SSc, although data are still emerging with regard to how this technology impacts the diagnosis and management of SSc-related esophageal disease.[42,43] Finally, formal reflux testing, via ambulatory pH impedance or prolonged wireless pH testing, has a clear role in the evaluation of select SSc patients with suspected reflux or continued symptoms despite therapy. Interestingly, data suggest that SSc patients may be less responsive to conventional reflux therapy, considering these tests may be helpful to optimize acid suppression.[44]

Treatment

The treatment of GI manifestations of SSc can be challenging. Available therapies directed at the slowing or reversal of SSc progression, including high-dose immunosuppression and stem cell transplantation, have not demonstrated efficacy from a GI perspective. Existing therapies are leveraged to manage the complications of dysmotility. Initial treatment often consists of lifestyle modification, including elevation of the head of the bed, avoidance of meals within 3 hours of lying supine, and avoidance of trigger foods. At present, acid suppressive therapy with PPI is the mainstay of therapy for SSc-related reflux. Although specific randomized controlled trials showing efficacy of PPI use in patients with SSc are lacking, expert consensus (European League against Rheumatism Scleroderma Trials and Research Group; UK Scleroderma Study Group) recommends PPI use to prevent reflux-induced complications.[45,46] These recommendations are supported by several small studies showing improvement in either symptoms or esophagitis with prolonged PPI use.[34,47,48] Data suggest that some SSc patients may require higher than typical PPI dosages, which is perhaps not surprising given the impairment of multiple physiologic determinants of reflux in SSc.[34,44] In addition, delayed gastric emptying and small intestinal bacterial overgrowth may also contribute to decreased PPI bioavailability, which may in turn impact decisions regarding PPI dose and formulation. For this reason, anecdotally, dexlansoprazole may be a nice option for reflux control in this population given its dual-release formulation. Other antireflux medical options, including antihistamines and alginates, have also been used in select patients, but their efficacy in the SSc population seems to be more limited than in the general population, and their additive benefit is likely modest at best.[49–52]

If symptoms progress despite high-dose acid suppressive therapy and lifestyle change, the next step is typically the addition of a prokinetic agent. Although the effects of prokinetics on the SSc esophagus are likely minimal, this class of agents has been shown to accelerate gastric emptying and potentially increase LES pressure. Limited data in SSc support at least short-term efficacy of cisapride, domperidone, erythromycin, metoclopramide, pyridostigmine, and prucalopride, although it should be emphasized that long-term data are largely lacking, and side effects with these therapies are not insignificant.[52–61] Nevertheless, given the severity of reflux in this population and the limited range of other therapeutic options, prokinetics are endorsed by expert consensus for the management of SSc-related symptomatic motility disturbances, including dysphagia and reflux.[45]

Other medical options used on occasion for select patients include buspirone and baclofen. Buspirone is an oral 5-HT$_{1A}$ agonist that is thought to affect receptors in the esophagus and fundus and by consequence enhance fundic accommodation.[62] Recently, investigators from Greece showed improvement in peristalsis and LES pressure in SSc patients treated with this agent for both acute and short-term administration.[63,64] Baclofen exerts action through modulation of GABA receptors and also has been found to increase LES pressure, although this agent has not been studied specifically in SSc.

For those patients with SSc with continued reflux symptoms or complications despite maximal medical therapy, surgical options can be considered. Care needs to be taken when making this decision, however, as the risk of postoperative dysphagia in the SSc population is significant, and the addition of even a minor degree of mechanical restriction at the esophagogastric junction in an SSc patient with absent esophageal peristalsis may result in the development of secondary achalasia. Early published series reported postoperative dysphagia rates ranging from 31% to 71%[65–68]; for this reason, surgical intervention has typically been reserved for either the most severe cases or patients with severe reflux and preserved peristalsis. Investigators from Pittsburgh reported on a series of SSc patients with reflux treated with a modified Roux-en-Y procedure with improved reflux and dysphagia rates as compared with fundoplication. This option may be considered in select cases, although the risk of malabsorption would have to be factored into the equation given the frequently tenuous nutritional circumstances of SSc patients.[69]

CONNECTIVE TISSUE DISEASES OTHER THAN SCLERODERMA
Mixed Connective Tissue Disease

MCTD was originally defined in 1972 as a connective tissue disorder characterized by the presence of high titers of anti-U1 ribonucleoprotein and as an overlap syndrome associated with antibodies in conjunction with selected clinical features of SSc, SLE, polymyositis, and/or rheumatoid arthritis.[70,71] Similar to other rheumatic disorders, MCTD can affect almost any organ system, and initial symptoms may be nonspecific. As MCTD represents an overlap disorder with features of both SSc and polymyositis, esophageal dysmotility can manifest proximally and distally because both striated and smooth muscle may be affected. By contrast, SSc affects the distal smooth muscle in the esophagus only.[72,73] GI involvement is frequent in MCTD and is viewed as the most common region of overlap with SSc.[72,74,75] Although esophageal dysmotility is common in MCTD, however, its onset tends to be more insidious and its severity less than is typically seen with SSc.[76,77] Moreover, although histopathologic changes of the esophagus are seen in greater than 90% of patients with MCTD,[75] symptoms are less prevalent, with reported ranges from 48% to 66% and initial presentations that are often subclinical.[72,77,78] Early evidence suggested potential benefit with steroids, although efficacy appears to be modest at best, and data are limited.[70,78]

Myositis

Inflammatory myopathies, also referred to as myositis, are a heterogeneous disease collection associated with immune-mediated skeletal muscle injury. From the vantage point of an esophagologist, the major disorders in this category are dermatomyositis, polymyositis, and inclusion body myositis. These disorders are associated with gradual onset of proximal skeletal muscle weakness with potential contractures and atrophy but preservation of sensation.[79] The inflammatory myopathies classically affect striated muscle. In the GI tract, these disorders classically present with dysphagia to solids and liquids, likely because of oropharyngeal and cricopharyngeal (CP) involvement, which results in poor oropharyngeal strength and coordination and insufficient relaxation of the upper esophageal sphincter. As smooth muscle is unaffected, patients with myositis typically do not have distal esophageal involvement. Dysphagia is reported in 32% to 84% of myositis patients.[79] Fluoroscopy is often the first diagnostic examination used and characteristically shows disordered and weak oropharyngeal function with a prominent CP, often referred to as a CP bar.[80–85] Manometric abnormalities have been reported,[79,86] but it is important to note that often findings may be subtle and that a normal study is not uncommon, particularly in early disease.

Treatment of dysphagia in the context of myositis consists of 3 approaches, often pursued in parallel. As dysphagia is a result of a systemic process, symptoms often respond in conjunction with disease manifestations outside the GI tract, and it is not uncommon to see dysphagia improve significantly or even resolve with systemic immune-modifying therapy. Second, as CP dysfunction is often a key driver of symptoms, endoscopic therapy directed at CP disruption has a key role in management, whether by dilation, botulinum toxin, or myotomy.[87–89] Even in cases of significant oropharyngeal dysfunction, alleviating CP resistance may be beneficial. Finally, focused swallow therapy may have a role, particularly in conjunction with the other measures detailed above.

Sjogren Syndrome

SS is a lymphocyte-mediated, infiltrative autoimmune disorder characterized by the destruction of exocrine glands leading to secretory dysfunction. Classically, SS is thought to predominantly affect the salivary glands, although extraglandular manifestations are common.[90,91] As SS affects salivary and lacrimal production, xerostomia and xerophthalmia are typical symptoms (referred to as sicca symptoms), affecting an estimated 80% of patients. In the oral cavity, these can result in mechanical complications, including dental caries, periodontal issues, angular cheilitis, nonspecific ulcerations, and lip dryness.

From an esophageal standpoint, both dysphagia and reflux symptoms appear to be increased. Although the exact mechanism is unclear, xerostomia certainly plays a role, as loss of saliva limits both lubrication for swallows and buffering of refluxate. Decreased salivary production alone may not be the whole explanation, however, as dysmotility and dysautonomia have also been implicated.[91–94] Cervical webs have also been reported in SS, but only in a minority of patients (approximately 10%).[95] Up to 80% of patients with SS report at least some degree of dysphagia. Typically, this symptom is more pronounced with solids than liquids and is subjectively localized in a proximal position.[92,96]

Diagnostic evaluation of SS is somewhat limited, although necessary to exclude other potential processes. Unlike other rheumatologic disorders addressed in this article, SS is not associated with any characteristic imaging or manometric abnormality. In practice, although we often pursue diagnostic evaluation for symptomatic patients with SS, results can be underwhelming. Treatment of esophageal symptoms related to SS is often focused on restoration of saliva via lifestyle measures like liquids in conjunction with solid food, lozenges, and chewing gum, and via pharmaceutical agents like pilocarpine and cevimeline. Endoscopy may have a role to exclude candidiasis and/or to dilate if there is an associated cervical web or peptic stricture.[90,91]

Systemic Lupus Erythematosus

SLE is a female-predominant multisystem disorder characterized by the presence of autoantibodies and typical symptoms. Esophageal involvement occurs in a minority of SLE patients, and associated symptoms are often less severe than with other rheumatic conditions detailed above. Dysphagia is reported in 2% to 25% of patients, and associated reflux symptoms and noncardiac chest pain may be prominent.[97–99] In many ways, SLE mimics other conditions and can overlap in phenotype with SSc, myositis, and SS.[100,101] Diagnostic testing is generally nonspecific and often normal.[102,103] Treatment of symptomatic esophageal patients with SLE is often symptomatic and via standard diagnostic algorithms. If sicca symptoms are prominent, lifestyle and pharmaceutical maneuvers may be used to improve lubrication and salivary production. If dysphagia is prominent, endoscopic evaluation and potential dilation are reasonable approaches, as is reflux therapy if indicated.

Fibromyalgia

FM is the second most common "rheumatic" disorder, with prevalence ranging from 2% to 8% of the population, and is associated with chronic widespread musculoskeletal pain.[104] It is often classified under the rubric of connective tissue disease, as prevailing theories in the twentieth century linked FM with soft tissue inflammation, termed fibrositis. More recent data have shown no evidence of significant inflammation, however,[104,105] such that FM is now considered to be a centralized pain state resulting in pain sensation out of proportion to peripheral nociceptive input.[104]

GI complaints are reported by many patients with FM.[106,107] Although irritable bowel syndrome is the classic manifestation, other regions of the gut can be affected. The hallmark of this disorder is symptom amplification. From an esophageal standpoint, reflux and chest pain are both thought to be more common than in the non-FM population; however, severe symptoms may be more commonly related to central sensory sensitization rather than abnormal motility or acid exposure per se.[107–109] Testing is often normal and useful primarily for reassurance and excluding alternative diagnoses. Common treatment modalities include education, lifestyle changes aimed at decreasing physiologic stressors (exercise, sleep hygiene, diet), complementary/alternative therapies, and neuromodulation. Therapeutic interventions, such as surgery, should only be considered after careful deliberation; as in the authors' experience, FM patients can be more sensitive to intervention.

Ehlers-Danlos Syndrome

The hypermobile form of EDS is a noninflammatory heritable disorder of connective tissue characterized by joint hyperflexibility, skin hyperelasticity, and musculoskeletal symptoms.[110–112] GI symptoms are almost universal in patients with EDS. In a recent survey of more than 600 EDS patients, nearly all (98%) met criteria for at least 1 Rome IV functional GI disorder (FGID), and the vast majority (84%) fulfilled criteria for at least 2 FGIDs.[113] The pathogenesis of GI symptoms is not entirely clear but likely relates to autonomic dysfunction, alterations in gut wall connective tissue compliance and mechanoreceptors, abnormal organ suspension within the abdominal cavity, alterations in organ mobility, changes in blood flow, alterations in gut motility, and/or abnormal pain thresholds.[112]

From an esophageal standpoint, reflux symptoms (heartburn and regurgitation), dysphagia, and chest pain all appear to be increased in prevalence in the EDS population. In several retrospective series, reflux symptoms were reported in 33% to 57% of patients, whereas dysphagia and chest pain were reported less frequently, although still at higher rates than in control populations.[112,114–116] In a recent series, almost half of patients with EDS with reported reflux symptoms were found to have either reflux hypersensitivity or functional heartburn on formal testing. Similarly, of those patients who reported dysphagia, 60% were thought to have a functional cause rather than a codified motility disorder after formal evaluation.[117] Endoscopy, manometry, and reflux testing are often normal but may help better define pathophysiology and potentially stratify therapy. With regard to treatment, standard therapy for reflux (diet, lifestyle, and acid-suppressive therapy) is an appropriate first step, whereas prokinetics can be considered in cases of concurrent delayed gastric emptying. As a high percentage of GI symptoms in EDS are functional, neuromodulatory and complementary therapies may be helpful and should be considered. Because these patients have connective tissue fragility, mechanical interventions and in particular surgeries should only be considered as a last resort.[118]

DISCLOSURE

J.O. Clarke has received honoraria for consulting from Alnylam, Isothrive, Medtronic, Regeneron, and Sanofi. N.K. Ahuja has served on advisory boards for Takeda and Laborie and has received honoraria for consulting from Medtronic and GlaxoSmithKline and research support from Nestle and Vanda. No conflicts of interest exist.

REFERENCES

1. Miller JB, Gandhi N, Clarke J, et al. Gastrointestinal involvement in systemic sclerosis: an update. J Clin Rheumatol 2018;24(6):328–37.
2. Roberts CG, Hummers LK, Ravich WJ, et al. A case-control study of the pathology of oesophageal disease in systemic sclerosis (scleroderma). Gut 2006; 55(12):1697–703.
3. Thoua NM, Bunce C, Brough G, et al. Assessment of gastrointestinal symptoms in patients with systemic sclerosis in a UK tertiary referral centre. Rheumatology (Oxford) 2010;49(9):1770–5.
4. Sjogren RW. Gastrointestinal motility disorders in scleroderma. Arthritis Rheum 1994;37(9):1265–82.
5. Howe S, Eaker EY, Sallustio JE, et al. Antimyenteric neuronal antibodies in scleroderma. J Clin Invest 1994;94(2):761–70.
6. Goldblatt F, Gordon TP, Waterman SA. Antibody-mediated gastrointestinal dysmotility in scleroderma. Gastroenterology 2002;123(4):1144–50.
7. Dessein PH, Joffe BI, Metz RM, et al. Autonomic dysfunction in systemic sclerosis: sympathetic overactivity and instability. Am J Med 1992;93(2):143–50.
8. Zuber-Jerger I, Müller A, Kullmann F, et al. Gastrointestinal manifestation of systemic sclerosis–thickening of the upper gastrointestinal wall detected by endoscopic ultrasound is a valid sign. Rheumatology (Oxford) 2010;49(2):368–72.
9. Taroni JN, Martyanov V, Huang CC, et al. Molecular characterization of systemic sclerosis esophageal pathology identifies inflammatory and proliferative signatures. Arthritis Res Ther 2015;17:194.
10. Taroni JN, Mahoney JM, Whitfield ML. The mechanistic implications of gene expression studies in SSc: insights from systems biology. Curr Treatm Opt Rheumatol 2017;3(3):181–92.
11. Ebert EC. Esophageal disease in progressive systemic sclerosis. Curr Treat Options Gastroenterol 2008;11(1):64–9.
12. Ebert EC. Esophageal disease in scleroderma. J Clin Gastroenterol 2006;40(9): 769–75.

13. Abu-Shakra M, Guillemin F, Lee P. Gastrointestinal manifestations of systemic sclerosis. Semin Arthritis Rheum 1994;24(1):29–39.
14. Ling TC, Johnston BT. Esophageal investigations in connective tissue disease: which tests are most appropriate? J Clin Gastroenterol 2001;32(1):33–6.
15. Kaye SA, Siraj QH, Agnew J, et al. Detection of early asymptomatic esophageal dysfunction in systemic sclerosis using a new scintigraphic grading method. J Rheumatol 1996;23(2):297–301.
16. Harper RA, Jackson DC. Progressive systemic sclerosis. Br J Radiol 1965; 38(455):825–34.
17. Weston S, Thumshirn M, Wiste J, et al. Clinical and upper gastrointestinal motility features in systemic sclerosis and related disorders. Am J Gastroenterol 1998;93(7):1085–9.
18. El-Serag HB, Sonnenberg A. Association of esophagitis and esophageal strictures with diseases treated with nonsteroidal anti-inflammatory drugs. Am J Gastroenterol 1997;92(1):52–6.
19. Zamost BJ, Hirschberg J, Ippoliti AF, et al. Esophagitis in scleroderma. Prevalence and risk factors. Gastroenterology 1987;92(2):421–8.
20. Katzka DA, Reynolds JC, Saul SH, et al. Barrett's metaplasia and adenocarcinoma of the esophagus in scleroderma. Am J Med 1987;82(1):46–52.
21. Segel MC, Campbell WL, Medsger TA, et al. Systemic sclerosis (scleroderma) and esophageal adenocarcinoma: is increased patient screening necessary? Gastroenterology 1985;89(3):485–8.
22. Denis P, Ducrotte P, Pasquis P, et al. Esophageal motility and pulmonary function in progressive systemic sclerosis. Respiration 1981;42(1):21–4.
23. Johnson DA, Drane WE, Curran J, et al. Pulmonary disease in progressive systemic sclerosis. A complication of gastroesophageal reflux and occult aspiration? Arch Intern Med 1989;149(3):589–93.
24. Lock G, Pfeifer M, Straub RH, et al. Association of esophageal dysfunction and pulmonary function impairment in systemic sclerosis. Am J Gastroenterol 1998; 93(3):341–5.
25. Marie I, Dominique S, Levesque H, et al. Esophageal involvement and pulmonary manifestations in systemic sclerosis. Arthritis Rheum 2001;45(4):346–54.
26. Kinuya K, Nakajima K, Kinuya S, et al. Esophageal hypomotility in systemic sclerosis: close relationship with pulmonary involvement. Ann Nucl Med 2001;15(2): 97–101.
27. Savarino E, Bazzica M, Zentilin P, et al. Gastroesophageal reflux and pulmonary fibrosis in scleroderma: a study using pH-impedance monitoring. Am J Respir Crit Care Med 2009;179(5):408–13.
28. Zhang XJ, Bonner A, Hudson M, et al. Association of gastroesophageal factors and worsening of forced vital capacity in systemic sclerosis. J Rheumatol 2013; 40(6):850–8.
29. Troshinsky MB, Kane GC, Varga J, et al. Pulmonary function and gastroesophageal reflux in systemic sclerosis. Ann Intern Med 1994;121(1):6–10.
30. Christmann RB, Wells AU, Capelozzi VL, et al. Gastroesophageal reflux incites interstitial lung disease in systemic sclerosis: clinical, radiologic, histopathologic, and treatment evidence. Semin Arthritis Rheum 2010;40(3):241–9.
31. Clements PJ, Kadell B, Ippoliti A, et al. Esophageal motility in progressive systemic sclerosis (PSS). Comparison of cine-radiographic and manometric evaluation. Dig Dis Sci 1979;24(8):639–44.
32. Madani G, Katz RD, Haddock JA, et al. The role of radiology in the management of systemic sclerosis. Clin Radiol 2008;63(9):959–67.

33. Arif T, Masood Q, Singh J, et al. Assessment of esophageal involvement in systemic sclerosis and morphea (localized scleroderma) by clinical, endoscopic, manometric and pH metric features: a prospective comparative hospital based study. BMC Gastroenterol 2015;15:24.

34. Marie I, Ducrotte P, Denis P, et al. Oesophageal mucosal involvement in patients with systemic sclerosis receiving proton pump inhibitor therapy. Aliment Pharmacol Ther 2006;24(11–12):1593–601.

35. Bassotti G, Battaglia E, Debernardi V, et al. Esophageal dysfunction in scleroderma: relationship with disease subsets. Arthritis Rheum 1997;40(12):2252–9.

36. Thonhofer R, Siegel C, Trummer M, et al. Early endoscopy in systemic sclerosis without gastrointestinal symptoms. Rheumatol Int 2012;32(1):165–8.

37. Lock G, Zeuner M, Straub RH, et al. Esophageal manometry in systemic sclerosis: screening procedure or confined to symptomatic patients? Rheumatol Int 1997;17(2):61–6.

38. Savarino E, Mei F, Parodi A, et al. Gastrointestinal motility disorder assessment in systemic sclerosis. Rheumatology (Oxford) 2013;52(6):1095–100.

39. Carlson DA, Crowell MD, Kimmel JN, et al. Loss of peristaltic reserve, determined by multiple rapid swallows, is the most frequent esophageal motility abnormality in patients with systemic sclerosis. Clin Gastroenterol Hepatol 2016; 14(10):1502–6.

40. Kimmel JN, Carlson DA, Hinchcliff M, et al. The association between systemic sclerosis disease manifestations and esophageal high-resolution manometry parameters. Neurogastroenterol Motil 2016;28(8):1157–65.

41. Carlson DA, Hinchcliff M, Pandolfino JE. Advances in the evaluation and management of esophageal disease of systemic sclerosis. Curr Rheumatol Rep 2015;17(1):475.

42. Fynne L, Liao D, Aksglaede K, et al. Esophagogastric junction in systemic sclerosis: a study with the functional lumen imaging probe. Neurogastroenterol Motil 2017;29(8). https://doi.org/10.1111/nmo.13073.

43. Gregersen H, Liao D, Pedersen J, et al. A new method for evaluation of intestinal muscle contraction properties: studies in normal subjects and in patients with systemic sclerosis. Neurogastroenterol Motil 2007;19(1):11–9.

44. Stern EK, Carlson DA, Falmagne S, et al. Abnormal esophageal acid exposure on high-dose proton pump inhibitor therapy is common in systemic sclerosis patients. Neurogastroenterol Motil 2018;30(2).

45. Kowal-Bielecka O, Landewé R, Avouac J, et al. EULAR recommendations for the treatment of systemic sclerosis: a report from the EULAR Scleroderma Trials and Research group (EUSTAR). Ann Rheum Dis 2009;68(5):620–8.

46. Hansi N, Thoua N, Carulli M, et al. Consensus best practice pathway of the UK scleroderma study group: gastrointestinal manifestations of systemic sclerosis. Clin Exp Rheumatol 2014;32(6 Suppl 86). S-214-21.

47. Olive A, Maddison PJ, Davis M. Treatment of oesophagitis in scleroderma with omeprazole. Br J Rheumatol 1989;28(6):553.

48. Hendel L. Hydroxyproline in the oesophageal mucosa of patients with progressive systemic sclerosis during omeprazole-induced healing of reflux oesophagitis. Aliment Pharmacol Ther 1991;5(5):471–80.

49. Hendel L, Aggestrup S, Stentoft P. Long-term ranitidine in progressive systemic sclerosis (scleroderma) with gastroesophageal reflux. Scand J Gastroenterol 1986;21(7):799–805.

50. Petrokubi RJ, Jeffries GH. Cimetidine versus antacid in scleroderma with reflux esophagitis. A randomized double-blind controlled study. Gastroenterology 1979;77(4 Pt 1):691–5.
51. Janiak P, Thumshirn M, Menne D, et al. Clinical trial: the effects of adding ranitidine at night to twice daily omeprazole therapy on nocturnal acid breakthrough and acid reflux in patients with systemic sclerosis–a randomized controlled, cross-over trial. Aliment Pharmacol Ther 2007;26(9):1259–65.
52. Foocharoen C, Chunlertrith K, Mairiang P, et al. Effectiveness of add-on therapy with domperidone vs alginic acid in proton pump inhibitor partial response gastro-oesophageal reflux disease in systemic sclerosis: randomized placebo-controlled trial. Rheumatology (Oxford) 2017;56(2):214–22.
53. Horowitz M, Maddern GJ, Maddox A, et al. Effects of cisapride on gastric and esophageal emptying in progressive systemic sclerosis. Gastroenterology 1987;93(2):311–5.
54. Wehrmann T, Caspary WF. [Effect of cisapride on esophageal motility in healthy probands and patients with progressive systemic scleroderma]. Klin Wochenschr 1990;68(12):602–7.
55. Kahan A, Chaussade S, Gaudric M, et al. The effect of cisapride on gastro-oesophageal dysfunction in systemic sclerosis: a controlled manometric study. Br J Clin Pharmacol 1991;31(6):683–7.
56. Wang SJ, La JL, Chen DY, et al. Effects of cisapride on oesophageal transit of solids in patients with progressive systemic sclerosis. Clin Rheumatol 2002; 21(1):43–5.
57. Johnson DA, Drane WE, Curran J, et al. Metoclopramide response in patients with progressive systemic sclerosis. Effect on esophageal and gastric motility abnormalities. Arch Intern Med 1987;147(9):1597–601.
58. Mercado U, Arroyo de Anda R, Avendaño L, et al. Metoclopramide response in patients with early diffuse systemic sclerosis. Effects on esophageal motility abnormalities. Clin Exp Rheumatol 2005;23(5):685–8.
59. Fiorucci S, Distrutti E, Bassotti G, et al. Effect of erythromycin administration on upper gastrointestinal motility in scleroderma patients. Scand J Gastroenterol 1994;29(9):807–13.
60. Ahuja NK, Mische L, Clarke JO, et al. Pyridostigmine for the treatment of gastrointestinal symptoms in systemic sclerosis. Semin Arthritis Rheum 2018;48(1): 111–6.
61. Vigone B, Caronni M, Severino A, et al. Preliminary safety and efficacy profile of prucalopride in the treatment of systemic sclerosis (SSc)-related intestinal involvement: results from the open label cross-over PROGASS study. Arthritis Res Ther 2017;19(1):145.
62. Tack J, Janssen P, Masaoka T, et al. Efficacy of buspirone, a fundus-relaxing drug, in patients with functional dyspepsia. Clin Gastroenterol Hepatol 2012; 10(11):1239–45.
63. Karamanolis GP, Panopoulos S, Denaxas K, et al. The 5-HT1A receptor agonist buspirone improves esophageal motor function and symptoms in systemic sclerosis: a 4-week, open-label trial. Arthritis Res Ther 2016;18:195.
64. Karamanolis GP, Panopoulos S, Karlaftis A, et al. Beneficial effect of the 5-HT1A receptor agonist buspirone on esophageal dysfunction associated with systemic sclerosis: a pilot study. United European Gastroenterol J 2015;3(3): 266–71.
65. Henderson RD, Pearson FG. Surgical management of esophageal scleroderma. J Thorac Cardiovasc Surg 1973;66(5):686–92.

66. Orringer MB, Orringer JS, Dabich L, et al. Combined Collis gastroplasty–fundo-plication operations for scleroderma reflux esophagitis. Surgery 1981;90(4): 624–30.

67. Mansour KA. 1988: surgery for scleroderma of the esophagus: a 12-year expe-rience. Updated in 1995. Ann Thorac Surg 1995;60(1):227.

68. Poirier NC, Taillefer R, Topart P, et al. Antireflux operations in patients with sclero-derma. Ann Thorac Surg 1994;58(1):66–72 [discussion 72–3].

69. Kent MS, Luketich JD, Irshad K, et al. Comparison of surgical approaches to recalcitrant gastroesophageal reflux disease in the patient with scleroderma. Ann Thorac Surg 2007;84(5):1710–5 [discussion 1715–6].

70. Sharp GC, Irvin WS, Tan EM, et al. Mixed connective tissue disease–an appar-ently distinct rheumatic disease syndrome associated with a specific antibody to an extractable nuclear antigen (ENA). Am J Med 1972;52(2):148–59.

71. Bennett RM, O'Connell DJ. Mixed connective tisssue disease: a clinicopatho-logic study of 20 cases. Semin Arthritis Rheum 1980;10(1):25–51.

72. Nica AE, Alexa LM, Ionescu AO, et al. Esophageal disorders in mixed connec-tive tissue diseases. J Med Life 2016;9(2):141–3.

73. LeRoy EC, Maricq HR, Kahaleh MB. Undifferentiated connective tissue syn-dromes. Arthritis Rheum 1980;23(3):341–3.

74. Fagundes MN, Caleiro MT, Navarro-Rodriguez T, et al. Esophageal involvement and interstitial lung disease in mixed connective tissue disease. Respir Med 2009;103(6):854–60.

75. Uzuki M, Kamataki A, Watanabe M, et al. Histological analysis of esophageal muscular layers from 27 autopsy cases with mixed connective tissue disease (MCTD). Pathol Res Pract 2011;207(6):383–90.

76. Kallenberg CG. Overlapping syndromes, undifferentiated connective tissue dis-ease, and other fibrosing conditions. Curr Opin Rheumatol 1995;7(6):568–73.

77. Doria A, Bonavina L, Anselmino M, et al. Esophageal involvement in mixed con-nective tissue disease. J Rheumatol 1991;18(5):685–90.

78. Marshall JB, Kretschmar JM, Gerhardt DC, et al. Gastrointestinal manifestations of mixed connective tissue disease. Gastroenterology 1990;98(5 Pt 1):1232–8.

79. Ebert EC. Review article: the gastrointestinal complications of myositis. Aliment Pharmacol Ther 2010;31(3):359–65.

80. O'Hara JM, Szemes G, Lowman RM. The esophageal lesions in dermatomyosi-tis. A correlation of radiologic and pathologic findings. Radiology 1967;89(1): 27–31.

81. Dietz F, Logeman JA, Sahgal V, et al. Cricopharyngeal muscle dysfunction in the differential diagnosis of dysphagia in polymyositis. Arthritis Rheum 1980;23(4): 491–5.

82. Jacob H, Berkowitz D, McDonald E, et al. The esophageal motility disorder of polymyositis. A prospective study. Arch Intern Med 1983;143(12):2262–4.

83. de Merieux P, Verity MA, Clements PJ, et al. Esophageal abnormalities and dysphagia in polymyositis and dermatomyositis. Arthritis Rheum 1983;26(8): 961–8.

84. Kagen LJ, Hochman RB, Strong EW. Cricopharyngeal obstruction in inflamma-tory myopathy (polymyositis/dermatomyositis). Report of three cases and review of the literature. Arthritis Rheum 1985;28(6):630–6.

85. Azola A, Mulheren R, Mckeon G, et al. Dysphagia in myositis: a study of the structural and physiologic changes resulting in disordered swallowing. Am J Phys Med Rehabil 2020;99(5):404–8.

86. Casal-Dominguez M, Pinal-Fernandez I, Mego M, et al. High-resolution manometry in patients with idiopathic inflammatory myopathy: elevated prevalence of esophageal involvement and differences according to autoantibody status and clinical subset. Muscle Nerve 2017;56(3):386–92.

87. Chandrasekhara V, Koh J, Lattimer L, et al. Endoscopic balloon catheter dilatation. World J Gastrointest Endosc 2017;9(4):183–8.

88. Schrey A, Airas L, Jokela M, et al. Botulinum toxin alleviates dysphagia of patients with inclusion body myositis. J Neurol Sci 2017;380:142–7.

89. Sanei-Moghaddam A, Kumar S, Jani P, et al. Cricopharyngeal myotomy for cricopharyngeus stricture in an inclusion body myositis patient with hiatus hernia: a learning experience. BMJ Case Rep 2013;2013. https://doi.org/10.1136/bcr-2012-008058.

90. Ebert EC. Gastrointestinal and hepatic manifestations of Sjogren syndrome. J Clin Gastroenterol 2012;46(1):25–30.

91. Popov Y, Salomon-Escoto K. Gastrointestinal and hepatic disease in Sjogren syndrome. Rheum Dis Clin North Am 2018;44(1):143–51.

92. Palma R, Freire A, Freitas J, et al. Esophageal motility disorders in patients with Sjögren's syndrome. Dig Dis Sci 1994;39(4):758–61.

93. Waterman SA. Multiple subtypes of voltage-gated calcium channel mediate transmitter release from parasympathetic neurons in the mouse bladder. J Neurosci 1996;16(13):4155–61.

94. Imrich R, Alevizos I, Bebris L, et al. Predominant glandular cholinergic dysautonomia in patients with primary Sjögren's syndrome. Arthritis Rheumatol 2015; 67(5):1345–52.

95. Kjellén G, Fransson SG, Lindström F, et al. Esophageal function, radiography, and dysphagia in Sjögren's syndrome. Dig Dis Sci 1986;31(3):225–9.

96. Pierce JL, Tanner K, Merrill RM, et al. Swallowing disorders in Sjögren's syndrome: prevalence, risk factors, and effects on quality of life. Dysphagia 2016;31(1):49–59.

97. Chua S, Dodd H, Saeed IT, et al. Dysphagia in a patient with lupus and review of the literature. Lupus 2002;11(5):322–4.

98. Ebert EC, Hagspiel KD. Gastrointestinal and hepatic manifestations of systemic lupus erythematosus. J Clin Gastroenterol 2011;45(5):436–41.

99. Peppercorn MA, Docken WP, Rosenberg S. Esophageal motor dysfunction in systemic lupus erythematosus. Two cases with unusual features. JAMA 1979; 242(17):1895–6.

100. ter Borg EJ, Groen H, Horst G, et al. Clinical associations of antiribonucleoprotein antibodies in patients with systemic lupus erythematosus. Semin Arthritis Rheum 1990;20(3):164–73.

101. Laique S, Singh T, Dornblaser D, et al. Clinical characteristics and associated systemic diseases in patients with esophageal "absent contractility"-a clinical algorithm. J Clin Gastroenterol 2019;53(3):184–90.

102. Gutierrez F, Valenzuela JE, Ehresmann GR, et al. Esophageal dysfunction in patients with mixed connective tissue diseases and systemic lupus erythematosus. Dig Dis Sci 1982;27(7):592–7.

103. Ramirez-Mata M, Reyes PA, Alarcon-Segovia D, et al. Esophageal motility in systemic lupus erythematosus. Am J Dig Dis 1974;19(2):132–6.

104. Clauw DJ. Fibromyalgia: a clinical review. JAMA 2014;311(15):1547–55.

105. Lund E, Kendall SA, Janerot-Sjøberg B, et al. Muscle metabolism in fibromyalgia studied by P-31 magnetic resonance spectroscopy during aerobic and anaerobic exercise. Scand J Rheumatol 2003;32(3):138–45.

106. Triadafilopoulos G, Simms RW, Goldenberg DL. Bowel dysfunction in fibromyalgia syndrome. Dig Dis Sci 1991;36(1):59–64.
107. Wallace DJ, Hallegua DS. Fibromyalgia: the gastrointestinal link. Curr Pain Headache Rep 2004;8(5):364–8.
108. Wang JC, Sung FC, Men M, et al. Bidirectional association between fibromyalgia and gastroesophageal reflux disease: two population-based retrospective cohort analysis. Pain 2017;158(10):1971–8.
109. Almansa C, Wang B, Achem SR. Noncardiac chest pain and fibromyalgia. Med Clin North Am 2010;94(2):275–89.
110. DiBaise JK, Harris LA, Goodman B. Postural tachycardia syndrome (POTS) and the GI tract: a primer for the gastroenterologist. Am J Gastroenterol 2018; 113(10):1458–67.
111. Beckers AB, Keszthelyi D, Fikree A, et al. Gastrointestinal disorders in joint hypermobility syndrome/Ehlers-Danlos syndrome hypermobility type: a review for the gastroenterologist. Neurogastroenterol Motil 2017;29(8). https://doi.org/10.1111/nmo.13013.
112. Botrus G, Baker O, Borrego E, et al. Spectrum of gastrointestinal manifestations in joint hypermobility syndromes. Am J Med Sci 2018;355(6):573–80.
113. Lam CY, Palsson OS, Whitehead WE, et al. Rome IV functional gastrointestinal disorders and health impairment in subjects with hypermobility spectrum disorders or hypermobile Ehlers-Danlos syndrome. Clin Gastroenterol Hepatol 2020. https://doi.org/10.1016/j.cgh.2020.02.034.
114. Fikree A, Grahame R, Aktar R, et al. A prospective evaluation of undiagnosed joint hypermobility syndrome in patients with gastrointestinal symptoms. Clin Gastroenterol Hepatol 2014;12(10):1680–7.e2.
115. Castori M, Camerota F, Celletti C, et al. Natural history and manifestations of the hypermobility type Ehlers-Danlos syndrome: a pilot study on 21 patients. Am J Med Genet A 2010;152A(3):556–64.
116. Nelson AD, Mouchli MA, Valentin N, et al. Ehlers Danlos syndrome and gastrointestinal manifestations: a 20-year experience at Mayo Clinic. Neurogastroenterol Motil 2015;27(11):1657–66.
117. Fikree A, Aziz Q, Sifrim D. Mechanisms underlying reflux symptoms and dysphagia in patients with joint hypermobility syndrome, with and without postural tachycardia syndrome. Neurogastroenterol Motil 2017;29(6). https://doi.org/10.1111/nmo.13029.
118. Burcharth J, Rosenberg J. Surgical recommendations in Ehlers-Danlos syndrome(s) need patient classification: the example of Ehlers-Danlos syndrome hypermobility type (a.k.a. joint hypermobility syndrome)—reply. Dig Surg 2012;29(6):456.

Sorting out the Relationship Between Esophageal and Pulmonary Disease

Noreen C. Okwara, MD[a,b], Walter W. Chan, MD, MPH[b,c],*

KEYWORDS

- Esophageal dysfunction • Aspiration • Pulmonary disease
- Gastroesophageal reflux disease (GERD) • Lung transplant

KEY POINTS

- The relationship between esophageal disease and pulmonary disease is bi-directional.
- Esophageal disease may influence the outcomes of pulmonary disease. The reflux and re-flex pathways explain the current understanding of physiological mechanisms through which esophageal diseases may impact pulmonary disease.
- The main pulmonary diseases that have been linked to esophageal syndromes include chronic conditions such as asthma, chronic obstructive pulmonary disorder (COPD), bronchiectasis, idiopathic pulmonary fibrosis (IPF) and cystic fibrosis.
- Aspiration pneumonia and lung transplant complications have also been linked to esophageal disease. Intervention for esophageal diseases, particularly anti-reflux therapies, have been shown to improve outcomes.
- Chronic lung diseases may impact esophageal disease through changes in trans-diaphragmatic pressure gradient and alterations in esophagogastric junction mechanics, leading to increase esophageal reflux and symptoms.

INTRODUCTION

There has been considerable interest in the relationship between esophageal and pulmonary diseases. Specifically, gastroesophageal reflux disease (GERD) has been speculated to play an important role in various chronic lung disorders. In the largest, population-based study to date of 101,366 patients, pulmonary disorders were shown to be more prevalent among individuals with GERD.[1] Specifically, lung diseases that

a Department of Medicine, Brigham and Women's Hospital, Boston, Massachusetts, USA;
b Harvard Medical School, Boston, Massachusetts, USA; c Division of Gastroenterology, Hepatology and Endoscopy, Brigham and Women's Hospital, 75 Francis Street, Boston, MA 02115, USA
* Corresponding author. Division of Gastroenterology, Hepatology and Endoscopy, Brigham and Women's Hospital, 75 Francis Street, Boston, MA 02115, USA.
E-mail address: wwchan@bwh.harvard.edu

Gastroenterol Clin N Am 50 (2021) 919–934
https://doi.org/10.1016/j.gtc.2021.08.006
0889-8553/21/© 2021 Elsevier Inc. All rights reserved.

have previously been linked to GERD include asthma[2,3], chronic obstructive pulmonary disorders (COPD),[3] pulmonary fibrosis,[4–7] bronchiectasis,[8] cystic fibrosis,[9,10] aspiration pneumonia,[11] and lung transplant complications.[12] However, despite this evidence, a direct, causal link between GERD and lung diseases could not be definitively established from these observational studies. Although GERD may result in microaspiration and cause lung dysfunction,[13] alteration in respiratory mechanics from chronic lung disorders may also predispose to increased reflux. However, given the significant morbidity and mortality often associated with these pulmonary disorders, an understanding of the potential relationships between esophageal disorders and lung diseases is important for both pulmonologists and gastroenterologists alike to identify candidates that may benefit from targeted esophageal interventions, such as antireflux therapy.

The potential relationships between the esophagus and the lungs are complex because of their developmental and organogenetic overlap.[14] Moreover, the shared intrathoracic cavity may have an impact and implications on the mechanics and physiology of the 2 organs. For the relationship between lung diseases and GERD, which has been the most investigated esophageal disorder for this correlation, 2 main pathophysiologic mechanisms have been hypothesized: reflux-induced lung injury (reflux theory) and changes in lung physiology due to reflux-mediated vagal stimulation (reflex theory).

The reflux pathway

The reflux theory proposes that gastric contents traveling up to the proximal esophagus are aspirated into the airway, leading to direct injury to airway tissue and potentially triggering bronchospasm and/or inflammation, ultimately resulting in pulmonary pathology. Gastroduodenal contents, such as pepsin and bile acids, have previously been found in the airway of patients with chronic lung disorders on both cytopathologic and radiographic studies, serving as evidence to support reflux with the aspiration of digestive contents as a pathway for GERD-related lung dysfunction.[15–17] The reflux pathway can further be divided into 2 main mechanisms in causing airway pathology: macroaspiration versus microaspiration.

Although macroaspiration, which involves large-volume gastric contents entering the airways as seen mostly in patients with neurologic or muscular diseases, undoubtedly contributes to reflux-related airway or lung injury, it is microaspiration that is believed to be the more common mechanism among patients with disorders of the aerodigestive tract. During microaspiration, gastroduodenal contents of any volume can reflux up to the proximal esophagus. With inappropriate relaxation of the upper esophageal sphincter (UES), the refluxate may accumulate in the hypopharynx, penetrate the larynx, and enter the upper and lower airways. This mechanism has been proposed to explain the association between GERD and multiple pulmonary disorders, including Idiopathic pulmonary fibrosis (IPF),[18] asthma,[19] and lung transplant allograft rejection.[20] Indeed, analyses of bronchoalveolar lavage fluid (BALF) obtained from patients with pulmonary diseases have identified markers for aspiration, including alimentary tract contents such as pepsin[16] and bile acids,[21] and lipid-laden alveolar macrophages,[22,23] which have been shown at higher levels among patients with evidence of aspiration.

Functional and structural esophageal disorders can further exacerbate microaspiration and macroaspiration, thus causing worsened pulmonary disease and symptoms. Specifically, lower esophageal dysfunction associated with hiatal hernia, obesity, and lower esophageal sphincter (LES) abnormalities has been shown to increase the risk of occult aspiration, leading to worsened GERD symptoms, airway abnormalities, and pulmonary fibrosis.[24]

The reflex pathway

The esophagus, stomach, and lower respiratory tract share the same embryonic origin, the foregut, with significant developmental overlap.[25] As a result, they share similar innervation and control through the vagus nerve. The mechanism underlying the reflex pathway of the esophago–pulmonary interaction normally serves to protect the airway from potential aspiration of any gastric contents that have refluxed into the esophagus. The presence of acid in the distal esophagus from the refluxate may trigger a vagal response, which may, in turn, lead to bronchospasm. This vaso–vagal esophageal–bronchial reflex has been demonstrated in multiple prior studies, both in animals and humans. In an animal study using dogs, acidification of the esophagus led to an increase in airway resistance—a response that was lost after bilateral vagotomy.[26] Several human studies demonstrated similar airway responses to intraesophageal acidification, both through the infusion of acid and through continuous pH monitoring.[27,28] Specifically, this vagally mediated airway response seemed to be mostly activated by the presence of acid in the distal esophagus alone in a study using dual-pH sensor monitoring.[28] In addition, this vaso–vagal esophago–bronchial reflex seems to be present in all individuals, regardless of the presence of underlying pulmonary/airway disease or pathologic reflux. Moreover, the use of antacids seemed to reverse the airway response to esophageal acidification in some studies,[27] supporting a potential pathway for intervention.

Reflux versus reflex theories

Prior studies have supported the role of both mechanisms in leading to airway changes. However, the relative significance and contributions of both pathways may differ. In an animal study using cats, Tuchman and colleagues found an increase in the total lung resistance from baseline associated with both tracheal and intraesophageal infusion of hydrochloric acid (HCl) that was pH dependent.[29] However, a much larger volume of HCl was needed to result in a smaller increase in the total lung resistance with intraesophageal than tracheal infusion. This suggests that the reflux theory, with direct exposure of airway to the refluxate, likely results in a stronger airway response and more severe pulmonary injury. On the other hand, given the higher prevalence of distal reflux alone and relative rarity of proximal or supraesophageal reflux, the reflex pathway may more frequently play a role in patients with GERD and pulmonary disorders. Nevertheless, given the possibility of both pathways, diagnosis and management of potential GERD-related pulmonary disorders should take into account both possibilities.

THE BIDIRECTIONAL RELATIONSHIP: IMPACT OF LUNG DISEASE ON THE ESOPHAGUS

Although the reflux and reflex theories support the role of esophageal disorders in causing pulmonary disease, studies have also shown a possible relationship in the opposite direction, given the shared intrathoracic cavity, vagal innervation, and embryonic origin. For instance, airway obstruction and chronic hyperinflation have been associated with decreased basal LES and UES pressures, as well as increased frequency of transient LES relaxation, likely due to the weakening of the crural pressure at the esophagogastric junction.[2,30] Conditions leading to a more negative intrathoracic pressure during inspiration may also create a higher transdiaphragmatic pressure gradient, thereby increasing the risk of reflux.[31–33] Changes in the intrathoracic pressure and diaphragmatic function may also predispose to the caudal displacement of the LES and formation of hiatal hernia, thereby increasing the risk of GERD. Esophageal body peristaltic dysfunction has also been identified in high prevalence in patients with advanced lung disease undergoing lung transplant evaluation.[34] Finally, medications used in the management of pulmonary diseases such as corticosteroids and beta-agonists have been found to decrease LES tone and esophageal body contractility[35,36] and may, therefore, contribute to and exacerbate esophageal dysfunction and GERD. Appreciating the bidirectional relationship between pulmonary disorders and esophageal dysfunction is important, as they may exacerbate the impact of each other, resulting in harder-to-treat and more poorly controlled diseases. Nevertheless, esophageal disorders, particularly GERD, represent a potentially modifiable etiologic factor to improve the severity and course of the lung diseases (**Fig. 1**).

DIAGNOSTIC APPROACHES

Traditionally, esophageal disorders, whether with typical or extraesophageal presentations, are first diagnosed based on clinical presentation and response to therapy. Patients with GERD typically present with heartburn, regurgitation, swallowing symptoms, dyspepsia, bloating, and abdominal discomfort.[37] Airway manifestations of esophageal disease may include chronic cough, wheezing, aspiration pneumonia, dyspnea, bronchitis, pulmonary fibrosis, and a general decline in lung function, including worsened pulmonary function test (PFT) results, increased oxygen requirement, and hospitalizations. Among the lung transplant population, GERD has also

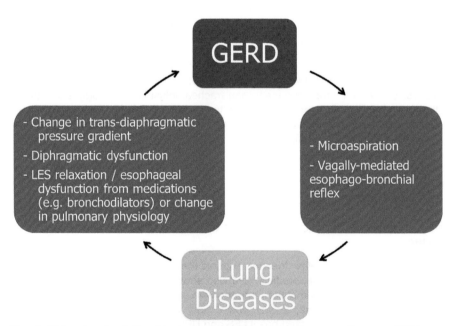

Fig. 1. Bidirectional relationship between GERD and pulmonary diseases. GERD may contribute to pulmonary disorders through direct injury to the airway from microaspiration or triggering the vagally mediated esophago–bronchial reflex. Lung diseases may also worsen GERD through an increase in transdiaphragmatic pressure gradient, diaphragmatic dysfunction leading to a weakened barrier at the esophagogastric junction or a hiatal hernia, or LES or esophageal dysfunction resulting from medications used for lung diseases or changes in pulmonary physiology.

been linked to a higher risk for allograft injury, acute and chronic rejection, and bronchiolitis obliterans syndrome (BOS).[12,38–41] Importantly, many patients with pulmonary complications of GERD may report no typical esophageal symptoms.[42] Accurate and timely diagnosis, therefore, requires a high degree of clinical suspicion and a standardized approach that includes the incorporation of esophageal function testing (EFT) (**Table 1**).

Empiric acid suppression

The diagnosis of GERD is typically made clinically and further supported by response to acid suppression therapy such as proton pump inhibitors (PPIs). The role and effectiveness of empirical acid suppression therapy in the diagnosis and management of pulmonary manifestations of reflux remain unclear, as data have been mixed and often limited by study design. Asthma represents the pulmonary condition with the most prospective data on the use of acid suppression. PPI therapy was found to result in improvement in the peak expiratory flow rate (PEFR) on PFTs compared with placebo in some randomized controlled studies, although the benefits were not consistently seen and seemed to be more pronounced among the subset of patients with asthma with GERD.[43–45] On a meta-analysis of randomized, placebo-controlled trials of PPIs for the treatment of asthma, PPI use was associated with a small, yet statistically significant, improvement in the morning PEFR (+8.683 L, $P = .007$) among the overall pooled population.[46] However, on subgroup analysis of studies including only patients with asthma with a concomitant diagnosis of GERD, a higher treatment effect was noted (+16.903 L, $P = .039$). These data suggest that PPIs may provide some small benefit in the treatment of asthma, particularly in those with concomitant GERD. Response to PPI therapy may, therefore, potentially help identify some patients with asthma in whom reflux may play a role. Some clinical factors to consider that may help increase suspicion for GERD among asthmatics include patients with adult-onset asthma, poor disease control with conventional therapies, onset of esophageal symptoms such as heartburn before asthma episodes, and worsening of asthma events with larger meals, ingestion of alcohol, or while lying in a supine position.

Data regarding the use of PPIs as a diagnostic or therapeutic tool in other pulmonary disorders remain much more limited. In the most recent Cochrane review on the use of PPIs for COPD published in 2020, only one randomized controlled trial was identified.[47] The study enrolled patients with COPD with no known symptoms or history of GERD and found a lower frequency of COPD exacerbations per patient per year among those treated with PPIs than among those receiving usual care alone.[48] For IPF, there has been no dedicated prospective, randomized trial to date. The largest controlled study comes from a pooled retrospective analysis of data from the placebo

Table 1		
Airway and pulmonary conditions associated with GERD		
Upper Airway	**Lower Airway**	
Chronic cough	Chronic cough	
Globus sensation	Asthma	
Throat clearing	Pulmonary fibrosis	
Hoarseness	Cystic fibrosis	
Dysphonia	Bronchiectasis	
Sore throat	Chronic obstructive pulmonary disorder	
	Lung transplant rejection	
	Recurrent aspiration pneumonia	

arms of 3 large randomized trials for antifibrotic therapy for IPF. In this analysis including 242 patients with IPF, among whom 124 (51%) were taking a PPI or a histamine-2-receptor antagonist (H2RA), the use of acid suppression medications was associated with a slower decline in forced vital capacity on PFTs and fewer exacerbations during the follow-up period.[49] In the most recent meta-analysis including 8 observational studies, medical therapy for GERD correlated with significantly decreased IPF-related mortality on time-to-event analyses, but not all-cause mortality.[50] Currently, the American Thoracic Society guidelines conditionally recommend an empirical trial of PPIs in the management of IPF, despite the currently limited evidence.[51] The data for the role of PPIs in the post–lung transplant population remain even more limited. In the only analysis to date of 188 lung transplant recipients, the persistent use of acid suppression, specifically PPIs, after transplant was associated with a lower risk of acute and chronic allograft rejections, independent of other clinical confounders.[52] Notably, prior animal studies have shown a potential antiinflammatory or antifibrotic effect of PPIs, which may also play a role in the protective effect seen in the studies for IPF and lung transplant allografts beyond reducing reflux alone.[53,54] Nevertheless, despite the inconsistent evidence, an empirical trial of PPIs seems to be a reasonable initial approach in the management of various pulmonary disorders, particularly when reflux is speculated to play an etiologic role.

Endoscopic assessment

Upper endoscopy plays an important part in the management algorithm of esophageal symptoms, including those related to GERD. It allows the identification of erosive esophagitis, an important marker for reflux-induced esophageal injury and other complications of GERD, such as peptic stricture, Barrett's esophagus, and malignancy. Anatomic features predisposing to GERD may also be identified on upper endoscopy, such as the presence of a hiatal hernia. Other etiologies for the esophageal symptoms, such as eosinophilic esophagitis, may also be assessed both endoscopically and histologically. However, the value of endoscopic evaluation in the assessment of pulmonary complications of GERD remains less clear. In a previous study of patients with asthma, those with more severe esophagitis reported worse symptoms and more frequent exacerbations than those with less severe or no esophagitis. However, nonerosive reflux disease (NERD) is common among those with esophageal symptoms and/or extraesophageal manifestations of GERD. In addition, a substantial proportion of pulmonary patients with reflux may not report any typical esophageal symptoms. NERD may still play an important role in the underlying pulmonary disorders, and a normal upper endoscopy alone would not be adequate in ruling out the potential effect of reflux in these patients.

Esophageal function testing

EFT is comprised of manometric assessment of esophageal peristaltic and contractile function, as well as objective reflux monitoring to quantify reflux burden and identify associations between reported symptoms and reflux. Numerous studies have investigated the associations between findings on EFT and the severity and clinical course of various pulmonary disorders. Nevertheless, the roles of EFT in the diagnosis and management of extraesophageal reflux are less established. Moreover, the optimal approach to objective testing, including the modality, testing protocol, and equipment, remains without a clear consensus. Specifically, the use of traditional ambulatory pH monitoring alone versus in combination with multichannel intraluminal impedance (MII) technology remains debated. Traditional pH monitoring identifies acid reflux events when the measured esophageal pH drops less than 4. However, this pH-based definition of acid reflux was established based on esophageal symptoms and complications of GERD. Refluxate with pH>4 (weakly acidic or nonacidic) may also play a role in airway complications if they reach more than the UES. Therefore, more recent studies have evaluated the value of combined MII and pH monitoring (MII–pH) in the evaluation of pulmonary manifestations of GERD.

Among patients with asthma, studies have demonstrated that increased acid reflux on ambulatory pH monitoring was associated with concomitant reflux symptoms, although 29% to 62% of those without reflux symptoms were also found to have abnormal acid reflux.[55,56] In a study of 257 patients with extraesophageal symptoms of reflux undergoing Bravo pH monitoring, asthma was an independent predictor for abnormal reflux, in addition to heartburn, increased body mass index, and hiatal hernia.[57] Increased acid reflux ambulatory pH monitoring has also been shown to correlate with more severe asthma disease activities. In a study of patients with asthma undergoing 24-h pH monitoring and PFTs, abnormal acid exposure was associated with worse asthma quality of life and more corticosteroid use.[58] MII–pH has also been evaluated in the asthma population. In a study of patients with chronic cough or asthma who completed both MII–pH and bronchoscopy, the number of nonacid reflux events on MII, but not any pH-based metrics, was the only parameter predictive of the presence of pepsin on BALF.[59] In another study of 31 patients with adult-onset asthma, abnormal proximal reflux exposure was found in 70% of the patients despite normal distal reflux parameters in most, suggesting a potentially increased sensitivity in identifying abnormal reflux using the MII–pH technology.[60] Despite these promising results, given the limited data with regards to treatment outcomes, the role of MII in the management of asthma requires further investigation.

Pulmonary fibrosis represents another condition for which the role of EFT has been evaluated. Given the high prevalence of GERD among patients with IPF despite only a minority reporting typical esophageal symptoms, a standardized approach using objective reflux monitoring may be of particular importance in the management of this population.[6,61] Moreover, both acid reflux and weakly acidic or nonacid reflux are common in this population, as demonstrated in prior studies using MII–pH and BALF. Specifically, total reflux on MII, but not acid reflux parameters on pH-only monitoring, correlated with the concentration of bile acids on BALF, degree of fibrosis on computer tomography (CT), and severity of decline on PFTs.[62,63] In addition to the cross-sectional associations, abnormal bolus reflux on MII also independently predicted worse pulmonary outcomes, defined by hospitalizations or death, over 1-year follow-up.[64] Again, pH-based metrics for acid reflux did not significantly correlate with IPF outcomes. These studies suggest that findings on reflux monitoring provide relevant information in the evaluation, prognostication, and management of IPF and that MII–pH may allow a more comprehensive evaluation than pH monitoring alone.

The role of EFT has been studied in the lung transplant population, given the association between GERD, potential microaspiration, and worse allograft outcomes. Among these patients, aspirated refluxate may cause direct chemical injury of the lung allograft, impairment of innate immunity, and release of proinflammatory cytokines, leading to rejection and allograft dysfunction.[65] Similar to the IPF population, many lung transplant patients with GERD, as identified on objective testing, do not report typical esophageal symptoms of reflux.[66] Therefore, a systemic approach to objective testing is needed to identify those with GERD and at increased risk for reflux-related allograft injury. However, a clear consensus algorithm for reflux evaluation in lung transplant patients has not been established, especially with regards to the optimal timing and modality of testing. Evidence of increased reflux on pretransplant reflux testing has been associated with worse posttransplant outcomes, including decreased allograft function on PFT, increased allograft injury, early rehospitalization, rejection, BOS, and shorter survival.[40,41,67,68] On the other hand, prior studies have also shown that increased reflux on posttransplant testing correlated with earlier acute rejection and BOS.[69,70] With regard to the modality of testing, impedance-based parameters for total reflux seemed to provide better sensitivity and stronger correlation with various transplant outcomes including early allograft injury, rejection, and BOS than pH-based metrics for acid reflux alone.[70,71] Therefore, routine objective testing for GERD may help identify lung transplant patients at a higher risk for reflux-related allograft injury and poorer transplant outcomes, and testing modalities that incorporate MII may provide additional diagnostic benefits over pH monitoring alone in this population.

The role of primary esophageal dysmotility in pulmonary disorders remains incompletely defined. Hypomotility, particularly ineffective esophageal motility, generally represents the most common manometric patterns observed among patients with chronic pulmonary disorders, including some with aperistalsis. The impact of impairment in esophageal peristaltic contractile function on airway diseases likely results from worsening of underlying reflux, increasing proximal reflux events, and reducing refluxate clearance.[72] Prior studies using esophageal manometry also found changes in the thoracoabdominal pressure gradient in patients with advanced lung disease, particularly those with restrictive physiology, thereby increasing the risk for reflux and reduced esophageal clearance.[73] The esophageal dysmotility observed may be secondary to the underlying cause of the lung disease, such as connective tissue disorders or scleroderma, or result from the altered pulmonary physiology. In studies of patients who underwent pre and postlung transplantation, esophageal manometry found general increases in esophageal contractile vigor after transplantation, suggesting a role of altered pulmonary and intrathoracic physiology in esophageal function.[74–76]

Biochemical testing

Assessing for the markers of aspiration in the airway has been studied as another modality to diagnose esophageal-related pulmonary diseases. Phagocytosis by alveolar macrophages leads to intracellular lipid accumulation and may serve as a marker for aspiration. Ozdemir and colleagues measured the amount of lipid-laden macrophages (LLMs) in the alveoli of 34 patients with a history of chronic cough and found that patients with increased reflux on MII–pH had higher levels of LLM in their BALF samples than those without reflux.[77] Other studies have established the LLM index (LLMI) to quantify the degree of alveolar intracellular lipid accumulation, which has been shown to differentiate patients with aspiration from normal controls with high sensitivity (100%) but only moderate specificity (57%).[22,23] Given the suboptimal specificity of LLM, as there are other non–aspiration-related causes of increased intracellular lipids, its role in the clinical evaluation of aspiration or reflux-related lung injury needs further assessment.

Direct detection of gastroduodenal contents in the airway serves as another modality of biochemical testing. The presence of pepsin and bile acids in BALF samples has been associated with pulmonary disease. Both pepsin, a proteolytic enzyme secreted in the stomach, and bile acids, released in the duodenum, are highly specific gastroduodenal contents whose presence in the airway serves as evidence for aspiration. In a study of children with chronic cough and asthma who underwent bronchoscopy and MII–pH, pepsin positivity on BALF positively correlated with the number of nonacid reflux events on MII–pH and the mean LLMI.[59] Among patients with IPF, increased levels of pepsin and bile acids were found in the BALF compared with patients with non-IPF lung disease and healthy controls. Both levels were also higher among those who tested positive for GERD on MII–pH and positively correlated with the severity of lung fibrosis on CT.[62] In another study, pepsin levels on BALF analysis were higher among patients with IPF during acute exacerbations than among those with stable disease.[78] In the lung transplant population, pepsin and bile acids identified on BALF have been associated with increased acute rejection and BOS.[12,38,39] The data for biochemical testing in other pulmonary conditions are more limited. In a study of 52 patients with COPD, no statistical difference in BALF bile acids or pepsin levels was noted between those with acute exacerbations and those without.[79]

Expectorated saliva pepsin testing has also been proposed as a cheaper and less invasive alternative to BALF analysis. A study showed increased levels of pepsin detection and concentration in the expectorated saliva samples of 93 patients with chronic cough compared with healthy, asymptomatic controls.[80] In another study of 25 patients with asthma, salivary pepsin was detected in 56% with good agreement between multiple samples collected. However, no significant associations were found between salivary pepsin and severity of asthma in this cohort.[81]

Although biochemical testing potentially represents a less invasive (samples obtained during routine bronchoscopy), cheaper, and less labor-intensive alternative for identifying reflux-related aspiration, there are currently several limitations associated with this technology. Chiefly, there have been questions regarding the specificity of these assays. Subtype C of pepsinogen is normally produced in alveolar cells, and there are concerns regarding potential cross-reactivity between pepsin subtypes C and A, which is the subtype currently measured as the marker for extraesophageal reflux.[82] In a recent study, pepsinogen/pepsin A genes and proteins have also been identified at multiple human tissue samples at different levels, including the lungs.[83] Therefore, biochemical testing of BALF and saliva for pepsin and bile acids in the assessment of pulmonary disorders related to gastroesophageal disorders requires further assessment and development. Nevertheless, they may represent a potentially promising adjustive diagnostic modality in the evaluation of this challenging patient population.

TREATMENT/CLINICAL MANAGEMENT

The treatment modalities for pulmonary manifestations of GERD are similar to those for typical esophageal symptoms of reflux. There are, however, several considerations specific to this population. Most importantly, properly identifying patients in whom GERD plays a role in their pulmonary conditions represents the crucial, yet often most challenging, step in the management. The aforementioned diagnostic modalities may help select those that are most likely to respond to antireflux therapy. Treatment options can be divided into 2 main categories: medical therapy, which chiefly consists of acid suppression, and surgical therapies, which may include various forms of fundoplications, magnetic sphincter augmentation, and bariatric surgery, if indicated. Given the high prevalence of weakly acidic or nonacidic reflux demonstrated in prior studies using MII–pH in this patient population, antireflux barrier therapies may be more effective than antisecretory therapy alone in improving pulmonary outcomes, particularly in those with poorly controlled diseases or postlung transplantation.

As the current evidence regarding acid suppression therapy has been discussed in the previous section on the diagnostic approach, this section will focus on reviewing antireflux therapy for managing pulmonary conditions related to GERD. Most evidence to date comes from the lung transplant population. Studies from early surgical literature showed that antireflux surgery may be associated with reduced or slowed progression to BOS, improved PFT findings, and better survival among lung transplant recipients with GERD.[84–86] In particular, antireflux surgery performed early (<6 months) after transplant has been shown to be significantly more protective against allograft injury than late antireflux surgery. Importantly, no significant difference in the transplant outcome was found between early posttransplant and pretransplant antireflux surgery.[87] Given the higher operative risk in patients with end-stage lung disease, the early (<6 months) posttransplant period may represent the optimal time for antireflux surgery to be performed among transplant recipients with GERD to help improve their allograft outcomes.

Evidence for antireflux surgery for the management of other chronic pulmonary disorders is more limited. In the asthma population, most published reports remain case series without control arms. Reductions in asthma symptoms and medication requirements have generally been noted in these reports, usually with limited improvement in PFT findings.[88] In the only randomized, controlled study to date, asthmatics with GERD on pH monitoring who underwent antireflux surgery had significantly more improvement in overall asthma status and symptom scores than those who received medical therapy alone.[89] However, no significant difference among the treatment arms was noted with regards to pulmonary function, medication needs, and survival on 2-year follow-up.[89] The current evidence for antireflux surgery in the IPF population is similarly limited. Results from the early case series were mixed with regards to the stabilization of pulmonary function and oxygen requirement. In the only randomized, controlled trial published to date of 58 patients with IPF, no significant differences were noted in PFT change or other secondary outcomes including hospitalization or death between the antireflux surgery and no surgery arms at the end of 48-week follow-up.[90] However, the power of the study to detect significant differences may have been limited by its study size, duration of follow-up, outcome chosen, and the mild to moderate severity population enrolled. Overall, antireflux surgery may provide clinical benefits in a carefully selected subset of patients in whom GERD plays a significant role in their pulmonary disorders. Identifying this subset of patients continues to pose the main clinical challenge. Further studies will be needed to provide guidance in selecting the optimal candidates that would benefit from surgical intervention for GERD.

Given the bidirectional relationship between esophageal disease and pulmonary disease, improvement in pulmonary status may also result in a reduction in reflux and improvement in esophageal motility. In a study of patients with advanced restrictive lung disease, improvement in reflux burden and measured thoracoabdominal pressure gradient were noted after undergoing lung transplantation.[76] Moreover, an increase in esophageal body peristaltic vigor after lung transplant has been reported in multiple studies.[74–76] Therefore, restoration of normal pulmonary physiology may also improve the underlying esophageal motility and reflux.

SUMMARY

- Evidence suggests a clear relationship between esophageal dysfunction and pulmonary disorders. Clinicians should, therefore, have a low threshold for suspecting and evaluating for esophageal disease in patients with chronic pulmonary disease or airway symptoms that do not respond to standard therapy, even in the absence of typical esophageal disease symptoms.
- A standardized approach to the evaluation and management of esophageal disorders among patients with chronic pulmonary diseases should be adopted, given the often lack of esophageal symptoms. For some conditions such as

asthma, an empirical trial of acid suppression medications may be reasonable as the initial step. For other conditions such as IPF and lung transplant recipients, a standardized protocol involving objective EFT should be undertaken.
- Given the prevalence of weakly acidic or nonacidic reflux and the potentially deleterious effects of nonacidic gastroduodenal contents on the airway or lungs, evaluation with MII–pH to include the assessment of all reflux events may be preferred over pH monitoring of acid reflux alone for the investigation of extrae-sophageal reflux.
- The relationship between pulmonary and esophageal disease is bidirectional. This means that while esophageal disorders such as GERD may contribute to the airway or pulmonary disorders, changes in pulmonary and intrathoracic phys-iology may also worsen esophageal function and reflux.
- Biochemical testing such as the detection of pepsin or bile acids in BALF or saliva has shown promise as a diagnostic tool for airway reflux and aspiration. Further studies are needed to address some limitations such as specificity and to better define the role of these tests in clinical management.
- Early detection of esophageal dysfunction and reflux in patients with pulmonary disease may allow early intervention, including surgery that may lead to improved disease outcomes.

CLINICS CARE POINTS

- Evaluation for esophageal disease should be considered in patients with chronic lung disease with either sub-optimal or no response to standard-of-care therapy, even in the absence of typical esophageal disease symptoms.

- Assessment for total reflux using multichannel intraluminal impedance technology may be preferred over pH-only monitor for acid reflux alone, as weakly or non-acidic reflux may also play a role in airway complications of gastroesophageal reflux disease.

- Newer adjunctive diagnostic tools may provide additional supportive evidence for airway reflux, including biochemical testing for pepsin or bile acid in saliva or bronchioalveolar fluid, and advanced metrics on impedance studies.

- In patients undergoing lung transplantation, evaluation and management for esophageal disease should be incorporated in the standard care algorithm. Early identification and treatment of esophageal disorders, particularly gastroesophageal reflux disease, may reduce the risk of allograft rejection.

DISCLOSURE

Noreen C. Okwara has nothing to disclose. Walter W. Chan served on the scientific advisory boards for Ironwood Pharmaceuticals and Takeda Pharmaceuticals.

REFERENCES

1. el-Serag HB, Sonnenberg A. Comorbid occurrence of laryngeal or pulmonary disease with esophagitis in United States military veterans. Gastroenterology 1997;113(3):755–60.
2. Field SK, Underwood M, Brant R, et al. Prevalence of gastroesophageal reflux symptoms in asthma. Chest 1996;109(2):316–22.

3. Broers C, Tack J, Pauwels A. Review article: gastro-oesophageal reflux disease in asthma and chronic obstructive pulmonary disease. Aliment Pharmacol Ther 2018;47(2):176–91.

4. Allaix ME, Fisichella PM, Noth I, et al. The pulmonary side of reflux disease: from heartburn to lung fibrosis. J Gastrointest Surg 2013;17(8):1526–35.

5. Hershcovici T, Jha LK, Johnson T, et al. Systematic review: the relationship between interstitial lung diseases and gastro-oesophageal reflux disease. Aliment Pharmacol Ther 2011;34(11–12):1295–305.

6. Tobin RW, Pope CE 2nd, Pellegrini CA, et al. Increased prevalence of gastro-esophageal reflux in patients with idiopathic pulmonary fibrosis. Am J Respir Crit Care Med 1998;158(6):1804–8.

7. Gavini S, Finn RT, Lo WK, et al. Idiopathic pulmonary fibrosis is associated with increased impedance measures of reflux compared to non-fibrotic disease among pre-lung transplant patients. Neurogastroenterol Motil 2015;27(9):1326–32.

8. Hu ZW, Wang ZG, Zhang Y, et al. Gastroesophageal reflux in bronchiectasis and the effect of anti-reflux treatment. BMC Pulm Med 2013;13:34.

9. Button BM, Roberts S, Kotsimbos TC, et al. Gastroesophageal reflux (symptomatic and silent): a potentially significant problem in patients with cystic fibrosis before and after lung transplantation. J Heart Lung Transpl 2005;24(10):1522–9.

10. Ledson MJ, Tran J, Walshaw MJ. Prevalence and mechanisms of gastro-oesophageal reflux in adult cystic fibrosis patients. J R Soc Med 1998;91(1):7–9.

11. Hsu WT, Lai CC, Wang YH, et al. Risk of pneumonia in patients with gastroesophageal reflux disease: a population-based cohort study. PLoS One 2017;12(8):e0183808.

12. Blondeau K, Mertens V, Vanaudenaerde BA, et al. Gastro-oesophageal reflux and gastric aspiration in lung transplant patients with or without chronic rejection. Eur Respir J 2008;31(4):707–13.

13. Lee AS, Lee JS, He Z, et al. Reflux-aspiration in chronic lung disease. Ann Am Thorac Soc 2020;17(2):155–64.

14. Morrisey EE, Rustgi AK. The lung and esophagus: developmental and regenerative overlap. Trends Cell Biol 2018;28(9):738–48.

15. Badellino MM, Buckman RF Jr, Malaspina PJ, et al. Detection of pulmonary aspiration of gastric contents in an animal model by assay of peptic activity in bronchoalveolar fluid. Crit Care Med 1996;24(11):1881–5.

16. Farrell S, McMaster C, Gibson D, et al. Pepsin in bronchoalveolar lavage fluid: a specific and sensitive method of diagnosing gastro-oesophageal reflux-related pulmonary aspiration. J Pediatr Surg 2006;41(2):289–93.

17. Ravelli AM, Panarotto MB, Verdoni L, et al. Pulmonary aspiration shown by scintigraphy in gastroesophageal reflux-related respiratory disease. Chest 2006;130(5):1520–6.

18. Lee JS. The role of gastroesophageal reflux and microaspiration in idiopathic pulmonary fibrosis. Clin Pulm Med 2014;21(2):81–5.

19. Harding SM, Allen JE, Blumin JH, et al. Respiratory manifestations of gastroesophageal reflux disease. Ann N Y Acad Sci 2013;1300:43–52.

20. Hathorn KE, Chan WW, Lo WK. Role of gastroesophageal reflux disease in lung transplantation. World J Transpl 2017;7(2):103–16.

21. Perng DW, Chang KT, Su KC, et al. Exposure of airway epithelium to bile acids associated with gastroesophageal reflux symptoms: a relation to transforming growth factor-beta1 production and fibroblast proliferation. Chest 2007;132(5):1548–56.

22. Knauer-Fischer S, Ratjen F. Lipid-laden macrophages in bronchoalveolar lavage fluid as a marker for pulmonary aspiration. Pediatr Pulmonol 1999;27(6):419–22.
23. Kazachkov MY, Muhlebach MS, Livasy CA, et al. Lipid-laden macrophage index and inflammation in bronchoalveolar lavage fluids in children. Eur Respir J 2001; 18(5):790–5.
24. Cardasis JJ, MacMahon H, Husain AN. The spectrum of lung disease due to chronic occult aspiration. Ann Am Thorac Soc 2014;11(6):865–73.
25. Mansfield LE. Embryonic origins of the relation of gastroesophageal reflux disease and airway disease. Am J Med 2001;111(Suppl):3S–7S.
26. Mansfield LE, Hameister HH, Spaulding HS, et al. The role of the vague nerve in airway narrowing caused by intraesophageal hydrochloric acid provocation and esophageal distention. Ann Allergy 1981;47(6):431–4.
27. Mansfield LE, Stein MR. Gastroesophageal reflux and asthma: a possible reflex mechanism. Ann Allergy 1978;41(4):224–6.
28. Schan CA, Harding SM, Haile JM, et al. Gastroesophageal reflux-induced bronchoconstriction. An intraesophageal acid infusion study using state-of-the-art technology. Chest 1994;106(3):731–7.
29. Tuchman DN, Boyle JT, Pack AI, et al. Comparison of airway responses following tracheal or esophageal acidification in the cat. Gastroenterology 1984;87(4): 872–81.
30. Gadel AA, Mostafa M, Younis A, et al. Esophageal motility pattern and gastroesophageal reflux in chronic obstructive pulmonary disease. Hepatogastroenterology 2012;59(120):2498–502.
31. Pauwels A, Blondeau K, Dupont LJ, et al. Mechanisms of increased gastroesophageal reflux in patients with cystic fibrosis. Am J Gastroenterol 2012;107(9): 1346–53.
32. Turbyville JC. Applying principles of physics to the airway to help explain the relationship between asthma and gastroesophageal reflux. Med Hypotheses 2010; 74(6):1075–80.
33. Holmes PW, Campbell AH, Barter CE. Acute changes of lung volumes and lung mechanics in asthma and in normal subjects. Thorax 1978;33(3):394–400.
34. Basseri B, Conklin JL, Pimentel M, et al. Esophageal motor dysfunction and gastroesophageal reflux are prevalent in lung transplant candidates. Ann Thorac Surg 2010;90(5):1630–6.
35. Lazenby JP, Guzzo MR, Harding SM, et al. Oral corticosteroids increase esophageal acid contact times in patients with stable asthma. Chest 2002;121(2): 625–34.
36. Crowell MD, Zayat EN, Lacy BE, et al. The effects of an inhaled beta(2)-adrenergic agonist on lower esophageal function: a dose-response study. Chest 2001;120(4):1184–9.
37. Richter JE, Rubenstein JH. Presentation and epidemiology of gastroesophageal reflux disease. Gastroenterology 2018;154(2):267–76.
38. Stovold R, Forrest IA, Corris PA, et al. Pepsin, a biomarker of gastric aspiration in lung allografts: a putative association with rejection. Am J Respir Crit Care Med 2007;175(12):1298–303.
39. D'Ovidio F, Mura M, Tsang M, et al. Bile acid aspiration and the development of bronchiolitis obliterans after lung transplantation. J Thorac Cardiovasc Surg 2005;129(5):1144–52.
40. Lo WK, Moniodis A, Goldberg HJ, et al. Increased acid exposure on pretransplant impedance-pH testing is associated with chronic rejection after lung

transplantation. J Clin Gastroenterol 2020. https://doi.org/10.1097/MCG. 0000000000001331.

41. Lo WK, Burakoff R, Goldberg HJ, et al. Pre-transplant impedance measures of reflux are associated with early allograft injury after lung transplantation. J Heart Lung Transpl 2015;34(1):26–35.

42. Posner S, Zheng J, Wood RK, et al. Gastroesophageal reflux symptoms are not sufficient to guide esophageal function testing in lung transplant candidates. Dis Esophagus 2018;31(5). https://doi.org/10.1093/dote/dox157.

43. American Lung Association Asthma Clinical Research C, Mastronarde JG, Anthonisen NR, Castro M, et al. Efficacy of esomeprazole for treatment of poorly controlled asthma. N Engl J Med 2009;360(15):1487–99.

44. Kiljander TO, Junghard O, Beckman O, et al. Effect of esomeprazole 40 mg once or twice daily on asthma: a randomized, placebo-controlled study. Am J Respir Crit Care Med 2010;181(10):1042–8.

45. Littner MR, Leung FW, Ballard ED 2nd, et al. Effects of 24 weeks of lansoprazole therapy on asthma symptoms, exacerbations, quality of life, and pulmonary function in adult asthmatic patients with acid reflux symptoms. Chest 2005;128(3): 1128–35.

46. Chan WW, Chiou E, Obstein KL, et al. The efficacy of proton pump inhibitors for the treatment of asthma in adults: a meta-analysis. Arch Intern Med 2011;171(7): 620–9.

47. Kikuchi S, Imai H, Tani Y, et al. Proton pump inhibitors for chronic obstructive pulmonary disease. Cochrane Database Syst Rev 2020;8:CD013113.

48. Sasaki T, Nakayama K, Yasuda H, et al. A randomized, single-blind study of lansoprazole for the prevention of exacerbations of chronic obstructive pulmonary disease in older patients. J Am Geriatr Soc 2009;57(8):1453–7.

49. Lee JS, Collard HR, Anstrom KJ, et al. Anti-acid treatment and disease progression in idiopathic pulmonary fibrosis: an analysis of data from three randomised controlled trials. Lancet Respir Med 2013;1(5):369–76.

50. Fidler L, Sitzer N, Shapera S, et al. Treatment of gastroesophageal reflux in patients with idiopathic pulmonary fibrosis: a systematic review and meta-analysis. Chest 2018;153(6):1405–15.

51. Raghu G, Collard HR, Egan JJ, et al. An official ATS/ERS/JRS/ALAT statement: idiopathic pulmonary fibrosis: evidence-based guidelines for diagnosis and management. Am J Respir Crit Care Med 2011;183(6):788–824.

52. Lo WK, Goldberg HJ, Boukedes S, et al. Proton pump inhibitors independently protect against early allograft injury or chronic rejection after lung transplantation. Dig Dis Sci 2018;63(2):403–10.

53. Ghebremariam YT, Cooke JP, Gerhart W, et al. Pleiotropic effect of the proton pump inhibitor esomeprazole leading to suppression of lung inflammation and fibrosis. J Transl Med 2015;13:249.

54. Ghebre YT, Raghu G. Idiopathic pulmonary fibrosis: novel concepts of proton pump inhibitors as antifibrotic drugs. Am J Respir Crit Care Med 2016;193(12): 1345–52.

55. Harding SM, Guzzo MR, Richter JE. The prevalence of gastroesophageal reflux in asthma patients without reflux symptoms. Am J Respir Crit Care Med 2000; 162(1):34–9.

56. Harding SM, Guzzo MR, Richter JE. 24-h esophageal pH testing in asthmatics: respiratory symptom correlation with esophageal acid events. Chest 1999; 115(3):654–9.

57. Patel DA, Sharda R, Choksi YA, et al. Model to select on-therapy vs off-therapy tests for patients with refractory esophageal or extraesophageal symptoms. Gastroenterology 2018;155(6):1729–1740 e1.

58. DiMango E, Holbrook JT, Simpson E, et al. Effects of asymptomatic proximal and distal gastroesophageal reflux on asthma severity. Am J Respir Crit Care Med 2009;180(9):809–16.

59. Rosen R, Johnston N, Hart K, et al. The presence of pepsin in the lung and its relationship to pathologic gastro-esophageal reflux. Neurogastroenterol Motil 2012;24(2):129–33, e84–5.

60. Komatsu Y, Hoppo T, Jobe BA. Proximal reflux as a cause of adult-onset asthma: the case for hypopharyngeal impedance testing to improve the sensitivity of diagnosis. JAMA Surg 2013;148(1):50–8.

61. Raghu G, Freudenberger TD, Yang S, et al. High prevalence of abnormal acid gastro-oesophageal reflux in idiopathic pulmonary fibrosis. Eur Respir J 2006; 27(1):136–42.

62. Savarino E, Carbone R, Marabotto E, et al. Gastro-oesophageal reflux and gastric aspiration in idiopathic pulmonary fibrosis patients. Eur Respir J 2013;42(5): 1322–31.

63. Gavini S, Borges LF, Finn RT, et al. Lung disease severity in idiopathic pulmonary fibrosis is more strongly associated with impedance measures of bolus reflux than pH parameters of acid reflux alone. Neurogastroenterol Motil 2017;29(5). https://doi.org/10.1111/nmo.13001.

64. Borges LF, Jagadeesan V, Goldberg H, et al. Abnormal bolus reflux is associated with poor pulmonary outcome in patients with idiopathic pulmonary fibrosis. J Neurogastroenterol Motil 2018;24(3):395–402.

65. Gulack BC, Meza JM, Lin SS, et al. Reflux and allograft dysfunction: is there a connection? Thorac Surg Clin 2015;25(1):97–105.

66. Sweet MP, Herbella FA, Leard L, et al. The prevalence of distal and proximal gastroesophageal reflux in patients awaiting lung transplantation. Ann Surg 2006;244(4):491–7.

67. Murthy SC, Nowicki ER, Mason DP, et al. Pretransplant gastroesophageal reflux compromises early outcomes after lung transplantation. J Thorac Cardiovasc Surg 2011;142(1):47–52.e3.

68. Lo WK, Goldberg HJ, Burakoff R, et al. Increased proximal acid reflux is associated with early readmission following lung transplantation. Neurogastroenterol Motil 2016;28(2):251–9.

69. Shah N, Force SD, Mitchell PO, et al. Gastroesophageal reflux disease is associated with an increased rate of acute rejection in lung transplant allografts. Transpl Proc 2010;42(7):2702–6.

70. King BJ, Iyer H, Leidi AA, et al. Gastroesophageal reflux in bronchiolitis obliterans syndrome: a new perspective. J Heart Lung Transpl 2009;28(9):870–5.

71. Lo WK, Burakoff R, Goldberg HJ, et al. Pre-lung transplant measures of reflux on impedance are superior to pH testing alone in predicting early allograft injury. World J Gastroenterol 2015;21(30):9111–7.

72. Cheah R, Chirnaksorn S, Abdelrahim AH, et al. The perils and pitfalls of esophageal dysmotility in idiopathic pulmonary fibrosis. Am J Gastroenterol 2021;116(6): 1189–200.

73. Masuda T, Mittal SK, Kovacs B, et al. Thoracoabdominal pressure gradient and gastroesophageal reflux: insights from lung transplant candidates. Dis Esophagus 2018;31(10). https://doi.org/10.1093/dote/doy025.

74. Posner S, Finn RT, Shimpi RA, et al. Esophageal contractility increases and gastroesophageal reflux does not worsen after lung transplantation. Dis Esophagus 2019;32(10):1–8.
75. Cangemi DJ, Flanagan R, Bailey A, et al. Jackhammer esophagus after lung transplantation: results of a retrospective multicenter study. J Clin Gastroenterol 2020;54(4):322–6.
76. Masuda T, Mittal SK, Kovacs B, et al. Foregut function before and after lung transplant. J Thorac Cardiovasc Surg 2019;158(2):619–29.
77. Ozdemir P, Erdinc M, Vardar R, et al. The role of microaspiration in the pathogenesis of gastroesophageal reflux-related chronic cough. J Neurogastroenterol Motil 2017;23(1):41–8.
78. Lee JS, Song JW, Wolters PJ, et al. Bronchoalveolar lavage pepsin in acute exacerbation of idiopathic pulmonary fibrosis. Eur Respir J 2012;39(2):352–8.
79. Hashemi-Bajgani SM, Abbasi F, Shafahi A, et al. Association of bile acid and pepsin micro-aspiration with chronic obstructive pulmonary disease exacerbation. Tanaffos 2019;18(1):52–7.
80. Strugala V, Woodcock AD, Dettmar PW, et al. Detection of pepsin in sputum: a rapid and objective measure of airways reflux. Eur Respir J 2016;47(1):339–41.
81. Marshall S, McCann AJ, Samuels TL, et al. Detection of pepsin and IL-8 in saliva of adult asthmatic patients. J Asthma Allergy 2019;12:155–61.
82. Bohman JK, Kor DJ, Kashyap R, et al. Airway pepsin levels in otherwise healthy surgical patients receiving general anesthesia with endotracheal intubation. Chest 2013;143(5):1407–13.
83. Rao YF, Wang J, Cheng DN, et al. The controversy of pepsinogen a/pepsin a in detecting extra-gastroesophageal reflux. J Voice 2021. https://doi.org/10.1016/j.jvoice.2021.04.009.
84. Cantu E 3rd, Appel JZ 3rd, Hartwig MG, et al. J. Maxwell Chamberlain Memorial Paper. Early fundoplication prevents chronic allograft dysfunction in patients with gastroesophageal reflux disease. Ann Thorac Surg 2004;78(4):1142–51 [discussion 1142–51].
85. Hartwig MG, Anderson DJ, Onaitis MW, et al. Fundoplication after lung transplantation prevents the allograft dysfunction associated with reflux. Ann Thorac Surg 2011;92(2):462–8 [discussion; 468–9].
86. Davis RD Jr, Lau CL, Eubanks S, et al. Improved lung allograft function after fundoplication in patients with gastroesophageal reflux disease undergoing lung transplantation. J Thorac Cardiovasc Surg 2003;125(3):533–42.
87. Lo WK, Goldberg HJ, Wee J, et al. Both pre-transplant and early post-transplant antireflux surgery prevent development of early allograft injury after lung transplantation. J Gastrointest Surg 2016;20(1):111–8 [discussion 118].
88. Field SK, Gelfand GA, McFadden SD. The effects of antireflux surgery on asthmatics with gastroesophageal reflux. Chest 1999;116(3):766–74.
89. Sontag SJ, O'Connell S, Khandelwal S, et al. Asthmatics with gastroesophageal reflux: long term results of a randomized trial of medical and surgical antireflux therapies. Am J Gastroenterol 2003;98(5):987–99.
90. Raghu G, Pellegrini CA, Yow E, et al. Laparoscopic anti-reflux surgery for the treatment of idiopathic pulmonary fibrosis (WRAP-IPF): a multicentre, randomised, controlled phase 2 trial. Lancet Respir Med 2018;6(9):707–14.

Therapeutic Endoscopy and the Esophagus
State of the Art and Future Directions

Linda Y. Zhang, MBBS[a], Anthony N. Kalloo, MD[b,c],
Saowanee Ngamruengphong, MD[d,*]

KEYWORDS

- Gastroesophageal reflux disease • Achalasia • Barrett's esophagus
- Peroral endoscopic myotomy • Transoral incisionless fundoplication
- Endoscopic submucosal dissection • Submucosal tunneling endoscopic resection
- Zenker diverticulum

KEY POINTS

- Peroral endoscopic myotomy (POEM) is an effective minimally invasive approach for treatment of achalasia with comparable efficacy to laparoscopic Heller myotomy, but the issue of post-POEM gastroesophageal reflux disease (GERD) still requires further evaluation
- Endoluminal therapies offer a minimally invasive option for treatment of early GERD with minimal crural defect
- The combination of ablative therapies (including radiofrequency ablation and cryotherapy) with endoscopic resection now allows treatment of the entire spectrum of Barrett's, related dysplasia, and early cancer
- Advancements in submucosal endoscopy have led to the conceptualization of techniques including submucosal tunneling endoscopic resection to expand the scope of therapeutic endoscopy

INTRODUCTION

Therapeutic gastrointestinal endoscopy is rapidly evolving, and this evolution is quite apparent for esophageal diseases. Minimally invasive endoluminal therapy can now be used to treat many esophageal diseases that have traditionally been managed surgically and are often performed in the outpatient setting. Peroral endoscopic myotomy (POEM) is now widely accepted for treatment of achalasia. The adaptation of POEM

[a] Division of Gastroenterology & Hepatology, Johns Hopkins Medicine, 1800 Orleans St, Sheikh Zayed Tower, Suite M2058, Baltimore, MD 21287, USA; [b] Department of Medicine, Maimonides Medical Center, 4802 Tenth Avenue, Brooklyn, NY 11219, USA; [c] Department of Medicine, Johns Hopkins Medicine, 1800 Orleans St, Sheikh Zayed Tower, Baltimore, MD 21287, USA; [d] Division of Gastroenterology & Hepatology, Johns Hopkins Medicine, 4940 Eastern Avenue, A Building, 5th Floor, A-501, Baltimore, MD 21224, USA
* Corresponding author.
E-mail address: sngamru1@jhmi.edu

Gastroenterol Clin N Am 50 (2021) 935–958
https://doi.org/10.1016/j.gtc.2021.08.007
0889-8553/21/© 2021 Elsevier Inc. All rights reserved.

for Zenker diverticulum (Z-POEM) has resulted in a resurgence in popularity of flexible endoscopic therapy, over open surgery or rigid endoscopic options. For gastroesophageal reflux disease (GERD), endoscopic fundoplication without the need for surgery is one of the novel technologies for effective treatment of selected patients with GERD. With regard to Barrett's esophagus, the combination of ablative therapies (including radiofrequency ablation and cryotherapy) with endoscopic mucosal resection or submucosal dissection now allows treatment of the entire spectrum of Barrett's, related dysplasia, and early cancer.

In this review article, we explore the previously mentioned conditions, discussing available literature, our personal takes, and future opportunities.

ACHALASIA

Achalasia is a primary esophageal motility disorder characterized by the absence of esophageal peristalsis and impaired relaxation of the lower esophageal sphincter (LES), resulting in esophageal dysphagia. The recent introduction of POEM has had significant impact on the management of this condition. The current state of achalasia evaluation and treatment is discussed, with a focus on recent changes.

Diagnosis

Achalasia should be considered in patients presenting with typical symptoms including dysphagia, regurgitation, heartburn, and chest pain. Esophagogastroduodenoscopy (EGD) is crucial to exclude alternate causes for mechanical obstruction and pseudo-achalasia secondary to malignancy. Typical findings include food or fluid retention, a "puckered" esophagogastric junction (EGJ) and a "popping" sensation when the endoscope is advanced past the EGJ. Barium esophagram may show a typical "bird beak" appearance at the EGJ with upstream esophageal dilation in later stages. Timed barium studies are helpful in documenting delayed rate of emptying and providing an objective measure to compare posttreatment outcomes. Finally, high-resolution manometry (HRM) is the gold standard for confirming a diagnosis and determining the subtype of achalasia. A disorder of EGJ outflow, including achalasia and esophagogastric junction outflow obstruction (EGJOO), is confirmed on HRM according to the recently updated Chicago Classification v4.0[1].

The novel endoluminal functional lumen imaging probe (FLIP) (EndoFLIP; Crospon, Galway, Ireland) has an evolving role in the assessment of achalasia and other motility disorders. Using impedance planimetry, FLIP simultaneously assesses cross-sectional area and pressure during volume-controlled distension. EGJ distensibility measured by FLIP is reduced in patients with achalasia (distensibility index <2.8 mm^2/mm Hg at 40 mL distension) compared with controls[2] (**Fig. 1**). FLIP may be a useful alternative in patients who cannot tolerate HRM, as FLIP is performed in sedated patients during endoscopy, to provide additional information in patients with equivocal HRM or confirmatory evidence in EGJOO. A further advantage is the ability to observe changes in real time with early data suggesting treatment can be tailored accordingly.[3]

Treatment

Patients should be managed with a tailored approach. All current therapies aim at weakening or disrupting the LES. Pharmacologic therapy is the least effective treatment option for achalasia and is limited by the short duration of action necessitating multiple dosages, which can result in adverse events (AEs). Botulinum toxin is a potent inhibitor of acetylcholine release from nerve endings. In achalasia treatment,

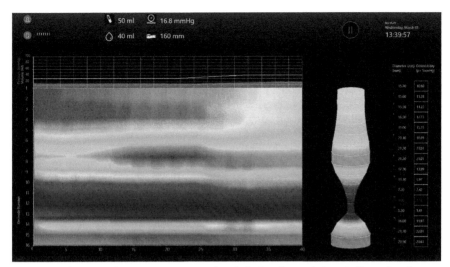

Fig. 1. Endoflip recording in a patient with achalasia. The real-time 3-dimensional recon-struction of the esophagus is seen on the right. In this image, the balloon is distended with 40 mL of ionic fluid. The hourglass shape with marked narrowing at the EGJ and reduced EGJ distensibility index of 1.12 mm²/mm Hg is highly suggestive of achalasia. The FLIP topography plot on the left shows a lack of contractile response, consistent with non-spastic achalasia.

botulinum toxin is delivered in a 4-quadrant injection above the squamocolumnar junction (SCJ). More widespread use is limited by durability, with 62.5% of patients re-lapsing within 12 months.[4] Further, repeated injections result in progressively weaker and briefer relief. Hence, it is usually reserved for patients with significant comorbid-ities or as a bridge to definitive therapy. There is a theoretic risk of scarring with repeated injections, although data on adverse effects on subsequent endoscopic or surgical therapy are conflicting.

Pneumatic dilation (PD) is based on the disruption of LES muscle fibers through distension of a rigid pressurized balloon (**Fig. 2**). The procedure is most commonly performed under fluoroscopic guidance with 3 available balloon sizes (30, 35, and 40 mm) often used sequentially in a graded fashion. The most serious complication

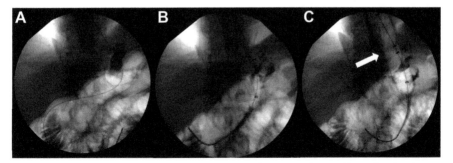

Fig. 2. Pneumatic balloon dilation. (*A*) A Savary guidewire is advanced into the duodenum. (*B*) The PD balloon is advanced over the guidewire until the midpoint (marked by the *dou-ble black lines*) is across the level of the gastroesophageal junction. (*C*) The balloon is dilated and a waist (*white arrow*) is seen at the level of the GEJ.

associated with PD is esophageal perforation, which can occur in up to 5%[5] of cases. Importantly, surgical repair may be needed, so patients must be warned and should be reasonably fit to proceed if needed. With graded dilation, short-term clinical success rates are high (up to 90% in the first year) but efficacy wanes over time.[5]

Surgical LES disruption, most commonly laparoscopic Heller myotomy (HM), causes disruption of the LES fibers through a surgical myotomy. HM is highly effective, with early clinical success rates of 91% in the first year.[6] Risk of postoperative GERD with HM alone is significant, and a concurrent partial fundoplication is now recommended and routinely performed.[7]

Peroral endoscopic myotomy (POEM) rapidly gained popularity by allowing a minimally invasive endoscopic approach to performing a controlled myotomy (**Fig. 3**). The creation of a submucosal tunnel maintains an intact mucosal layer while exposing the underlying muscle for myotomy. POEM is a highly effective option for all types of achalasia,[8] and has been shown to be noninferior to HM.[9] A systematic review showed a clinical success of 98% (95% confidence interval [CI] 97%–100%) with a preoperative Eckardt score of 6.9 $\pm$ 0.15 reducing to 0.77 $\pm$ 1.0 post-procedure.[10] Further, emerging long-term outcomes data support durability beyond at least 4 years.[11] Importantly, POEM remains effective in type III achalasia, a subtype in which prior treatments have traditionally been mediocre.[8] A major advantage of POEM is the ability to adjust myotomy length. Generally, a standard myotomy extends at least 5 cm into the esophageal body and 2 cm below the LES into the gastric cardia. In type III

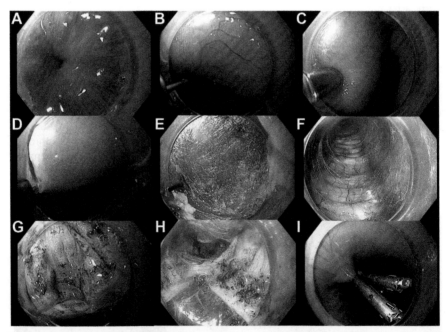

Fig. 3. Esophageal POEM. (A) A puckered GEJ is seen on entry. (B) A point 8 to 10 cm (depending on the planned myotomy length) proximal to the GEJ is selected for mucosal entry. (C) A submucosal injection is performed. (D) A mucosal incision is made, usually longitudinally oriented. (E) The submucosal space is entered. (F) The submucosal tunnel is completed. (G) A selective circular myotomy is performed in the esophagus. (H) A full-thickness myotomy is performed at the GEJ and extending into the gastric cardia. (I) Closure of the mucosal incision is performed with through-the-scope clips.

achalasia, where there is spastic contractility of the distal esophagus, myotomy can be extended proximally to include the obstructive contractile segment of the distal esophagus. POEM is safe, with rates of both esophageal perforation and significant bleeding requiring intervention at 0.2%.[10] Although post-POEM GERD is usually responsive to proton pump inhibitors (PPIs), up to 13% (95% CI 5%–25%) of patients have endoscopy-proven esophagitis and 47% (95% CI 21%–74%) have abnormal acid exposure.[10] Combined POEM with endoscopic fundoplication has been demonstrated in case series with excellent technical success and reduction in PPI use and symptoms,[12,13] but requires further evaluation. It is therefore prudent to screen appropriately for GERD preoperatively.

Although outcomes data are still limited by the lack of head-to-head comparison trials and long-term data, currently available data suggest that PD, HM, and POEM result in comparable symptom improvement in patients with type I and II achalasia; however, POEM may be more effective for type III disease. We therefore propose a treatment algorithm for achalasia in **Fig. 4**.

Management of Treatment Failures

Although early clinical success is high with available treatment modalities, up to a third of patients managed with HM or PD will require repeat treatment after 5 years.[14,15] These data are not yet available for POEM, but one recent study reported clinical success (Eckardt score <3 and freedom from additional interventions) in 79% at 5 years.[11] There are no consensus guidelines to guide management of treatment failures or recurrent achalasia. Notwithstanding the lack of comparative head-to-head trials, POEM is often preferred and has been safely used as rescue therapy in the setting of failed HM[16] or even POEM.[17]

Future Directions

Although POEM is arising as a first-line modality, widespread uptake will remain limited by availability of local expertise. POEM is now just reaching beyond a decade

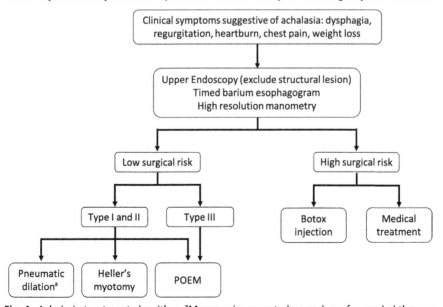

Fig. 4. Achalasia treatment algorithm. [a]May require repeated procedures for graded therapy.

since its introduction, and evidence to support its use is mounting. The excellent efficacy seen in studies to date, however, are somewhat clouded by significant rates of post-POEM GERD. Further research into the ability to combine POEM with an endoscopic antireflux treatment[18] will be of critical importance if POEM is to become the gold standard treatment for achalasia.

DISORDERS OF THE CRICOPHARYNGEUS

Disorders involving the upper esophageal sphincter (UES) can arise from either failure of UES relaxation or a structural disorder of the cricopharyngeal (CP) muscle. This review focuses on Zenker diverticulum (ZD) due to the significant advances in its management.

Zenker Diverticulum

ZD is a rare condition characterized by herniation through an area of relative muscular weakness (Killian dehiscence) just proximal to the upper margin of the CP muscle. It is believed that a poorly compliant but normally relaxing CP underlies ZD. Accordingly, the mainstay of treatment is disruption of the CP muscle. Traditional approaches included open surgery (transcervical diverticulectomy, diverticuloplexy, or diverticular inversion) and rigid endoscopic CP myotomy. However, the elderly and often comorbid population that makes up most patients with ZD requires a minimally invasive approach. Flexible endoscopic CP myotomy (FECM) quickly became widely accepted as a minimally invasive first-line therapy for most small to moderate-sized ZD. In this procedure, the septum (including the CP muscle) is commonly divided (**Fig. 5**). A major limitation to this procedure was difficulty ensuring a complete myotomy while avoiding perforation or leak. As a result, a small residual septum was often left, leading to variable recurrence rates of 0% to 32%.[18] A Zenker myectomy, consisting of double parallel incisions on the septum followed by wedge-shaped snare resection at the base (**Fig. 6**), was proposed to reduce recurrence rates,[19] but is limited to a few small-scale studies.[20,21]

Z-POEM has rapidly gained interest because of high rates of clinical success and low rates of AEs.[22] The initial technique started with a mucosal incision proximal to the diverticular septum, followed by submucosal tunneling to expose the septum before dividing it[23] (**Fig. 7**). Mucosal closure followed, most commonly with clips. More recently, an over-the-septum modification was introduced[24] (**Fig. 8**), reducing technical difficulty and procedural time due to improved working space and shorter tunnel, while still allowing direct access to the CP muscle. The advantage of mucosal

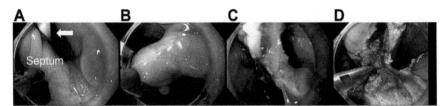

Fig. 5. Flexible endoscopic cricopharyngeal myotomy. (*A*) An orogastric tube (*white arrow*) is placed into the stomach to delineate the true esophageal lumen. The ZD is seen on the other side of the septum. (*B*) The SB knife is used to divide the septum, including the cricopharyngeal muscle. (*C*) Division is continued until the base of the diverticulum is reached and no further muscle fibers are seen. (*D*) Through-the-scope clips can be applied to the apex of the defect on completion.

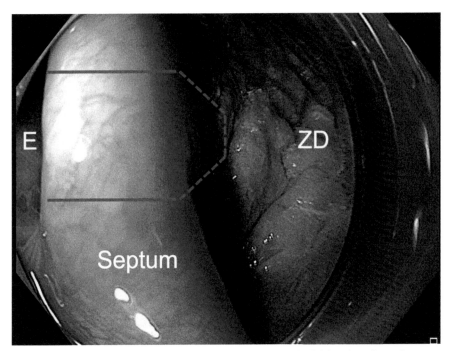

Fig. 6. Zenker myectomy. Two parallel incisions are made (*solid lines*) and a subsequent snare resection is performed to the incision base (*dashed lines*). E, esophagus.

preservation in Z-POEM allows complete CP myotomy and transection of the surrounding high-pressure zone under direct visualization, while protecting against leak.

Most published literature on endoscopic ZD management consists of retrospective observational studies with heterogeneity of procedural technique, instrumentation, and outcome measures. A review of FECM reported composite technical success,

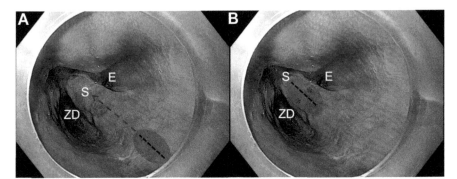

Fig. 7. Comparison between the original Z-POEM and over-the-septum Z-POEM. (*A*) Original Z-POEM in which submucosal injection (*blue oval*) and mucosal incision (*black dotted line*) is performed a few centimeters proximal to the Zenker septum. Tunneling is then performed until the septum is exposed (*blue dotted line*). (*B*) In the modified Z-POEM (over-the-septum Z-POEM), submucosal injection (*blue oval*) and mucosal incision (*black dotted line*) are performed directly over the septum. Tunneling is then performed to expose the septum on both sides (*blue asterisks*). E, esophagus; S, septum.

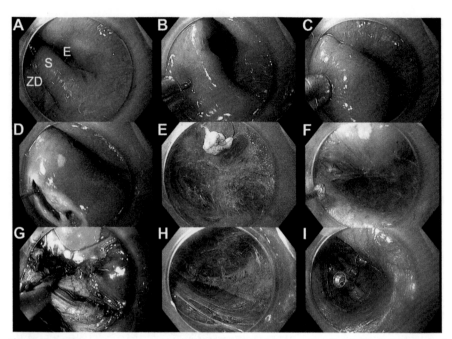

Fig. 8. Over-the-septum Z-POEM. (*A*) The ZD and septum are visualized. (*B, C*) Submucosal injection is performed at the level of the septum to create a mucosal bleb. (*D*) Mucosal incision is performed. (*E*) Submucosal tunnel is performed on both sides of the septum. (*F*) The septum is exposed. (*G*) Myotomy is performed to divide the septum (including the cricopharyngeal muscle). (*H*) The septum is divided and myotomy is continued into the esophageal muscle. (*I*) Mucosal closure with through-the-scope clips. E, esophagus; S, septum.

clinical success, and recurrence rate of 99.4%, 87.9%, and 13.6%, respectively.[24] Perforation occurred in 5.3%, although only 0.9% required invasive management. Bleeding occurred in 6.6%, and all were managed conservatively or endoscopically. Z-POEM theoretically lowers the rate of recurrence, although long-term data and head-to-head comparative trials are still awaited. Retrospective studies have reported clinical success rates in excess of 90%.[22,25,26] Further, Z-POEM remains effective in patients with prior endoscopic and/or surgical intervention for ZD, with technical success achieved in 93.8% in a cohort of 32 previously treated patients.[27] Clinical success was achieved in 96.7% with 12.5% AE rate (mucosotomies or leaks, all managed endoscopically). A recent retrospective analysis of FECM versus Z-POEM found no significant difference in technical or clinical success (97.1% vs 95.8%, $P = .56$ and 75.2% vs 90.9%, $P = .16$, respectively), although the Z-POEM cohort was much smaller (n = 137 vs n = 24).[28]

Cricopharyngeal Bar

A CP bar is a frequent incidentally noted anomaly, seen as a posterior indentation of the cervical esophageal lumen. Although often asymptomatic, a small proportion can cause dysphagia and recurrent aspiration. Similar to ZD, CP bar is thought to arise from reduced compliance due to fibrosis, and therefore CP disruption is also the mainstay of treatment. Although botulinum toxin A injection and cricopharyngeal dilation have both been used to treat CP bar, they are preferred for conditions with failed CP relaxation (rather than reduced compliance). Further, despite good short-term response, repeat procedures are often required to maintain relief.[29] During endoscopic myotomy, in contrast to a ZD in which the diverticulum and adjacent septum provide a visible target, the CP can be more difficult to delineate in the absence of a diverticulum. Studies addressing endoscopic CP myotomy for CP bar alone are significantly limited. Recently, cricopharyngeal POEM (C-POEM) was introduced,[30,31] which, by proximal submucosal tunneling, allows exposure, identification, and complete transection of the CP muscle while keeping the mucosal layer intact. Data regarding this are still limited to case reports.

Future Directions

It is clear that flexible endoscopic treatment of ZD and other esophageal diverticula is safe and highly effective. However, procedures are far from standardized and significant variation exists between institutions. Long-term outcomes following Z-POEM or C-POEM are eagerly awaited. In addition, robust prospective comparative trials with standardized outcome measures are needed.

GASTROESOPHAGEAL REFLUX DISEASE

GERD is one of the most common chronic conditions affecting adults in Western countries. Although PPIs can be highly effective, a significant number of patients continue to experience troublesome symptoms despite maximal medical therapy. Further, there has been increased recognition of the AEs of chronic PPI use. Laparoscopic antireflux surgery (LARS) remains the gold standard treatment for patients who have failed medical therapy or have complicated GERD. However, more widespread use is limited by the invasiveness of the procedure, postsurgical risks (albeit low), and AEs including de novo dysphagia and gas bloat. Endoscopic therapies have the potential to bridge the gap between medications and surgery, thus providing a minimally invasive option for patients unwilling or unable to continue indefinite medical therapy.

This review focuses on the most widely used devices and recent advances in endoscopic GERD treatment: radiofrequency treatment, transoral incisionless fundoplication (TIF), endoscopic suturing, and antireflux mucosectomy (ARM).

Pre-procedure Evaluation

Pre-procedure evaluation should include diagnostic EGD to evaluate for structural abnormalities, including hiatal hernia, Hill grade, and any GERD complications including esophagitis or Barrett's esophagus (BE). When assessing for suitability for endoscopic GERD treatment, accurate assessment of (1) the presence of a hiatal hernia, and (2) the crural opening, is of utmost importance. The Hill classification provides an endoscopic grading system for the EGJ, specifically assessing the gastroesophageal flap valve (**Fig. 9**). Grading from 1 to 4, the Hill classification shows a consistent association with symptomatic GERD and erosive esophagitis.[32] Unfortunately, it is often underestimated because of insufficient time and insufflation, or a fat pad filling the open hiatus, creating a "stuffing" effect. We recommend at least 45 seconds be spent in retroflexion with active insufflation before determining the Hill classification. A Hill grade of ≥3 contraindicates pure endoluminal therapy and an underestimated Hill grade is a common reason for failure of endoluminal therapy.

Transoral Incisionless Fundoplication

TIF is a minimally invasive antireflux procedure, most commonly performed using the EsophyX (EndoGastric Solutions, Inc, Redmond, WA) device. The all-inclusive system has evolved through several iterations to arrive at TIF2.0, which achieves outcomes

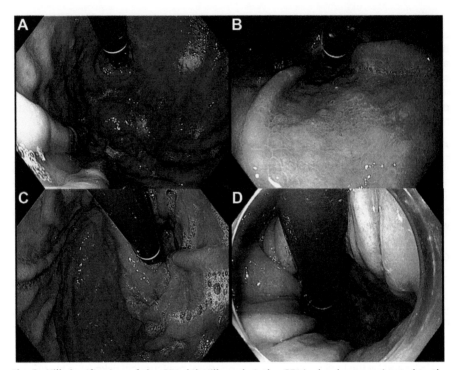

Fig. 9. Hill classification of the GEJ. (*A*) Hill grade I, the GEJ is closely approximated to the scope. (*B*) Hill grade II, the adherence of the GEJ to the scope is less well defined. (*C*) Hill grade III, there is incomplete closure of the GEJ around the scope. Esophageal mucosa is frequency visible. (*D*) Hill grade IV, the hiatus is wide open and displaced axially. A hiatal hernia is always present.

morphologically and physiologically comparable to the gold standard laparoscopic Nissen fundoplication (LNF). During the procedure, polypropylene fasteners are placed to create a 2-cm to 4-cm length valve and 270° partial fundoplication (**Fig. 10**). In doing so, this procedure accentuates the cardiac notch, steepens the angle of His, and reestablishes the flap valve mechanism.

The 3 major prospective trials evaluating TIF2.0[33–35] demonstrated improved esophageal pH, decreased PPI utilization, and improved quality of life. In contrast to surgical fundoplication, patients did not report gas-bloat symptoms. Further, TIF is durable out to at least 5 years[36,37] and does not negate the performance of repeat TIF or LARS should the need arise.[38,39] Serious AEs are low since TIF2.0 was introduced, occurring in 0.41%.[40]

Although TIF is limited to small crural defects (hiatal hernias of axial length $\leq$2 cm and Hill grade $\leq$2), the introduction of concomitant surgical hernia repair and TIF (cTIF) allows the inclusion of patients with larger crural defects. Several studies have demonstrated the feasibility, safety, and efficacy of cTIF,[41,42] which now allows a greater population of patients to undergo LARS without traditional AEs such as gas bloat or dysphagia.

MUSE (Medigus Ltd, Omer, Israel) is a newer device for TIF, gaining Food and Drug Administration (FDA) approval in 2015. Although the surgical and anatomic principles are similar to that of TIF2.0, the technique differs significantly. The device creates a

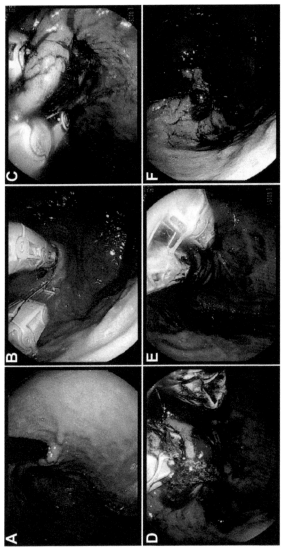

Fig. 10. TIF. (*A*) The GEJ is inspected to ensure Hill grade 1 and the absence of a hiatal hernia >2 cm. (*B*) The EsophyX device (EndoGastric Solutions, Inc) is advanced into the stomach under direct vision with the scope within the device. The scope is then retroflexed to allow a view of the GEJ. The helical retractor is then advanced. (*C*) While desufflating, the retractor is pulled into the device (hence providing length for the valve). Once fully retracted, the entire device is rotated (to provide the wrap). Once in position, the device is fired, and 2 polypropylene fasteners create a full-thickness plication of the esophagus and stomach. (*D, E*) The process is repeated such that plications are made in (usually) 4 points around the GEJ to create a 270° wrap and a 3-cm-long valve. (*F*) Post-TIF.

180° fundoplication by stapling the gastric fundus to the esophagus below the diaphragm under ultrasound guidance. MUSE is safe and effective out to 4 years.[43]

A recent systematic review and meta-analysis captured long-term outcomes following TIF with either device.[44] The pooled rate of patients completely off or on occasional PPI was 53.8% (95% CI 42.0%–65.1%) and 75.8% (95% CI 67.6–82.6), respectively. There are no direct comparisons to surgical fundoplication; however, a meta-analysis comparing TIF with PPI and LNF showed that although health-related quality of life improved post-TIF, LNF was more effective in increasing LES pressure and decreasing esophageal acid exposure.[45]

Radiofrequency Energy Treatment (Stretta)

Stretta (Restech, Houston, TX) is an endoluminal radiofrequency energy delivery system. Although the mechanism of effect is not entirely understood, it is believed that by applying radiofrequency energy to the LES and gastric cardia, tissue compliance is decreased along with transient lower esophageal relaxations. Similar to TIF, Stretta is appropriate for patients with GERD who have a hiatal hernia ≤2 cm and Hill grade ≤2. Stretta significantly improves GERD symptoms, GERD quality of life, and esophageal acid exposure.[46,47] Further, Stretta is durable out to 10 years, although long-term outcomes data are limited.[48] Stretta is safe, with an overall AE rate of 0.93%.[49] Serious AEs are rare, including esophageal perforation in 3 patients and 2 deaths due to aspiration pneumonia. All of these occurred before 2002 and since then there have been changes to the protocol and equipment with no further serious AEs reported to the FDA. Stretta has been effectively used in patients with refractory LNF,[50] with effect lasting out to 10 years and no significant difference in outcome when compared with nonoperated patients with refractory GERD.

Endoscopic Suturing for Gastroesophageal Reflux Disease

Endoscopic full-thickness plication devices have existed in various forms for the past 2 decades. The OverStitch endoscopic suturing system (Apollo Endosurgery, Austin, TX) allows performance of full-thickness sutures and has been used in a variety of settings including primary endoscopic obesity surgery and closure of perforations, leaks, or fistulae. Use in GERD is limited to case series,[51] with early follow-up demonstrating promising results and minimal AEs. Notably, the cohort included several patients with prior surgical fundoplication, esophagectomy, and sleeve gastrectomy, suggesting a potential role in altered anatomy.

Modified suturing techniques have been proposed to improve durability of tissue plication including Mucosal Ablation and Suturing of the EGJ (MASE)[52] and Resection and Plication (RAP).[53] The rationale behind these procedures is to induce a mucosal inflammatory response for better adherence when the tissue is subsequently plicated, MASE using mucosal ablation and RAP with mucosal resection. Both are potentially effective antireflux options, with pilot studies indicating significant improvements in GERD-related quality of life, and PPI usage.[52,53]

Antireflux Mucosectomy

Inoue and colleagues[54] first described ARM as a possible GERD treatment in 2014, after incidentally noting some patients had improved GERD symptoms after mucosectomy for cardia lesions. In this technique, a hemi-circumferential mucosectomy is performed around the gastroesophageal junction (GEJ) by endoscopic mucosal resection (EMR) or endoscopic submucosal dissection (ESD). The rationale is that healing would result in shrinkage and scarring of the area, thereby reducing the opening and sharpening the angle of His. The original pilot study reported significantly improved esophageal pH and GERD symptoms.[54] Several further studies have confirmed these findings[55,56]; however, wider uptake is limited by the required technical ability for such extensive resection. Recently, a modified antireflux mucosal ablation (ARMA) was reported,[57] using a similar technique with ablation instead of mucosectomy. Like endoscopic suturing, these additional techniques likely have a role in patients with GERD with altered anatomy in whom options for other antireflux surgeries or endoscopies are limited.

Future Directions

There has been significant progress in endoscopic therapies for GERD. GERD is a spectrum disorder, and it is likely that endoluminal therapies are most appropriate early in the spectrum. Although multiple endoscopic GERD therapies have been tried and tested, TIF has potentially the most promising future as the minimally invasive technique that most closely mimics LARS. Further, collaboration of endoscopic GERD treatment, such as TIF, with LARS allows minimally invasive treatment of even patients with large crural defects and is truly an exciting space to follow.

BARRETT'S ESOPHAGUS

The incidence of esophageal adenocarcinoma (EAC) is rapidly rising in Western populations, and a significant proportion of patients are still diagnosed with advanced disease, which portends a poor prognosis. The stepwise BE follows a stepwise progression through intestinal metaplasia or nondysplastic BE (NDBE), low-grade dysplasia (LGD), to high-grade dysplasia (HGD), intramucosal carcinoma (IMC), and finally to invasive EAC. This forms the basis for screening and surveillance. However, to date there is no definite evidence that surveillance leads to a reduction in the proportion of patients with advanced-stage EAC or EAC-related/all-cause mortality.

Nondysplastic Barrett's Esophagus

The overall rate of progression to EAC in patients with NDBE is low. Importantly, as patients who underwent endoscopic eradication therapy (EET) would still require regular surveillance, a cost-effectiveness analysis did not support upfront EET for NDBE.[58] However, despite a lack of strong supporting evidence, most guidelines recommend surveillance for patients with NDBE.[59,60]

Low-Grade Dysplasia

LGD is commonly diagnosed in the community; however, this is frequently downgraded following review by expert gastrointestinal pathologists. When LGD is confirmed by an expert pathologist, the risk of progression to HGD/EAC is significant at 13.4% per person-year.[61] Hence, the diagnosis of LGD always should be reviewed by expert gastrointestinal pathologists. EET reduces the risk of progression to HGD/EAC by 9% to 25%.[62,63] Consequently, updated guidelines are increasingly recommending EET as the preferred approach over continued surveillance.[59,60]

High-Grade Dysplasia or Intramucosal Carcinoma

Patients with HGD and IMC have a low risk of lymph node metastasis (HGD 0%, IMC up to 2%).[64] EET for treatment of HGD/IMC is cost-effective,[58] and is now widely accepted as the preferred option over esophagectomy,[59,60] although there is no high-quality randomized controlled trial (RCT) evidence to support this. Thorough inspection by an expert endoscopist is crucial, as early neoplastic lesions can present as subtle mucosal irregularities. In patients referred for EET, expert endoscopists can find a suspicious lesion in 76% of cases referred for evaluation of HGD/IMC in random biopsies without a reported visible abnormality.[65]

Methods of Endoscopic Eradication Therapy

EET is widely established as first-line in the management of BE and associated neoplasia.[59,60] The rationale is for resection of all visible lesions followed by ablative therapies until complete eradication of dysplasia (CE-D) and complete eradication of intestinal metaplasia (CE-IM) are achieved.

Endoscopic mucosal resection and endoscopic submucosal dissection

EMR is an established treatment for visible BE neoplasia that allows for en bloc resection of lesions up to 20 mm in diameter. Larger lesions require either multiple resections (piecemeal) or ESD. A significant limitation with piecemeal resection is the inability to assess for histologically complete resection (R0) due to disruption of the lateral borders. The most common EMR technique is using a modified variceal band ligator with a transparent cap, with or without prior submucosal lifting (**Fig. 11**). The largest retrospective study of EMR for HGD/IMC achieved remission of neoplasia in 96%.[66] Recurrent or metachronous lesions developed in 15%, but 82% of these were successfully endoscopically retreated. The overall long-term complete remission rate was 94%, and only 0.2% died due to metastatic EAC during follow-up. EMR is safe, with a reported perforation rate of 0.9% (95% CI 0.31%–2.62%) and late bleeding in 1.5% (95% CI 0.65%–3.48%).[67]

In contrast, ESD allows en bloc resection of even large lesions, preserving margins and allowing for accurate assessment of neoplastic grade. A recent systematic review and meta-analysis[68] demonstrated pooled R0 and curative resection rates of 74.5% (95% CI 66.3%–81.9%) and 64.9% (95% CI 55.7%–73.6%) respectively, with a low incidence of recurrence of 0.17% (95% CI 0%–3%) at a mean follow-up of 22.9 (95% CI 17.5–28.3) months. The pooled incidence of bleeding and perforation were 1.7% (95% CI 0.6%–3.4%) and 1.5% (95% CI 0.4%–3.0%), respectively. One small RCT[69] compared cap-based EMR and ESD in patients with early Barrett's neoplasia. Although the en bloc resection rate (100% vs 15%, P<.001) and curative resection rate (53% vs 12%, P = .03) were significantly higher with ESD than EMR, there was no difference in complete remission at 3 months. Hence, ESD has not been shown to be superior to EMR for treatment of BE dysplasia or superficial EAC in this short-term

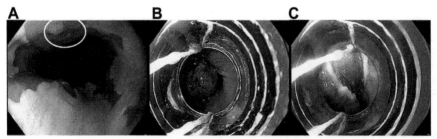

Fig. 11. EMR for Barrett's dysplasia. (*A*) Nodular friable mucosa is seen at the 12 o'clock position (*circled*). Prior biopsies had demonstrated intramucosal carcinoma. (*B*) The band ligator system is loaded on to the distal tip of the endoscope. After a submucosal injection, the lesion is suctioned into the cap and a band is deployed. The pseudopolyp created by the band is seen here. (*C*) A snare is placed over the pseudopolyp and closed under the rubber band. The pseudopolyp is then resected. The immediate post-resection appearance is shown.

follow-up study. Further large, randomized trials with long-term outcomes are warranted to determine roles of EMR and ESD for BE-associated neoplasia. Suggested indications for ESD include recurrent dysplasia, strong suspicion of submucosal invasion, poorly lifting lesions, and those with a large intraluminal component.[70]

Ablative therapies

Currently available ablative techniques include radiofrequency ablation (RFA), argon plasma coagulation (APC), and cryotherapy. RFA is the most widely studied and adopted. The 3 major prospective trials (AIM dysplasia, EURO II, and the SURF trial) showed CE-D between 81% and 95% and CE-IM between 77% and 87%.[62,63,71] An improvement in CE-IM, CE-D, and need for rescue EMR after RFA can be appreciated over time, coinciding with an increase in EMR before RFA.[70] Another trial showed the use of EMR before RFA also significantly reduced the risk of treatment failure.[72] Hence, a low threshold for EMR before RFA is key to its success. For focal ablation (**Fig. 12**), 3×12 J/cm^2 is performed without cleaning, which has been shown to be noninferior to a classic 2 sessions of 2×15 J/cm^2 with a clean in-between while reducing on average 7 minutes of procedure time.[73] For circumferential ablation (**Fig. 13**), however, a 10 J/cm^2 setting is used for a single hit, followed by a clean before a further ablation at the same energy.[74]

APC is broadly available and offers a lower cost compared with the other modalities.[75] Although some trials suggest similar efficacy to RFA,[75] others report modest efficacy and/or significant recurrence rate.[76–78] Further, the ideal power setting is not yet known, and distribution of energy may not be even, especially when treating long-segment BE. The use of hybrid APC, in which a submucosal fluid injection is performed before ablation, may reduce the depth of tissue damage with a low reported rate of posttreatment stricture formation (2%).[79] We reserve the use of APC for those with small burden of BE disease, such as in the setting of residual BE islands following prior ablation (**Fig. 14**).

In contrast to heat-based ablation techniques, cryotherapy is believed to preserve the extracellular matrix architecture,[80] which may enable deeper ablation without increasing stricture risk. Further, cryotherapy is associated with lower post-procedure pain when compared with RFA.[81] Cryotherapy is delivered with the C2 CryoBalloon system (Pentax Medical, Redwood City, CA) with a cryogen dose of

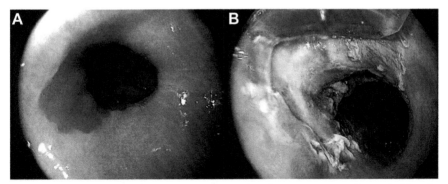

Fig. 12. Focal RFA using the Barrx Halo 90 system (Medtronic, Minneapolis, MN). (*A*) A flat Barrett's tongue is seen at the 9 o'clock position. (*B*) The Halo 90 device is mounted on to the distal tip of the endoscope. The electrode (seen at the 12 o'clock position) is placed in contact with the target epithelium and energy is delivered. Postablation appearance is seen here.

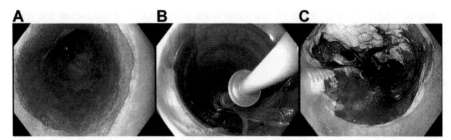

Fig. 13. Circumferential RFA using the Barrx Halo 360 system. (*A*) A circumferential segment of flat BE is seen. (*B*) The self-sizing balloon is distended across the segment of Barrett's. (*C*) Immediate postablation appearance.

10 seconds for each ablation site (**Fig. 15**). Cryotherapy results in CE-D and CE-IM of up to 97% and 91%, respectively.[82] Despite the theoretic advantages, the largest prospective trial to date reports a stricture rate of 12.5%,[82] which is comparable to RFA (6%–11.8%).[80] Esophageal perforation has not been reported with the CryoBalloon system.

Follow-up

CE-IM is most commonly defined as the absence of IM on biopsies obtained from the entire pretreatment BE segment, gastric cardia, and squamocolumnar junction after 2 consecutive surveillance endoscopies following EET, although variations in this definition are seen. Notably, higher rates of IM are reported on gastric cardia biopsies and may not represent a true BE recurrence.[83] After CE-IM is achieved, the annual rate of recurrence of IM and dysplasia is estimated at 8% to 10% and 2% to 3%, respectively.[84] Buried BE after treatment can occur and carcinoma developing from these sub-squamous BE glands have been described.[85] Hence, careful inspection of the GEJ and neo-squamous epithelium within prior BE territory is critical.

In addition to surveillance, aggressive reflux control is key. Poor acid suppression post-CE-IM is linked to BE recurrence[86] and high-dose PPI has been shown to reduce overall mortality and progression to HGD/cancer.[87]

Refractory Barrett Esophagus

Fewer than 15% of patients with dysplastic BE are refractory to EET.[88] Validated risk factors for refractory BE include lack of long-term reflux control, presence of a hiatal hernia, and length of BE segment >5 cm.[88] The optimal management of these patients is unknown. Wide-field salvage EMR of the entire BE segment has an eradication rate

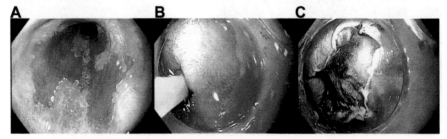

Fig. 14. Hybrid APC. (*A*) Endoscopic view of flat Barrett's tongues. (*B*) Submucosal injection is performed with the hybrid APC probe. (*C*) Following ablation with APC.

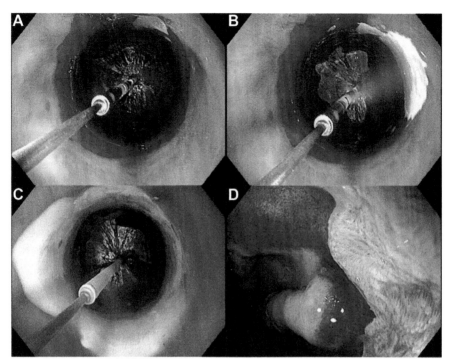

Fig. 15. Cryoablation for BE. (*A*) BE is seen through the cryoballoon. (*B*) Nitrous oxide is released resulting in an ice patch on the target mucosa. (*C*) The GEJ and Barrett's segment are circumferentially ablated. (*D*) Immediate postablation appearance.

of up to 96% for HGD and EAC but carries a significant risk of stricturing and perforation of up to 2%, especially with increasing length of the affected segment.[88] Other options, yet to be fully explored include cryoablation and APC.

Treatment of Recurrence

Risk factors for recurrence include longer BE segment (>3 cm), tobacco use, increased EET sessions to achieve CE-IM, higher grade dysplasia at baseline histology, presence of hiatal hernia, older age, and non-White race. The vast majority of recurrence after CE-IM, even those with dysplasia or EAC, can be managed endoscopically.[89] We recommend a similar strategy to the general principles of EET for BE; that is, areas of nodular recurrence should be resected followed by ablation of flat BE. ESD may be required for nodular recurrence in the presence of underlying scarring.

Future Directions

Data directly comparing BE ablative techniques are very limited, with no large-scale prospective studies or direct head-to-head comparisons. Hence, the ideal position for each within the BE treatment algorithm is unknown. More data are needed to identify the optimal treatment for those with refractory or recurrent BE.

ESOPHAGEAL SUBEPITHELIAL LESION

Esophageal subepithelial lesions (SELs), such as gastrointestinal stromal tumors (GISTs), pancreatic rests, lipomas, neuroendocrine tumors, schwannomas, and leiomyomas, are usually incidental findings. SELs <2 cm are often benign; however, some, such as GISTs, can become malignant at smaller sizes. Resection options include surgery (open, laparoscopic, or video-assisted thoracoscopic) or endoscopy, including endoscopic mucosal excavation, full-thickness resection (FTR), ESD, and more recently submucosal tunneling endoscopic resection (STER). Preoperative evaluation often includes EUS for lesion characterization, determination of structural origin, and, if indicated, fine-needle biopsy to determine risk of malignancy.

Inspired by POEM and ESD, STER uses a submucosal tunnel to serve as a working space for introducing the endoscope and resecting the tumor. The preservation of the mucosal layer theoretically results in lower perforation risk and allows better healing.

STER is usually performed under general anesthesia with the following key steps: (1) tumor identification; (2) submucosal tunneling; (3) tumor dissection (aiming to keep the capsule intact) starting from the mucosal aspect, before the tumor is enucleated from the muscle layer by gradual dissection and division of muscle fibers; (4) tumor resection; and (5) mucosal closure using either TTS clips or endoscopic suturing. Carbon dioxide insufflation is critical, as pneumoperitoneum is not uncommon.

STER is indicated for SELs that originate from the muscularis propria layer. STER should not be used in the setting of advanced lesions, as suggested by irregular margins, vascular invasion, or abundance of vascular supply within the SEL or any evidence of metastasis. STER has been used on large lesions; however, tumor transverse diameter is a significant risk factor for piecemeal resection, AEs, and technical difficulties.[90] To assist with lesion retrieval, benign tumors can be cut into pieces with a snare. Alternatively, combined STER with thoracoscopic enucleation has been reported,[91] as has the formation of a second mucosal incision distal to the lesion.[92]

STER results in en bloc resection rates of 83% to 90% but was still able to achieve curative resection of 100% with no evidence of local recurrence.[90,93] Notably, STER offers a shorter procedure time, and reduced postoperative pain and hospital stay when compared with thoracoscopic resection.[90,93] A recent series demonstrated en bloc resection rate of 91.9%, 4.7% intraprocedural AE (all mucosal injuries managed conservatively) with no recurrence to a median of 44 (10–96) months.[94] The investigators proposed limiting STER to lesions smaller than 30 mm or tumor mass index (product of the major and minor axes in millimeters) <1000 mm^2 to avoid needing to intentionally divide the tumor for peroral extraction. Notably, should the patient require further treatment, STER does not preclude further surgical or medical treatment.

SUMMARY

In this review article, we have summarized the newest advances in endoscopic treatment of esophageal conditions. We are truly at an exciting time in this field as the spectrum of esophageal conditions treatable by endoluminal therapy continues to grow. The future is full of opportunities for innovation that will significantly impact the management of many conditions.

CLINICS CARE POINTS

- POEM, laparoscopic Heller myotomy, and PD are comparable treatment options for management of patients with achalasia types I and II; however, POEM is the preferred treatment for achalasia type III.
- Patients undergoing peroral endoscopic myotomy should be counseled regarding the risk of post-procedure reflux compared with PD and laparoscopic Heller myotomy.

- Zenker peroral endoscopic myotomy is safe and effective for management of ZD; however, long-term data and comparative trials are awaited.
- TIF is a minimally invasive therapy that closely mimics LARS, which is safe, effective, and durable in a select cohort of patients with GERD and minimal crural defect.
- Nondysplastic BE should be followed by surveillance.
- BE with dysplasia should be referred to expert centers and managed with EET as first-line.

DISCLOSURE

L.Y. Zhang: None. S. Ngamruengphong: consultant for Boston Scientific. A.N. Kalloo: A.N. Kalloo is a founding member, equity holder, and consultant for Apollo Endosurgery.

REFERENCES

1. Yadlapati R, Pandolfino JE, Fox MR, et al. What is new in Chicago Classification version 4.0? Neurogastroenterol Motil 2020;33(1):e14053.
2. Pandolfino JE, de Ruigh A, Nicodème F, et al. Distensibility of the esophagogastric junction assessed with the functional lumen imaging probe (FLIP™) in achalasia patients. Neurogastroenterol Motil 2013;25:496–501.
3. Wu PI, Szczesniak MM, Craig PI, et al. Novel intra-procedural distensibility measurement accurately predicts immediate outcome of pneumatic dilatation for idiopathic achalasia. Am J Gastroenterol 2018;113:205–12.
4. Leyden JE, Moss AC, MacMathuna P. Endoscopic pneumatic dilation versus botulinum toxin injection in the management of primary achalasia. Cochrane Database Syst Rev 2014;(12):CD005046.
5. Moonen A, Annese V, Belmans A, et al. Long-term results of the European achalasia trial: a multicentre randomised controlled trial comparing pneumatic dilation versus laparoscopic Heller myotomy. Gut 2016;65:732–9.
6. Vela MF, Richter JE, Khandwala F, et al. The long-term efficacy of pneumatic dilatation and Heller myotomy for the treatment of achalasia. Clin Gastroenterol Hepatol 2006;4:580–7.
7. Vaezi MF, Pandolfino JE, Yadlapati RH, et al. ACG clinical guidelines: diagnosis and management of achalasia. Am J Gastroenterol 2020;115:1393–411.
8. Andolfi C, Fisichella PM. Meta-analysis of clinical outcome after treatment for achalasia based on manometric subtypes. Br J Surg 2019;106:332–41.
9. Werner YB, Hakanson B, Martinek J, et al. Endoscopic or surgical myotomy in patients with idiopathic achalasia. N Engl J Med 2019;381:2219–29.
10. Akintoye E, Kumar N, Obaitan I, et al. Peroral endoscopic myotomy: a meta-analysis. Endoscopy 2016;48:1059–68.
11. McKay SC, Dunst CM, Sharata AM, et al. POEM: clinical outcomes beyond 5 years. Surg Endosc 2021. https://doi.org/10.1007/s00464-020-08031-3.
12. Tyberg A, Choi A, Gaidhane M, et al. Transoral incisional fundoplication for reflux after peroral endoscopic myotomy: a crucial addition to our arsenal. Endosc Int Open 2018;6:E549–52.
13. Inoue H, Ueno A, Shimamura Y, et al. Peroral endoscopic myotomy and fundoplication: a novel NOTES procedure. Endoscopy 2019;51:161–4.
14. Bonatti H, Hinder RA, Klocker J, et al. Long-term results of laparoscopic Heller myotomy with partial fundoplication for the treatment of achalasia. Am J Surg 2005;190:874–8.

15. Hulselmans M, Vanuytsel T, Degreef T, et al. Long-term outcome of pneumatic dilation in the treatment of achalasia. Clin Gastroenterol Hepatol 2010;8:30–5.

16. Ngamruengphong S, Inoue H, Ujiki MB, et al. Efficacy and safety of peroral endoscopic myotomy for treatment of achalasia after failed Heller myotomy. Clin Gastroenterol Hepatol 2017;15:1531–7.e3.

17. Tyberg A, Seewald S, Sharaiha RZ, et al. A multicenter international registry of redo per-oral endoscopic myotomy (POEM) after failed POEM. Gastrointest Endosc 2017;85:1208–11.

18. Brewer Gutierrez OI, Benias PC, Khashab MA. Same-session per-oral endoscopic myotomy followed by transoral incisionless fundoplication in achalasia: are we there yet? Am J Gastroenterol 2020;115:162.

19. Pang M, Koop A, Brahmbhatt B, et al. Comparison of flexible endoscopic cricopharyngeal myectomy and myotomy approaches for Zenker diverticulum repair. Gastrointest Endosc 2019;89:880–6.

20. Gölder SK, Brueckner J, Ebigbo A, et al. Double incision and snare resection in symptomatic Zenker's diverticulum: a modification of the stag beetle knife technique. Endoscopy 2018;50:137–41.

21. Battaglia G, Antonello A, Realdon S, et al. Flexible endoscopic treatment for Zenker's diverticulum with the SB Knife. Preliminary results from a single-center experience. Dig Endosc 2015;27:728–33.

22. Yang J, Novak S, Ujiki M, et al. An international study on the use of peroral endoscopic myotomy in the management of Zenker's diverticulum. Gastrointest Endosc 2020;91:163–8.

23. Li QL, Chen WF, Zhang XC, et al. Submucosal tunneling endoscopic septum division: a novel technique for treating Zenker's diverticulum. Gastroenterology 2016;151:1071–4.

24. Jain D, Sharma A, Shah M, et al. Efficacy and safety of flexible endoscopic management of Zenker's diverticulum. J Clin Gastroenterol 2018;52:369–85.

25. Elkholy S, El-Sherbiny M, Delano-Alonso R, et al. Peroral endoscopic myotomy as treatment for Zenker's diverticulum (Z-POEM): a multi-center international study. Esophagus 2021;18(3):693–9. https://doi.org/10.1007/s10388-020-00809-7.

26. Budnicka A, Januszewicz W, Białek AB, et al. Peroral endoscopic myotomy in the management of Zenker's diverticulum: a retrospective multicenter study. J Clin Med 2021;10:187.

27. Sanaei O, Ichkhanian Y, Mondragón OVH, et al. Impact of prior treatment on feasibility and outcomes of Zenker's peroral endoscopic myotomy (Z-POEM). Endoscopy 2021;53(7):722–6. https://doi.org/10.1055/a-1276-0219.

28. Mittal C, Diehl DL, Draganov PV, et al. Practice patterns, techniques, and outcomes of flexible endoscopic myotomy for Zenker's diverticulum: a retrospective multicenter study. Endoscopy 2021;53(4):346–53. https://doi.org/10.1055/a-1219-4516.

29. Marston AP, Maldonado FJ, Ravi K, et al. Treatment of oropharyngeal dysphagia secondary to idiopathic cricopharyngeal bar: surgical cricopharyngeal muscle myotomy versus dilation. Am J Otolaryngol 2016;37:507–12.

30. Al Ghamdi SS, Farha J, Runge TM, et al. PMC7332726; No pouch, no problem: successful endoscopic division of a symptomatic cricopharyngeal bar using a modified peroral endoscopic myotomy technique for Zenker's diverticulum. VideoGIE 2020;5:281–2.

31. Elmunzer BJ, Moran RA. Peroral endoscopic myotomy for cricopharyngeal bar. VideoGIE 2020;5:378–9.

32. Osman A, Albashir MM, Nandipati K, et al. Esophagogastric junction morphology on hill's classification predicts gastroesophageal reflux with good accuracy and consistency. Dig Dis Sci 2021;66:151–9.

33. Håkansson B, Montgomery M, Cadiere GB, et al. Randomised clinical trial: transoral incisionless fundoplication vs. sham intervention to control chronic GERD. Aliment Pharmacol Ther 2015;42:1261–70.

34. Hunter JG, Kahrilas PJ, Bell RC, et al. Efficacy of transoral fundoplication vs omeprazole for treatment of regurgitation in a randomized controlled trial. Gastroenterology 2015;148:324–33.e5.

35. Trad KS, Barnes WE, Simoni G, et al. Transoral incisionless fundoplication effective in eliminating GERD symptoms in partial responders to proton pump inhibitor therapy at 6 months: the TEMPO Randomized Clinical Trial. Surg Innov 2015;22: 26–40.

36. Trad KS, Barnes WE, Prevou ER, et al. The TEMPO trial at 5 years: transoral fundoplication (TIF 2.0) is safe, durable, and cost-effective. Surg Innov 2018;25: 149–57.

37. Testoni PA, Testoni S, Distefano G, et al. Transoral incisionless fundoplication with EsophyX for gastroesophageal reflux disease: clinical efficacy is maintained up to 10 years. Endosc Int Open 2019;7:E647–54.

38. Perry KA, Linn JG, Eakin JL, et al. Transoral incisionless fundoplication does not significantly increase morbidity of subsequent laparoscopic Nissen fundoplication. J Laparoendosc Adv Surg Tech A 2013;23:456–8.

39. Bell RC, Kurian AA, Freeman KD. Laparoscopic anti-reflux revision surgery after transoral incisionless fundoplication is safe and effective. Surg Endosc 2015;29: 1746–52.

40. Ihde GM. PMC7243382; The evolution of TIF: transoral incisionless fundoplication. Therap Adv Gastroenterol 2020;13. 1756284820924206.

41. Janu P, Shughoury AB, Venkat K, et al. Laparoscopic hiatal hernia repair followed by transoral incisionless fundoplication with EsophyX device (HH + TIF): efficacy and safety in two community hospitals. Surg Innov 2019;26:675–86.

42. Choi AY, Roccato MK, Samarasena JB, et al. Novel Interdisciplinary Approach to GERD: Concomitant Laparoscopic Hiatal Hernia Repair with Transoral Incisionless Fundoplication. J Am Coll Surg 2021;232(3):309–18. https://doi.org/10.1016/j.jamcollsurg.2020.11.021.

43. Kim HJ, Kwon CI, Kessler WR, et al. Long-term follow-up results of endoscopic treatment of gastroesophageal reflux disease with the MUSE™ endoscopic stapling device. Surg Endosc 2016;30:3402–8.

44. Testoni S, Hassan C, Mazzoleni G, et al. Long-term outcomes of transoral incisionless fundoplication for gastro-esophageal reflux disease: systematic-review and meta-analysis. Endosc Int Open 2021;9:E239–46.

45. Richter JE, Kumar A, Lipka S, et al. Efficacy of laparoscopic nissen fundoplication vs transoral incisionless fundoplication or proton pump inhibitors in patients with gastroesophageal reflux disease: a systematic review and network meta-analysis. Gastroenterology 2018;154:1298–308.e7.

46. Aziz AM, El-Khayat HR, Sadek A, et al. A prospective randomized trial of sham, single-dose Stretta, and double-dose Stretta for the treatment of gastroesophageal reflux disease. Surg Endosc 2010;24:818–25.

47. Triadafilopoulos G, DiBaise JK, Nostrant TT, et al. The Stretta procedure for the treatment of GERD: 6 and 12 month follow-up of the U.S. open label trial. Gastrointest Endosc 2002;55:149–56.

48. Noar M, Squires P, Noar E, et al. Long-term maintenance effect of radiofrequency energy delivery for refractory GERD: a decade later. Surg Endosc 2014;28: 2323–33.

49. Fass R, Cahn F, Scotti DJ, et al. Systematic review and meta-analysis of controlled and prospective cohort efficacy studies of endoscopic radiofrequency for treatment of gastroesophageal reflux disease. Surg Endosc 2017;31:4865–82.

50. Noar M, Squires P, Khan S. Radiofrequency energy delivery to the lower esophageal sphincter improves gastroesophageal reflux patient-reported outcomes in failed laparoscopic Nissen fundoplication cohort. Surg Endosc 2017;31:2854–62.

51. Han J, Chin M, Fortinsky KJ, et al. Endoscopic augmentation of gastroesophageal junction using a full-thickness endoscopic suturing device. Endosc Int Open 2018;6:E1120–5.

52. Fortinsky KJ, Shimizu T, Chin MA, et al. Tu1168 Mucosal ablation and suturing at the esophagogastric junction (MASE): a novel procedure for the management of patients with gastroesophageal reflux disease. Gastrointest Endosc 2018;87: AB552.

53. Benias PC, D'Souza L, Lan G, et al. Initial experience with a novel resection and plication (RAP) method for acid reflux: a pilot study. Endosc Int Open 2018;6: E443–9.

54. Inoue H, Ito H, Ikeda H, et al. Anti-reflux mucosectomy for gastroesophageal reflux disease in the absence of hiatus hernia: a pilot study. Ann Gastroenterol 2014;27:346–51.

55. Wong HJ, Su B, Attaar M, et al. Anti-reflux mucosectomy (ARMS) results in improved recovery and similar reflux quality of life outcomes compared to laparoscopic Nissen fundoplication. Surg Endosc 2020. https://doi.org/10.1007/s00464-020-08144-9.

56. Sumi K, Inoue H, Kobayashi Y, et al. Endoscopic treatment of proton pump inhibitor-refractory gastroesophageal reflux disease with anti-reflux mucosectomy: Experience of 109 cases. Dig Endosc 2021;33(3):347–54. https://doi.org/10.1111/den.13727.

57. Inoue H, Tanabe M, de Santiago ER, et al. Anti-reflux mucosal ablation (ARMA) as a new treatment for gastroesophageal reflux refractory to proton pump inhibitors: a pilot study. Endosc Int Open 2020;8:E133–8.

58. Rubenstein JH, Inadomi JM. Cost-effectiveness of screening, surveillance, and endoscopic eradication therapies for managing the burden of esophageal adenocarcinoma. Gastrointest Endosc Clin N Am 2021;31:77–90.

59. Shaheen NJ, Falk GW, Iyer PG, et al. ACG clinical guideline: diagnosis and management of Barrett's esophagus. Am J Gastroenterol 2016;111:30–50 [quiz 51].

60. Weusten B, Bisschops R, Coron E, et al. Endoscopic management of Barrett's esophagus: European Society of Gastrointestinal Endoscopy (ESGE) Position Statement. Endoscopy 2017;49:191–8.

61. Curvers WL, ten Kate FJ, Krishnadath KK, et al. Low-grade dysplasia in Barrett's esophagus: overdiagnosed and underestimated. Am J Gastroenterol 2010;105: 1523–30.

62. Shaheen NJ, Sharma P, Overholt BF, et al. Radiofrequency ablation in Barrett's esophagus with dysplasia. N Engl J Med 2009;360:2277–88.

63. Phoa KN, van Vilsteren FG, Weusten BL, et al. Radiofrequency ablation vs endoscopic surveillance for patients with Barrett esophagus and low-grade dysplasia: a randomized clinical trial. JAMA 2014;311:1209–17.

64. Dunbar KB, Spechler SJ. The risk of lymph-node metastases in patients with high-grade dysplasia or intramucosal carcinoma in Barrett's esophagus: a systematic review. Am J Gastroenterol 2012;107:850–62 [quiz 863].

65. Schölvinck DW, van der Meulen K, Bergman JJ, et al. Detection of lesions in dysplastic Barrett's esophagus by community and expert endoscopists. Endoscopy 2017;49:113–20.

66. Pech O, May A, Manner H, et al. Long-term efficacy and safety of endoscopic resection for patients with mucosal adenocarcinoma of the esophagus. Gastroenterology 2014;146:652–60.e1.

67. Pouw RE, Beyna T, Belghazi K, et al. A prospective multicenter study using a new multiband mucosectomy device for endoscopic resection of early neoplasia in Barrett's esophagus. Gastrointest Endosc 2018;88:647–54.

68. Yang D, Zou F, Xiong S, et al. Endoscopic submucosal dissection for early Barrett's neoplasia: a meta-analysis. Gastrointest Endosc 2018;87:1383–93.

69. Terheggen G, Horn EM, Vieth M, et al. A randomised trial of endoscopic submucosal dissection versus endoscopic mucosal resection for early Barrett's neoplasia. Gut 2017;66:783–93.

70. Haidry RJ, Butt MA, Dunn JM, et al. Improvement over time in outcomes for patients undergoing endoscopic therapy for Barrett's oesophagus-related neoplasia: 6-year experience from the first 500 patients treated in the UK patient registry. Gut 2015;64:1192–9.

71. Phoa KN, Pouw RE, Bisschops R, et al. Multimodality endoscopic eradication for neoplastic Barrett oesophagus: results of an European multicentre study (EURO-II). Gut 2016;65:555–62.

72. Agoston AT, Strauss AC, Dulai PS, et al. Predictors of treatment failure after radiofrequency ablation for intramucosal adenocarcinoma in barrett esophagus: a multi-institutional retrospective cohort study. Am J Surg Pathol 2016;40:554–62.

73. Pouw RE, Künzli HT, Bisschops R, et al. Simplified versus standard regimen for focal radiofrequency ablation of dysplastic Barrett's oesophagus: a multicentre randomised controlled trial. Lancet Gastroenterol Hepatol 2018;3:566–74.

74. Belghazi K, Pouw RE, Koch AD, et al. Self-sizing radiofrequency ablation balloon for eradication of Barrett's esophagus: results of an international multicenter randomized trial comparing 3 different treatment regimens. Gastrointest Endosc 2019;90:415–23.

75. Peerally MF, Bhandari P, Ragunath K, et al. Radiofrequency ablation compared with argon plasma coagulation after endoscopic resection of high-grade dysplasia or stage T1 adenocarcinoma in Barrett's esophagus: a randomized pilot study (BRIDE). Gastrointest Endosc 2019;89:680–9.

76. Dulai GS, Jensen DM, Cortina G, et al. Randomized trial of argon plasma coagulation vs. multipolar electrocoagulation for ablation of Barrett's esophagus. Gastrointest Endosc 2005;61:232–40.

77. Sharma P, Wani S, Weston AP, et al. A randomised controlled trial of ablation of Barrett's oesophagus with multipolar electrocoagulation versus argon plasma coagulation in combination with acid suppression: long term results. Gut 2006;55:1233–9.

78. Sie C, Bright T, Schoeman M, et al. Argon plasma coagulation ablation versus endoscopic surveillance of Barrett's esophagus: late outcomes from two randomized trials. Endoscopy 2013;45:859–65.

79. Manner H, May A, Kouti I, et al. Efficacy and safety of Hybrid-APC for the ablation of Barrett's esophagus. Surg Endosc 2016;30:1364–70.

80. Frederiks CN, Canto MI, Weusten BL. Updates in cryotherapy for Barrett's esophagus. Gastrointest Endosc Clin N Am 2021;31:155–70.
81. van Munster SN, Overwater A, Haidry R, et al. Focal cryoballoon versus radiofrequency ablation of dysplastic Barrett's esophagus: impact on treatment response and postprocedural pain. Gastrointest Endosc 2018;88:795–803.e2.
82. Canto MI, Trindade AJ, Abrams J, et al. Multifocal cryoballoon ablation for eradication of Barrett's Esophagus-related neoplasia: a prospective multicenter clinical trial. Am J Gastroenterol 2020;115:1879–90.
83. Eluri S, Earasi AG, Moist SE, et al. Prevalence and incidence of intestinal metaplasia and dysplasia of gastric cardia in patients with Barrett's esophagus after endoscopic therapy. Clin Gastroenterol Hepatol 2020;18:82–8.e1.
84. Kahn A, Shaheen NJ, Iyer PG. Approach to the post-ablation Barrett's esophagus patient. Am J Gastroenterol 2020;115:823–31.
85. Lee JK, Cameron RG, Binmoeller KF, et al. Recurrence of subsquamous dysplasia and carcinoma after successful endoscopic and radiofrequency ablation therapy for dysplastic Barrett's Esophagus. Endoscopy 2013;45:571–4.
86. Komanduri S, Kahrilas PJ, Krishnan K, et al. Recurrence of Barrett's esophagus is rare following endoscopic eradication therapy coupled with effective reflux control. Am J Gastroenterol 2017;112:556–66.
87. Jankowski JAZ, de Caestecker J, Love SB, et al. Esomeprazole and aspirin in Barrett's oesophagus (AspECT): a randomised factorial trial. Lancet 2018;392:400–8.
88. Farina DA, Condon A, Komanduri S, et al. A practical approach to refractory and recurrent Barrett's esophagus. Gastrointest Endosc Clin N Am 2021;31:183–203.
89. Wolf WA, Pasricha S, Cotton C, et al. Incidence of esophageal adenocarcinoma and causes of mortality after radiofrequency ablation of Barrett's esophagus. Gastroenterology 2015;149:1752–61.e1.
90. Chen T, Lin ZW, Zhang YQ, et al. Submucosal tunneling endoscopic resection vs thoracoscopic enucleation for large submucosal tumors in the esophagus and the esophagogastric junction. J Am Coll Surg 2017;225:806–16.
91. Zhong YS, Shi Q, Guo WG, et al. Thoracoscope assisted tunnel endoscopic resection for esophageal SMT from the muscularis propria. Zhonghua Weichang Waike Zazhi 2012;15:404–5.
92. Zhang Q, Cai JQ, Xiang L, et al. Modified submucosal tunneling endoscopic resection for submucosal tumors in the esophagus and gastric fundus near the cardia. Endoscopy 2017;49:784–91.
93. Chai N, Du C, Gao Y, et al. Comparison between submucosal tunneling endoscopic resection and video-assisted thoracoscopic enucleation for esophageal submucosal tumors originating from the muscularis propria layer: a randomized controlled trial. Surg Endosc 2018;32:3364–72.
94. Onimaru M, Inoue H, Bechara R, et al. Clinical outcomes of per-oral endoscopic tumor resection for submucosal tumors in the esophagus and gastric cardia. Dig Endosc 2020;32:328–36.

Using Diet to Treat Diseases of Esophagus: Back to the Basics

Carolyn Newberry, MD[a], Kristle Lynch, MD[b],*

KEYWORDS

- Esophageal diseases • Dietary therapy • Elimination diet • GERD • Dysphagia
- Eosinophilic esophagitis • Barrett's esophagus • Esophageal cancer

KEY POINTS

- The relationship between dietary intake and pathogenesis and management of esophageal diseases continues to evolve.
- Dietary therapy is an increasingly common therapeutic option for patients with esophageal diseases, serving as primary or augmentative treatment.
- Diet can reduce symptom burden in patients with dysphagia and reflux disease and serve as a primary therapy for those with eosinophilic esophagitis.
- Dietary patterns have been linked to esophageal adenocarcinoma and squamous cell carcinoma; thus diet alterations may play an important role in risk mitigation.

INTRODUCTION

The esophagus is the entryway into the gastrointestinal tract, serving as a crucial gatekeeper for all orally ingested nutrients. As such, diet and esophageal disease are intimately related. The following is a comprehensive review of dietary therapies used in treating diseases of the esophagus. In particular, diet and its relationship to swallowing dysfunction, motility disorders, malignancies, and inflammatory mucosal diseases such as gastroesophageal reflux disease (GERD) and eosinophilic esophagitis (EoE) is highlighted.

Dysphagia

Pathophysiology of swallowing

Deglutition occurs through 3 separate phases: oral, pharyngeal, and esophageal. These phases can be affected by medical conditions, medications, and aging.[1] The oral phase of swallowing is characterized by the introduction of food into the mouth

The authors do not have any relevant conflicts of interest to report.

[a] Division of Gastroenterology, Weill Cornell Medical Center, 1305 York Avenue, 4th Floor, New York, NY 10021, USA; [b] Division of Gastroenterology, University of Pennsylvania Perelman School of Medicine, 3400 Civic Center Boulevard, 7th Floor, South Tower, Philadelphia, PA 19104, USA
* Corresponding author.
E-mail address: Kristle.lynch@pennmedicine.upenn.edu

with subsequent mastication and lubrication via salivary secretions. The resultant food bolus is propelled to the back of the pharynx by the tongue in order to enter the next phase of swallowing, the pharyngeal phase. This first phase is voluntary and can be affected by efficacy and efficiency of oral musculature; salivary gland health; and texture, size, and intrinsic properties of the food being ingested. The second phase of swallowing known as the pharyngeal phase is involuntary and includes projection of the food bolus into the esophagus through a now open upper esophageal sphincter.[2] This is the phase where the esophageal phase of swallowing occurs, which includes involuntary propagation of the bolus through the esophagus via primary peristalsis and then into the stomach after adequate relaxation of the lower esophageal sphincter.

Types of dysphagia

Considering the complex process of swallowing, problems can arise in any stage of the process. Oropharyngeal dysphagia occurs when there is failure during the early phases of swallowing. The condition can occur with a variety of neurologic and muscular diseases as well as anatomic variants and iatrogenic causes, which alter the function and efficacy of swallowing musculature (**Fig. 1**).[3] This condition increases in prevalance with aging, with nearly one-fifth of community-dwelling persons older than 50 years and half of those in assisted care reporting feeding difficulties.[4] Esophageal dysphagia is intuitively defined by dysfunction at any point in the esophageal phase of swallowing. Common causes include motility disorders, mucosal diseases, and structural abnormalities (**Fig. 2**).[3] Accurate diagnosis is based on thorough history taking that determines which further investigations are of highest diagnostic and potentially therapeutic yield. These examinations typically include imaging, endoscopic evaluation, and often motility testing.[5]

Dietary therapy in dysphagia

Although the main method of treating dysphagia is addressing the underlying cause, dietary and speech-language therapy are important augmentative treatments and may become primary therapy if the underlying disease process is not amenable to

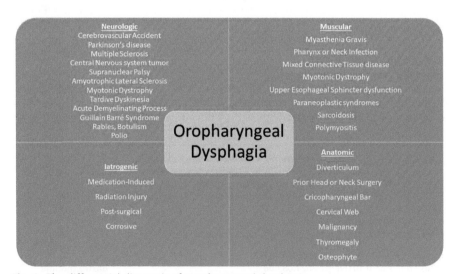

Fig. 1. The differential diagnosis of oropharyngeal dysphagia.

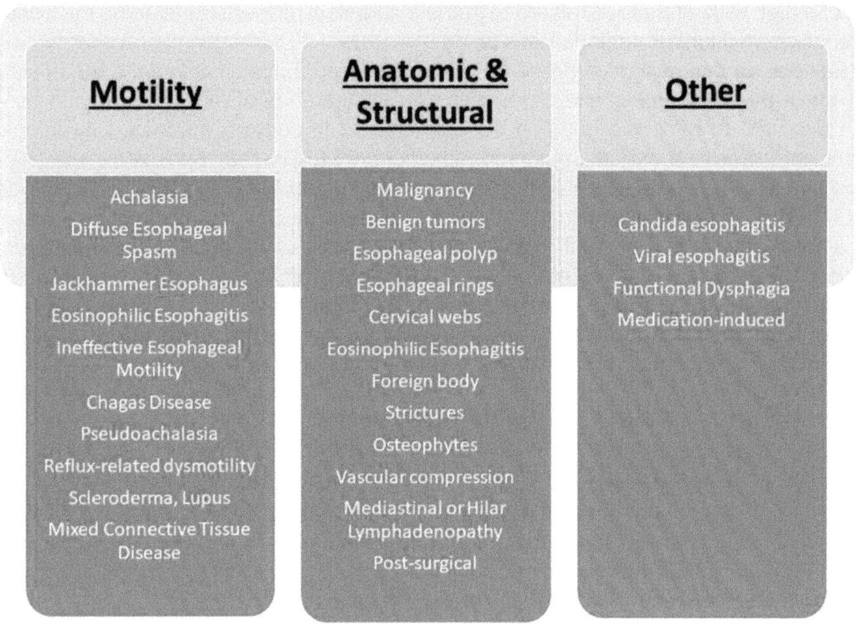

Fig. 2. The differential diagnosis of esophageal dysphagia.

medical or surgical intervention. Dietary therapy relies on the modification of food and liquid consistency, which became standardized after the publication of the National Dysphagia Diet in 2002 by the National Dysphagia Diet Task Force[6]; this was further clarified in 2013 with the adoption of an updated International Dysphagia Diet Standardization Initiative Framework. Using these published frameworks, solid food texture is now defined by markers of adhesiveness/cohesiveness, firmness/hardness, fracturability, and springiness—and adjusted based on degree of swallowing dysfunction.[7] Severe dysfunction may require significant alteration (ie, liquidized/pureed food), whereas milder dysfunction is typically amenable to the avoidance of large food boluses and hard, sticky, or crunchy foods. Liquids similarly are systematically altered in terms of viscosity, with the following consistencies defined: thin, nectarlike, honeylike, and spoon-thick (pudding).[8] In addition to the alteration of food consistency, patients may benefit from adaptative eating behaviors such as postural adjustments and swallowing maneuvers as well as supervised and hand-feeding tactics (especially in the elderly).[9]

Gastroesophageal Reflux Disease

Epidemiology and pathophysiology

GERD is one of the most commonly reported esophageal diseases worldwide, with estimated prevalence ranging from 2.5% to 33.1% across all locations.[10] GERD is defined by troublesome symptoms and/or complications arising from increased esophageal exposure to refluxed stomach contents.[11] The disease is often further classified based on presence or absence of reflux esophagitis. Underlying pathophysiologic mechanisms of this disease include a compromised esophagogastric barrier and/or inadequate clearance of acidic fluid.[12] Lower esophageal sphincter tone is mediated by multiple factors, including neural, hormonal, and paracrine signaling molecules that maintain intrinsic contraction. These signaling pathways can be affected by oral diet, with alterations related to nutrient chemical properties including macronutrient composition and caloric density.[13]

Besides barrier protection provided by the lower esophageal sphincter (LES) in concert with the angle of His and crural diaphragm, clearance of refluxed stomach contents is vital to minimize irritation and damage to underlying mucosa. Physiologic transient lower esophageal sphincter relaxations (TLESRs) may release excess trapped air in healthy persons, although an increase in frequency and duration can illicit GER (**Fig. 3**). This change in timing may occur with increasing gastric distention, which is additionally associated with dietary choices as well as medications.[14] Peristalsis, along with gravity, drives refluxed fluid back into the stomach. The amplitude and frequency of peristaltic contractions is mediated by intrinsic factors as well as size and density of ingested food. It is inhibited by elevation of intraabdominal pressure, which can occur in the setting of food and gas retention in the stomach.[15]

Dietary Therapy in Gastroesophageal Reflux Disease

General principles
Although pharmacotherapy via acid suppressants is typically the mainstay of treatment of GERD, recent literature has alluded to the increasing importance of lifestyle modifications including dietary therapy in controlling disease symptom and progression. Enthusiasm for this approach has been demonstrated in the community, with recent literature noting high efficacy rates of lifestyle approaches.[16]

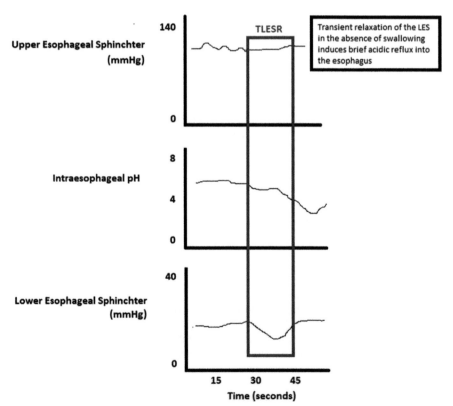

Fig. 3. Physiologic transient lower esophageal sphincter relaxations can illicit gastroesophageal reflux disease.

Individual elimination diets

Initial dietary approaches to GERD often include specific elimination diets that remove common triggering foods, beverages, and spices. Overall, this approach may be effective in individuals within the general population, although requires personalization and close follow-up. For example, a recent study of 100 patients with positive GERD symptoms by standardized questionnaire were asked to identify and reduce or eliminate triggering foods. This study found statistically significant reduction in classic heartburn and regurgitation after 2 weeks of therapy.[17] The importance of self-identification of culprit foods is highlighted, as epidemiologic studies do not support blanket recommendations for populations due to lack of evidence. Commonly implicated foods include those with excessive added spices, coffee and caffeinated drinks, chocolate, mint, citrus, tomato-based products, and carbonated beverages. Individual response to these food types, however, is variable. For instance, although mint and cacao (a primary ingredient in chocolate) have been found in physiologic studies to enhance relaxation of the LES, correlation with GERD symptoms is not routinely reported in large population studies.[18–20] Similarly, carbonated and caffeinated beverages have also been found to alter esophageal pathophysiological through increases in intraabdominal pressure and alterations in LES tone and TLESR frequency; however, large meta-analyses show a limited association between beverage intake and GERD,[21–23] and this may reflect personalized physiologic responses to ingested foods as well as lack of clinical translation of transient changes in sphincter and intraabdominal pressures. Interestingly, degree of intake may also play a role in symptom induction. A large study conducted on the Nurses' Health Study II cohort showed that among 7961 women who reported GERD symptoms at least once weekly and were not on acid suppressing therapy, those who consumed at least 6 servings of coffee, tea, or soda per day showed increased hazard ratios for GERD (1.34, 1.26, and 1.29, respectively) when compared with those who consumed no servings.[24] **Table 1** summarizes these dietary therapies and proposed underlying mechanisms.

Macronutrient manipulation and specific dietary patterns

Prescribed eating patterns that alter macronutrient intake and promote particular eating habits have recently become of interest to GERD researchers, sometimes with more evidence backing their use than specific elimination diets. For instance,

Table 1
Dietary therapies for gastroesophageal reflux disease and proposed underlying mechanisms

	Increased Gastric Distention/ TLESR	Reduction in LES Tone	Reduction in Gastric Motility	Increased Gastric Acid Production	Direct Esophageal Irritant
Fats	X	X			
Carbohydrates	X				
Late Night Eating				X	
Large/Calorie Dense Meal	X				
Carbonation	X				
Alcohol		X	X		
Coffee		X			
Mint		X			
Acidic Foods					X
Spicy Foods					X

manipulating the type of carbohydrate intake (ie, replacing monosaccharides, disaccharides, and starches with fiber) may be more beneficial in controlling reflux symptoms than cutting out specific foods. The proposed mechanism of this approach includes enhanced colonic fermentation of partially digested sugars (ie, nonfiber carbohydrates), leading to altered neurohormonal pathways, enhancement of LES relaxation, and increased esophageal acid exposure.[25] This theory has now been tested in several small prospective trials that have randomized patients to both higher and lower carbohydrate diets, with manipulation of simple sugar and starch intake in relation to fiber. For instance, a study of 130 patients with reflux disease who followed a low glycemic diet for 2 weeks noted improvement of symptoms during this time period.[26] Another study of 144 women with elevated body mass index (BMI) demonstrated near symptom resolution after reduction in starch and simple sugar intake in favor of fiber.[27] Whether fiber supplementation alone is helpful for GERD management is still unknown, although a recent publication investigating the addition of daily psyllium to the diet of 30 patients with nonerosive reflux disease noted statistical improvement of reported symptoms in 40% to 93% of participants.[28]

The relationship of reflux symptoms to fat ingestion is less clearly defined. Fat is calorically dense and slows gastric emptying as well as induces secretion of esophageal irritants such as bile salts. Observational studies have been mixed in correlating symptoms with total fat intake, with some reporting positive association and others noting little or no relationship.[29–31] Potential confounding factors include total daily calories ingested, overall BMI, and weight fluctuations. A prospective trial in 15 GERD patients with mixed BMIs noted no change in esophageal acid exposure in those following a high-fat diet (50% of calories) versus those on a low-fat diet (25% of calories), although those on a high-fat diet did report increase in symptom frequency.[30] Overall reduction in fat intake may be beneficial in controlling reflux symptoms in some patients, although this relationship warrants further investigation. The relationship between protein intake and reflux disease similarly merits further exploration, with a recent analysis noting that children who consumed higher amounts of protein reported lower rates of GERD symptoms.[32]

Timing of meal ingestion as well as meal size are also important in GERD management in select patients. In terms of timing, increasing the interval between dinner and bedtime does reduce nocturnal esophageal acid exposure time and supine reflux episodes that may correlate to symptom improvement in some patients.[33–35] Because gastric clearance of solid meals can take around 4 hours, meals can be timed to be ~3 hours before sleep to mitigate effects. Meal size may also influence esophageal acid exposure, with several physiologic studies confirming that increased size, caloric density, and resultant gastric distention increase TLESRs and reflux.[36,37] Whether this correlates to consistent improvement in reflux symptoms is less clear and may be patient dependent.

Malignancies of the Esophagus

Barrett's esophagus and esophageal adenocarcinoma

Esophageal adenocarcinoma (EAC) (**Fig. 4**) is one of the more common types of digestive cancers and now represents the main histologic subtype of esophageal malignancy in westernized countries, with a reported incidence of 0.7 cases per 100,000 person-years.[38] The prevalence of Barrett's esophagus (BE) (see **Fig. 4**), a precursor state to EAC defined by a change in normal squamous epithelial cells to columnar-lined intestinal metaplasia in the distal esophagus, is also currently on the increase.[39] Although greater than 90% of EAC is diagnosed in patients without prior BE history, early diagnosis and mitigation of risk factors including diet and lifestyle habits can

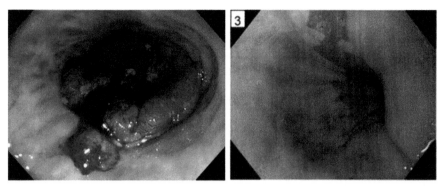

Fig. 4. Esophageal adenocarcinoma (*left*) and Barrett's esophagus (*right*) are seen here.

reduce disease progression and improve outcomes.[40,41] Metaplastic and dysplastic changes to distal esophageal mucosa occur most commonly in the setting of GERD, where continued esophageal acid exposure induces inflammation and cellular changes. In the United States, approximately 5% to 15% of patients with GERD will be diagnosed with BE on endoscopic examination, and annual risk of conversion of BE to EAC is 0.1% to 0.5%. Risk factors for the development and progression of BE include GERD, caucasian race, male gender, central adiposity, tobacco use, a family history of EAC or BE, and increasing age.[39]

Esophageal squamous cell carcinoma

Esophageal squamous cell carcinoma (ESCC) is the most common form of esophageal cancer worldwide, accounting for 90% of incident esophageal malignancies. It occurs most frequently in Eastern Europe, Asia, Central and South America, and sub-Saharan Africa, with marked reduction in incidence in western countries such as the United States, Europe, and Australia in favor of EAC.[42] Risk factors for the development and progression of ESCC include tobacco use, alcohol use, and lower socioeconomic status.[42] Dietary factors have also been studied and will be reviewed in more detail.

Diet and esophageal malignancy

Specific food components. Several food components have been implicated in esophageal cancer risk calculations, varying based on cancer type. For example, N-nitroso–containing foods, such as found in chewing quid and pickled foods, have been correlated with higher risk of ESCC. Chewing "quid mixtures," which consist of betel nuts, areca leaves, and tobacco, is a common practice in the Asia-Pacific region. Carcinogenic nitrosamines are derived when mixed with saliva and induce development of both oral and esophageal squamous cell carcinomas. In a recent meta-analysis of greater than 12,000 Asian patients, chewing areca nuts alone was significantly and independently associated with ESCC (odds ratio [OR] 3.05), with even higher risk noted when mixed with tobacco products (OR 6.79).[43] Considering widespread use of chewing quid, global initiatives have been developed to discourage this historical practice.[44] Pickled vegetables are produced by enclosing moist produce in tightly packed jars, thereby promoting fermentation and growth of yeasts and fungi over time. This process can also produce N-nitroso compounds as well as carcinogenic mycotoxins.[45] A meta-analysis of 34 studies mainly conducted in China found that pickled vegetable consumption was associated with a 2-fold increase in ESCC, although notably with heterogeneity in study protocol and design.[46] Although prospective data are still forthcoming, intake reduction of pickled produce is recommended in high-risk populations.

In contrast, protective effects of fruits, vegetables, and other fiber sources have been reported for both ESCC and EAC. Mechanistically, fruits and vegetables contain increased levels of antioxidants and flavones, which have anticarcinogenic properties. In a meta-analysis of 12 studies of EAC, higher intake of vegetables (risk ratio [RR] 0.76) and fruits (RR 0.73) was correlated with reduced rates of incident cancers.[47] Similar findings have been noted on meta-analysis in relationship to fruit and vegetable intake and ESCC.[48] Although red and processed meats have also been studied as possible culprit foods, data regarding their association with cancers of the esophagus have been less robust than with gastric and colonic malignancies.

Food preparation. In addition to specific food components, consumption of particular food and beverage types has been analyzed. For example, very hot beverages and foods may increase ESCC risk, as reported by a large meta-analysis of 56,286 patients, which showed a pooled OR of 1.60. The opposite was found in EAC, with reported pooled OR of 0.79. Interestingly, risk was higher in Asian and South American populations (OR 2.06, OR 1.52) compared with European populations (OR 0.95), indicating there may also be genetic factors playing a role.[49]

Eosinophilic Esophagitis

Epidemiology and pathophysiology

EoE is chronic immune-mediated condition most often manifested with swallowing dysfunction in the presence of elevated esophageal eosinophil count (at least 15 eosinophils per high-powered field) without other identifiable cause.[50] Its relationship with GERD continues to evolve, with the most recently published clinical guidelines indicating there is considerable overlap between the 2 conditions.[51] Pathogenesis of disease includes a combination of genetic and environmental factors including exposure to specific dietary antigens. As such, considerable research has been conducted to define dietary treatment algorithms, which are considered first-line therapy in children and adults along with proton pump inhibitors and swallowed topical steroids.[50]

Dietary therapy for eosinophilic esophagitis

Considering that food antigen exposure is one of the proposed culprit causes of EoE, identifying and removing dietary triggers in motivated patients has considerable therapeutic potential. Continued research has defined several approaches to dietary therapy in EoE, including use of an elemental diet, allergen-directed diet, and empirical food allergen elimination diet (**Table 2**).

Elemental diet

The elemental diet (ELED) consists entirely of single amino acid–based enteral formulas that have limited antigenic properties. This dietary approach was first studied in pediatric patients diagnosed with EoE, with the hope that eliminating food antigen exposures would minimize eosinophilic inflammation and disease complications. In 1995, a landmark trial following 10 children with refractory GERD symptoms and evidence of eosinophilic infiltration on esophageal biopsy placed on an elemental formula diet for a minimum of 6 weeks was published. Most of the children in this study (8/10) had resolution of symptoms with significant reduction in intraepithelial eosinophil counts on subsequent endoscopy.[52] Additional prospective trials using ELED were later conducted in mostly pediatric populations, with recent meta-analysis of 13 trials and 429 patients (411 children, 18 adults) reporting a 90.8% histologic remission rate.[53] Notably, the single study conducted in adults found a lower

Table 2		
Dietary treatment options for eosinophilic esophagitis and efficacy rates		
Diet	Description	% Efficacy (95% CI)[53]
Elemental Diet	Amino acid–based enteral formula provides total nutrition	90.8 (84.7–95.5)
Allergen-Directed Diet	Avoidance of allergens identified by allergy patch testing and skin prick testing	45.5 (35.4–55.7)
Six-Food Elimination Diet	Avoidance of the 6 most common food allergens (wheat, milk, soy, eggs, nuts, seafood/shellfish) with sequential reintroduction	72.1 (65.8–78.1)

Abbreviation: CI, confidence interval.
Data from Arias Á, González-Cervera J, Tenias JM, Lucendo AJ. Efficacy of dietary interventions for inducing histologic remission in Patients with eosinophilic esophagitis: A systematic review and meta-analysis. Gastroenterology. 2014;146(7):1639-1648.

efficacy rate (72%) and higher rates of nonadherence (38% of initially enrolled subjects did not follow the diet as prescribed).[54] Despite its proved clinical effectiveness, this diet is rarely used in adults due to inherent limitations that include formula intolerance, high cost secondary to lack of insurance coverage, and social barriers.[55] Although its role in pediatric populations may also be limited due to similar factors, it may be an option for select children and caregivers.

Targeted elimination diets
Targeted elimination diets based on diagnostic allergy testing including skin prick testing (SPT) and allergy patch testing (APT) are of continued interest in this population, but data are not consistent in terms of their overall efficacy. Clinical trials in pediatric patients have noted histologic remission rates of 13% to 77%, depending on patient population and allergy testing used.[56–58] In the most comprehensive study reporting a 77% efficacy rate in 146 children undergoing both SPT and APT, the most commonly implicated allergens were eggs, milk, soy, peanuts, chicken, wheat, beef, corn, rice, and potatoes. The investigators noted only 7% (57/810) of foods were positive by both testing modalities, instead the majority required identification by SPT or APT. Notably, the 25 children who did respond had to transition to elemental diets due to nutritional deficiencies in the setting of multiple food eliminations. Thus, although this approach may be effective in some pediatric population, it may not be appropriate for all patients depending on the restrictiveness of intervention.[57] Similar to ELED, this diet also has scant evidence of efficacy and feasibility in adult populations, although several small trials have reported histologic remission rates of 26% to 54%.[59,60] Most recently, newer approaches to allergen selection are being analyzed to streamline identification. For example, 24 adult EoE patients responsive to a 6-food elimination diet (SFED) were asked to provide blood samples for development of a CD4+ T-cell proliferation assay and esophageal biopsy samples to assess food-specific tissue immunoglobulin G4 levels. Although correlation with either the blood or esophageal tissue test yielded accuracy rates of 53% to 75% depending on food allergen, only 4 of 22 patients in a separate clinical trial achieved histologic remission after assay-directed elimination diets.[61] Testing for food components is also being explored as reported by a study of 12 patients undergoing expanded APT for chemicals, dyes, preservatives, and additives. This study noted a 92% adherence rate to the strict elimination diet and 57% histologic remission in the 7 patients who underwent follow-up endoscopy.[62]

Six-food elimination diet

The most common diet used in EoE patients is the SFED, which can be approached via either a step-down or a step-up approach. This diet eliminates the 6 most common food allergens, including cow's milk, wheat, peanuts and tree nuts, eggs, soy, and fish and shellfish.[63] Consistent with other dietary therapies, this approach was first evaluated in a pediatric population. There were 60 children treated with SFED or ELED for 6 weeks noting similar efficacy rates (74% in SFED vs 88% in ELED).[64] A meta-analysis of 7 additional studies analyzing both pediatric and adult patients (75 children, 122 adults) noted high efficacy rates in both populations, 72.8% and 71.3% respectively.[53] Although this diet is effective, standardization of dietary implementation has yet to be established. Classically, patients have been asked to avoid all 6 food allergen categories for a minimum of 6 weeks, confirm histologic remission on endoscopy, and then complete serial endoscopies approximately every 6 weeks after reintroduction of food categories, and this allows for gradual broadening of the diet and reduced restrictiveness. In one analysis of 49 patients who initially responded to SFED, 35.7% eventually narrowed down to 1 trigger allergen, 31.0% identified 2, and 33.3% identified 3 or more.[65] More recent studies have tested alternative approaches including starting with elimination of 2 (milk, wheat) or 4 (milk, wheat, soy, eggs) of the most common triggers and expanding the diet as needed (ie, a "step-up" approach). For example, 130 adult and pediatric patients were started on a 2-food elimination diet including all milk products (cow, goat, sheep) and gluten (wheat, barley, and rye) to reduce possibility of cross-contamination. Almost half (43%) of the patients had confirmation of histologic remission after 6 weeks, and the remaining patients were offered the 4-food elimination diet with step up to SFED if needed. Of those who agreed to continue with dietary therapy after failing the 2-food elimination diet, an additional 22% of patients responded histologically with the 4-food or 6-food elimination approach.[66] Overall, empirical elimination diets are effective and algorithms can be tailored to patient preference. However, significant limitations exist including increased cost, frequent endoscopies, and the challenges associated with grocery shopping and dining outside the home.[67,68]

SUMMARY

The knowledge regarding the relationship between diet and esophageal diseases, including abnormal swallowing patterns, mucosal diseases, and malignancies, continues to evolve. For many esophageal conditions, dietary intervention can both improve patient experience and serve as either primary or augmentative therapy. With continued patient interest in avoiding medical and procedural interventions, an understanding of how to use diet to treat diseases of the esophagus is crucial.

CLINICS CARE POINTS

- Commonly implicated foods in GERD include those with excessive added spices, coffee and caffeinated drinks, chocolate, mint, citrus, tomato-based products, and carbonated beverages. Although elimination of these foods has been shown to alter esophageal pathophysiology, meta-analyses show a limited association between specific elimination diets and response to GERD symptoms.

- Small prospective trials have revealed that diets lower in carbohydrates and higher in fiber correlate with symptoms resolution in GERD. Further investigations into this area are ongoing.

- Elimination diets are critical in the treatment of eosinophilic esophagitis; the SFED and other empirical elimination diets are superior to the allergy-guided diet.

REFERENCES

1. Cook IJ. Oropharyngeal dysphagia. Gastroenterol Clin North Am 2009;38(3): 411–31.
2. Engmann J, Burbidge AS. Fluid mechanics of eating, swallowing and digestion - overview and perspectives. Food Funct 2013;4(3):443–7.
3. Nierengarten MB. Evaluating dysphagia: Current approaches. Oncol times 2009; 31(14):29–30.
4. Khan A, Carmona R, Traube M. Dysphagia in the elderly. Clin Geriatr Med 2014; 30(1):43–53.
5. Cook IJ. Diagnostic evaluation of dysphagia. Nat Clin Pract Gastroenterol Hepatol 2008;5(7):393–403.
6. American Dietetic Association. National dysphagia diet task force. National dysphagia diet: standardization for optimal care. Chicago. 2002.
7. Cichero J, Steele C, Duivestein J, et al. The need for international terminology and definitions for texture-modified foods and thickened liquids used in dysphagia management: Foundations of a global initiative. Curr Phys Med Rehabil Rep 2013;1(4):280–91.
8. Mertz Garcia J, Chambers E. Managing dysphagia through diet modifications. The Am J Nurs 2010;110(11):26–35.
9. Sura L, Madhavan A, Carnaby G, et al. Dysphagia in the elderly: management and nutritional considerations. Clin Interventions Aging 2012;7:287–98.
10. El-Serag HB, Sweet S, Winchester CC, et al. Update on the epidemiology of gastro-oesophageal reflux disease: A systematic review. Gut 2014;63(6):871–80.
11. Vakil N, van Zanten SV, Kahrilas P, et al. The montreal definition and classification of gastroesophageal reflux disease: A global evidence-based consensus. The Am J Gastroenterol 2006;101(8):1900–20.
12. Katzka DA, Pandolfino JE, Kahrilas PJ. Phenotypes of gastroesophageal reflux disease: Where rome, lyon, and montreal meet. Clin Gastroenterol Hepatol 2020;18(4):767–76.
13. Lentle RG, Janssen PWM. The physical processes of digestion. New York: Springer; 2011.
14. Kim HI, Hong SJ, Han JP, et al. Specific movement of esophagus during transient lower esophageal sphincter relaxation in gastroesophageal reflux disease. J neurogastroenterology Motil 2013;19(3):332–7.
15. Shaker R, Belafsky PC, Postma GN, et al. Principles of deglutition. New York: Springer; 2013.
16. Mehta RS, Nguyen LH, Ma W, et al. Association of diet and lifestyle with the risk of gastroesophageal reflux disease symptoms in US women. JAMA Intern Med 2021. https://doi.org/10.1001/jamainternmed.2020.7238. Available at: https://jamanetwork.com/journals/jamainternalmedicine/article-abstract/2774728.
17. Tosetti C, Savarino E, Benedeto E, et al. Elimination of Dietary Triggers is Successful in Treating Symptoms of Gastroesophageal Reflux Disease. Digetive Diseases and Sciences 2020. https://doi.org/10.1007/s10620-020-06414-z. Available at: https://link.springer.com/article/10.1007%2Fs10620-020-06414-z.
18. Kaltenbach T, Crockett S, Gerson LB. Are lifestyle measures effective in patients with gastroesophageal reflux disease?: An evidence-based approach. Arch Intern Med 2006;166(9):965–71.
19. Babka JC, Castell DO. On the genesis of heartburn. the effects of specific foods on the lower esophageal sphincter. The Am J Dig Dis 1973;18(5):391–7.

20. Benamouzig R, Airinei G. Diet and reflux. J Clin Gastroenterol 2007;41(Suppl 2): S64–71.
21. Zhang Y, Chen S. Effect of coffee on gastroesophageal reflux disease. Food Sci Technology Res 2013;19(1):1–6.
22. Kim J, Oh S-, Myung S-, et al. Association between coffee intake and gastro-esophageal reflux disease: A meta-analysis. Dis Esophagus 2014;27(4):311–7.
23. Johnson T, Gerson L, Hershcovici T, et al. Systematic review: The effects of carbonated beverages on gastro-oesophageal reflux disease. Aliment Pharmacol Ther 2010;31(6):607–14.
24. Mehta RS, Song M, Staller K, et al. Association between beverage intake and incidence of gastroesophageal reflux symptoms. Clin Gastroenterol Hepatol 2020;18(10):2226–33.e4.
25. Piche T, des Varannes SB, Sacher-Huvelin S, et al. Colonic fermentation influences lower esophageal sphincter function in gastroesophageal reflux disease. Gastroenterology 2003;124(4):894–902.
26. Langella C, Naviglio D, Marino M, et al. New food approaches to reduce and/or eliminate increased gastric acidity related to gastroesophageal pathologies. Nutrition 2018;54:26–32.
27. Pointer SD, Rickstrew J, Slaughter JC, et al. Dietary carbohydrate intake, insulin resistance and gastro-oesophageal reflux disease: A pilot study in european- and African-American obese women. Aliment Pharmacol Ther 2016;44(9):976–88.
28. Morozov S, Isakov V, Konovalova M. Fiber-enriched diet helps to control symptoms and improves esophageal motility in patients with non-erosive gastroesophageal reflux disease. World J Gastroenterol : WJG 2018;24(21):2291–9.
29. El-Serag HB, Satia JA, Rabeneck L. Dietary intake and the risk of gastro-oesophageal reflux disease: A cross sectional study in volunteers. Gut 2005; 54(1):11–7.
30. Fox M, Barr C, Nolan S, et al. The effects of dietary fat and calorie density on esophageal acid exposure and reflux symptoms. Clin Gastroenterol Hepatol 2007;5(4):439–44.e1.
31. Ruhl CE, Everhart JE. Overweight, but not high dietary fat intake, increases risk of gastroesophageal reflux disease hospitalization: The NHANES I epidemiologic followup study. Ann Epidemiol 1999;9(7):424–35.
32. Borodina G, Morozov S. Children with gastroesophageal reflux disease consume more calories and fat compared to controls of same weight and age. J Pediatr Gastroenterol Nutr 2020;70(6):808–14.
33. Fujiwara Y, Machida A, Watanabe Y, et al. Association between dinner-to-bed time and gastro-esophageal reflux disease. The Am J Gastroenterol 2005; 100(12):2633–6.
34. Piesman M, Hwang I, Maydonovitch C, et al. Nocturnal reflux episodes following the administration of a standardized meal. does timing matter. The Am J Gastroenterol 2007;102(10):2128–34.
35. Duroux PH, Bauerfeind P, Emde C, et al. Early dinner reduces nocturnal gastric acidity. Gut 1989;30:1063–7.
36. Holloway RH, Kocyan P, Dent J. Provocation of transient lower esophageal sphincter relaxations by meals in patients with symptomatic gastroesophageal reflux. Dig Dis Sci 1991;36(8):1034–9.
37. Hunt JN, Stubbs DF. The volume and energy content of meals as determinants of gastric emptying. J Physiol 1975;245:209–25.
38. Coleman HG, Xie S, Lagergren J. The epidemiology of esophageal adenocarcinoma. Gastroenterology (New York, N.Y. 1943) 2018;154(2):390–405.

39. Runge TM, Abrams JA, Shaheen NJ. Epidemiology of barrett's esophagus and esophageal adenocarcinoma. Gastroenterol Clin North Am 2015;44(2):203–31.

40. Hvid-Jensen F, Pedersen L, Drewes M, et al. Incidence Adenocarcinoma among Patients with Barrett's Esophagus. The New Engl J Med 2011;365(15):1375–83.

41. Shaheen NJ, Falk GW, Iyer PG, et al. ACG clinical guideline: Diagnosis and management of barrett's esophagus. The Am J Gastroenterol 2016;111(1):30–50.

42. Abnet CC, Arnold M, Wei W. Epidemiology of esophageal squamous cell carcinoma. Gastroenterology 2018;154(2):360–73.

43. Akhtar S. Areca nut chewing and esophageal squamous-cell carcinoma risk in asians: A meta-analysis of case–control studies. Cancer Causes Control 2013; 24(2):257–65.

44. Mehrtash H, Duncan K, Parascandola M, et al. Defining a global research and policy agenda for betel quid and areca nut. The Lancet Oncol 2017;18(12):e767.

45. Abnet CC, Corley DA, Freedman ND, et al. Diet and upper gastrointestinal malignancies. Gastroenterology (New York, N.Y. 1943) 2015;148(6):1234–43.e4.

46. Islami F, Ren J, Taylor PR, et al. Pickled vegetables and the risk of oesophageal cancer: A meta-analysis. Br J Cancer 2009;101(9):1641–7.

47. Li B, Jiang G, Zhang G, et al. Intake of vegetables and fruit and risk of esophageal adenocarcinoma: A meta-analysis of observational studies. Eur J Nutr 2014; 53(7):1511–21.

48. Liu J, Wang J, Leng Y, et al. Intake of fruit and vegetables and risk of esophageal squamous cell carcinoma: A meta-analysis of observational studies. Int J Cancer 2013;133(2):473–85.

49. Chen Y, Tong Y, Yang C, et al. Consumption of hot beverages and foods and the risk of esophageal cancer: A meta-analysis of observational studies. BMC cancer 2015;15(1):449.

50. Furuta GT, Katzka DA. Eosinophilic esophagitis. The New Engl J Med 2015; 373(17):1640–8.

51. Hirano I, Chan ES, Rank MA, et al. American gastroenterological association and the joint task force on allergy-immunology practice parameters clinical guidelines for the management of eosinophilic esophagitis acknowledgements. Ann Allergy Asthma Immunol 2020;124(5):416–23.

52. Kelly KJ, Lazenby AJ, Rowe PC, et al. Eosinophilic esophagitis attributed to gastroesophageal reflux: Improvement with an amino acid-based formula. Gastroenterology (New York, N.Y. 1943) 1995;109(5):1503–12.

53. Arias Á, González-Cervera J, Tenias JM, et al. Efficacy of dietary interventions for inducing histologic remission in Patients with eosinophilic esophagitis: A systematic review and meta-analysis. Gastroenterology (New York, N.Y. 1943) 2014; 146(7):1639–48.

54. Peterson KA, Byrne KR, Vinson LA, et al. Elemental diet induces histologic response in adult eosinophilic esophagitis. Am J Gastroenterol 2013;108(5): 759–66.

55. Cotton CC, Durban R, Dellon ES. Illuminating elimination diets: Controversies regarding dietary treatment of eosinophilic esophagitis. Dig Dis Sci 2019;64(6): 1401.

56. Liacouras CA, Spergel JM, Ruchelli E, et al. Eosinophilic esophagitis: A 10-year experience in 381 children. Clin Gastroenterol Hepatol 2005;3(12):1198–206.

57. Spergel JM, Andrews T, Brown-Whitehorn TF, et al. Treatment of eosinophilic esophagitis with specific food elimination diet directed by a combination of skin prick and patch tests. Ann Allergy Asthma Immunol 2005;95(4):336–43.

58. Al-Hussaini A, Al-Idressi E, Al-Zahrani M. The role of allergy evaluation in children with eosinophilic esophagitis. J Gastroenterol 2013;48(11):1205–12.

59. Wolf WA, Jerath MR, Sperry SLW, et al. Dietary elimination therapy is an effective option for adults with eosinophilic esophagitis. Clin Gastroenterol Hepatol 2014; 12(8):1272–9.

60. Molina-Infante J, Martin-Noguerol E, Alvarado-Arenas M, et al. Selective elimination diet based on skin testing has suboptimal efficacy for adult EoE. J Allergy Clin Immunol 2012;130(5):P1200–2.

61. Paquet B, Egin PB, Paradis L, et al. Variable yield of allergy patch testing in children with EoE. J Allergy Clin Immunol 2013;131(2):613.

62. Ghosh G, Parra C, Cressey B, et al. Clinical, endoscopic, and histologic benefit with comprehensive type IV hypersensitivity patch testing in adults with eosinophilic esophagitis. Clin Gastroenterol Hepatol 2020. https://doi.org/10.1016/j.cgh.2020.10.044.

63. Gonsalves N, Kagalwalla AF. Dietary treatment of eosinophilic esophagitis. Gastroenterol Clin North Am 2014;43(2):375–83.

64. Kagalwalla AF, Sentongo TA, Ritz S, et al. Effect of six-food elimination diet on clinical and histologic outcomes in eosinophilic esophagitis. Clin Gastroenterol Hepatol 2006;4(9):1097–102.

65. Lucendo AJ, Arias Á, González-Cervera J, et al. Empiric 6-food elimination diet induced and maintained prolonged remission in patients with adult eosinophilic esophagitis: A prospective study on the food cause of the disease. J Allergy Clin Immunol 2013;131(3):797–804.

66. Molina-Infante J, Arias Á, Alcedo J, et al. Step-up empiric elimination diet for pediatric and adult eosinophilic esophagitis: The 2-4-6 study. J Allergy Clin Immunol 2018;141(4):1365–72.

67. Asher Wolf W, Huang K, Durban R, et al. The six-food elimination diet for eosinophilic esophagitis increases grocery shopping cost and complexity. Dysphagia 2016;31(6):765–70.

68. Wang R, Hirano I, Doerfler B, et al. Assessing adherence and barriers to long-term elimination diet therapy in adults with eosinophilic esophagitis. Dig Dis Sci 2018;63(7):1756–62.

UNITED STATES POSTAL SERVICE®

Statement of Ownership, Management, and Circulation
(All Periodicals Publications Except Requester Publications)

1. Publication Title	2. Publication Number	3. Filing Date
GASTROENTEROLOGY CLINICS OF NORTH AMERICA	000 – 279	9/18/21

4. Issue Frequency	5. Number of Issues Published Annually	6. Annual Subscription Price
MAR, JUN, SEP, DEC	4	$395.00

7. Complete Mailing Address of Known Office of Publication (Not printer) (Street, city, county, state, and ZIP+4®)

ELSEVIER INC.
230 Park Avenue, Suite 800
New York, NY 10169

Contact Person
Malathi Samayan

Telephone (Include area code)
91-44-4299-4507

8. Complete Mailing Address of Headquarters or General Business Office of Publisher (Not printer)

ELSEVIER INC.
230 Park Avenue, Suite 800
New York, NY 10169

9. Full Names and Complete Mailing Addresses of Publisher, Editor, and Managing Editor (Do not leave blank)

Publisher (Name and complete mailing address)

DOLORES MELONI, ELSEVIER INC.
1600 JOHN F KENNEDY BLVD. SUITE 1800
PHILADELPHIA, PA 19103-2899

Editor (Name and complete mailing address)

KERRY HOLLAND, ELSEVIER INC.
1600 JOHN F KENNEDY BLVD. SUITE 1800
PHILADELPHIA, PA 19103-2899

Managing Editor (Name and complete mailing address)

PATRICK MANLEY, ELSEVIER INC.
1600 JOHN F KENNEDY BLVD. SUITE 1800
PHILADELPHIA, PA 19103-2899

10. Owner (Do not leave blank. If the publication is owned by a corporation, give the name and address of the corporation immediately followed by the names and addresses of all stockholders owning or holding 1 percent or more of the total amount of stock. If not owned by a corporation, give the names and addresses of the individual owners. If owned by a partnership or other unincorporated firm, give its name and address as well as those of each individual owner. If the publication is published by a nonprofit organization, give its name and address.)

Full Name	Complete Mailing Address
WHOLLY OWNED SUBSIDIARY OF REED/ELSEVIER, US HOLDINGS	1600 JOHN F KENNEDY BLVD, SUITE 1800 PHILADELPHIA, PA 19103-2899

11. Known Bondholders, Mortgagees, and Other Security Holders Owning or Holding 1 Percent or More of Total Amount of Bonds, Mortgages, or Other Securities. If none, check box ▶ ☐ None

Full Name	Complete Mailing Address
N/A	

12. Tax Status (For completion by nonprofit organizations authorized to mail at nonprofit rates) (Check one)
The purpose, function, and nonprofit status of this organization and the exempt status for federal income tax purposes:
☒ Has Not Changed During Preceding 12 Months
☐ Has Changed During Preceding 12 Months (Publisher must submit explanation of change with this statement)

PS Form **3526**, July 2014 [Page 1 of 4 (see instructions page 4)] PSN: 7530-01-000-9931 PRIVACY NOTICE: See our privacy policy on www.usps.com

13. Publication Title	14. Issue Date for Circulation Data Below
GASTROENTEROLOGY CLINICS OF NORTH AMERICA	JUNE 2021

15. Extent and Nature of Circulation			Average No. Copies Each Issue During Preceding 12 Months	No. Copies of Single Issue Published Nearest to Filing Date
a. Total Number of Copies (Net press run)			213	172
b. Paid Circulation (By Mail and Outside the Mail)	(1)	Mailed Outside-County Paid Subscriptions Stated on PS Form 3541 (Include paid distribution above nominal rate, advertiser's proof copies, and exchange copies)	82	66
	(2)	Mailed In-County Paid Subscriptions Stated on PS Form 3541 (Include paid distribution above nominal rate, advertiser's proof copies, and exchange copies)	0	0
	(3)	Paid Distribution Outside the Mails Including Sales Through Dealers and Carriers, Street Vendors, Counter Sales, and Other Paid Distribution Outside USPS®	69	60
	(4)	Paid Distribution by Other Classes of Mail Through the USPS (e.g., First-Class Mail®)	0	0
c. Total Paid Distribution [Sum of 15b (1), (2), (3), and (4)]			151	126
d. Free or Nominal Rate Distribution (By Mail and Outside the Mail)	(1)	Free or Nominal Rate Outside-County Copies included on PS Form 3541	45	33
	(2)	Free or Nominal Rate In-County Copies Included on PS Form 3541	0	0
	(3)	Free or Nominal Rate Copies Mailed at Other Classes Through the USPS (e.g., First-Class Mail)	0	0
	(4)	Free or Nominal Rate Distribution Outside the Mail (Carriers or other means)	0	0
e. Total Free or Nominal Rate Distribution (Sum of 15d (1), (2), (3) and (4))			45	33
f. Total Distribution (Sum of 15c and 15e)			196	159
g. Copies not Distributed (See Instructions to Publishers #4 (page #3))			17	13
h. Total (Sum of 15f and g)			213	172
i. Percent Paid (15c divided by 15f times 100)			77.04%	79.24%

* If you are claiming electronic copies, go to line 16 on page 3. If you are not claiming electronic copies, skip to line 17 on page 3.

16. Electronic Copy Circulation		Average No. Copies Each Issue During Preceding 12 Months	No. Copies of Single Issue Published Nearest to Filing Date
a. Paid Electronic Copies	▲		
b. Total Paid Print Copies (Line 15c) + Paid Electronic Copies (Line 16a)	▲		
c. Total Print Distribution (Line 15f) + Paid Electronic Copies (Line 16a)	▲		
d. Percent Paid (Both Print & Electronic Copies) (16b divided by 16c × 100)	▲		

☒ I certify that 50% of all my distributed copies (electronic and print) are paid above a nominal price.

17. Publication of Statement of Ownership

☒ If the publication is a general publication, publication of this statement is required. Will be printed
in the DECEMBER 2021 issue of this publication. ☐ Publication not required.

18. Signature and Title of Editor, Publisher, Business Manager, or Owner		Date
Malathi Samayan - Distribution Controller	*Malathi Samayan*	9/18/21

I certify that all information furnished on this form is true and complete. I understand that anyone who furnishes false or misleading information on this form or who omits material or information requested on the form may be subject to criminal sanctions (including fines and imprisonment) and/or civil sanctions (including civil penalties).

PS Form **3526**, July 2014 (Page 3 of 4) PRIVACY NOTICE: See our privacy policy on www.usps.com